# Current Topics in Pathology
# 85

Nobuaki Sasano (Ed.)

# Gynecological Tumors

## Recent Progress in Diagnostic Pathology

Contributors

D. A. Bell · G. Dallenbach-Hellweg · Y. Furuhashi
C. T. Garrett · S. Goto · T. Ishizuka · R. Kudo
K. Noda · T. Okagaki · H. Sasano · R. E. Scully
M. K. Sidaway · S. G. Silverberg · A. Talerman
Y. Tomoda · G. Ueda · M. Yamasaki · R. H. Young

Springer-Verlag
Berlin Heidelberg NewYork
London Paris Tokyo
Hong Kong Barcelona
Budapest

Nobuaki Sasano, MD
Professor Emeritus, Tohoku University School of Medicine
3-6-12 Kuromatsu
Izumi-ku
Sendai 981
Japan

With 168 Figures and 28 Tables

ISBN-13:978-3-642-75943-7 e-ISBN-13:978-3-642-75941-3
DOI: 10.1007/978-3-642-75941-3

Library of Congress Cataloging-in-Publication Data
Gynecological tumors : recent progress in diagnostic pathology / Nobuaki Sasano, (ed) : contributors D.A. Bell ... [et al.]. (Current topics in pathology : 85)
Includes index.
ISBN-13:978-3-642-75943-7
1. Generative organs, Female--Cancer--Histopathology. I. Sasano, Nobuak i. II. Series. III. Series: Current topics in pathology : v. 85.
[DNLM: 1. Genital Neoplasma, Female--Pathology. W1 CU821H v. 85 / WP 145 G9997] RB1. E6 vol. 85 [RC 280.G5] 616.07 s--dc20 [616.99'265] DNLM/DLC


Softcover reprint of the hardcover 1st edition 1992



Typesetting: Thomson Press (India) Ltd, New Delhi

13/3020-543210 – Printed on acid-free paper

# List of Contributors


| | |
|---|---|
| BELL, D.A., MD<br>Assistant Professor | Department of Pathology, Harvard Medical School and the James Homer Wright Pathology Laboratories of the Massachusetts General Hospital, Boston, MA 02114, USA |
| DALLENBACH-HELLWEG, G.<br>Prof. Dr. med. | Institut für Pathologie, A 2, 2, W-6800 Mannheim, Germany |
| FURUHASHI, Y., MD<br>Assistant Professor | Department of Obstetrics and Gynecology, School of Medicine, Nagoya University, 65 Tsurumai-cho, Showa-ku, Nagoya 466, Japan |
| GARRETT, C.T., MD<br>Professor | Department of Pathology, The George Washington University Medical Center, 2300 Eye Street, N.W., Washington, D.C. 20037, USA |
| GOTO, S., MD<br>Assistant Professor | Department of Obstetrics and Gynecology, School of Medicine, Nagoya University, 65 Tsurumai-cho, Show-ku, Nagoya 466, Japan |
| ISHIZUKA, T., MD<br>Assistant Professor | Department of Obstetrics and Gynecology, School of Medicine, Nagoya University, 65 Tsurumai-cho, Showa-ku,<br>Nagoya 466, Japan |
| KUDO, R., MD<br>Professor | Department of Obstetrics and Gynecology, Sapporo Medical College, Minami 1, Nishi 16, Chuo-ku, Sapporo 060, Japan |

| | |
|---|---|
| Noda, K., MD<br>Professor | Department of Obstetrics and Gynecology, Kinki University School of Medicine, 377-2, Ohno-Higashi, Osaka-Sayama 589, Japan |
| Okagaki, T., MD, PhD<br>Professor | Departments of Laboratory Medicine and Pathology, and Obstetrics and Gynecology, University of Minnesota Medical School, Minneapolis, MN 55455-0385, USA |
| Sasano, H., MD<br>Assistant Professor | Department of Pathology, Tohoku University School of Medicine, 2-1 Seiryomachi, Aoba-ku, Sendai 980, Japan |
| Scully, R.E., MD<br>Professor | Department of Pathology, Harvard Medical School and the James Homer Wright Pathology Laboratories of the Massachusetts General Hospital, Boston, MA 02114, USA |
| Sidawy, M.K., MD<br>Assistant Professor | Department of Pathology, The George Washington University Medical Center, 2300 Eye Street, N.W., Washington, D.C. 20037, USA |
| Silverberg, S.G., MD<br>Professor | Department of Pathology, The George Washington University Medical Center, 2300 Eye Street, N.W., Washington, D.C. 20037, USA |
| Talerman, A., MD, F.R.C. Path.<br>Professor | Department of Pathology and Cell Biology, Thomas Jefferson University, 11th and Walnut Streets, Philadelphia, PA 19107-5244, USA |
| Tomoda, Y., MD<br>Professor | Department of Obstetrics and Gynecology, School of Medicine, Nagoya University, 65 Tsurumai-cho, Showa-ku, Nagoya 466, Japan |
| Ueda, G., MD<br>Associate Professor | Department of Obstetrics and Gynecology, Osaka University Medical School, 1-1-50 Fukushima, Fukushima-ku, Osaka 553, Japan |

YAMASAKI, M., MD
Director

Department of Obstetrics and Gynecology, Osaka Rosai Hospital, 1179-3 Nagasonemachi, Sakai 591, Japan

YOUNG, R.H., MD, M.R.C. Path.
Associate Professor

Department of Pathology, Harvard Medical School and the James Homer Wright Pathology Laboratories of the Massachusetts General Hospital, Boston, MA 02114, USA

# Preface

During the past ten years numerous new findings have been documented in the field of gynecological pathology, especially in respect of neoplasms. These findings have been generated by the application of recently developed techniques of immunology and molecular biology. However, clinicopathologic examinations are still an absolute requirement for the morphologic evaluation of neoplasms, including gynecological tumors.

The International Society of Gynecological Pathologists (ISGYP) has contributed greatly to the progress within gynecological pathology. The ISGYP Nomenclature Committee has promoted the *International Histological Classification of Gynecological Tumors* under the auspices of the World Health Organization. A new edition of the classification of tumors and tumor-like conditions of trophoblastic disease, uterine corpus, cervix, vagina, and vulva is currently in press. A second volume covering the ovaries, fallopian tubes, broad ligament, and female peritoneum will be published later.

Organization of scientific symposia and seminars has also been an important activity of the ISGYP. The present editor organized and chaired a symposium entitled "Recent Progress in Diagnostic Pathology of Gynecological Tumors" held in Sendai, Japan on 11 April 1986 in close cooperation with Prof. T. Okagaki, University of Minnesota Medical School, and under the joint auspices of the ISGYP and the Japanese Society of Pathology. The following topics were discussed at this symposium:

—Immunocytochemistry of gestational trophoblastic disease (Dr. R.J. Kurman)
—Mesenchymal tumors of the uterus (Dr. S.G. Silverberg)
—Germ cell tumors of the ovary (Dr. A. Talerman)
—Endometrial carcinoma and its precursors: histogenesis and classification (Dr. G. Dallenbach-Hellweg)
—Sex cord tumors of the ovary (Dr. J. Prat)
—Adenocarcinoma with argyrophil cells (Dr. G. Ueda)
—In vitro and in vivo differentiation of germ-cell tumors (Dr. T. Motoyama)

In each subject area, current knowledge and new findings relevant to diagnostic pathology were presented and discussed.

Now five years have elapsed since the ISGYP Sendai Symposium. During these years diagnostic pathology of gynecological tumors has undergone rapid development with the aid of immunohistochemistry and molecular pathology. Application of various monoclonal antibodies to morphologic study has made immunohistochemistry a very useful ancillary diagnostic procedure in anatomic pathology.

Gynecological patholgoy is a particular field of human pathology dealing with female reproductive and genital tissues, which are characterized by either the production of sex hormones or the site of their receptors. Therefore, modern techniques of biology and biochemistry are particularly useful for the analysis of various diagnostic problems in the field of gynecological pathology. The effect of endocrine and paracrine activities may be remarkable in gynecological tumors.

Immunohistochemistry provides accuracy at the diagnostic level in general and in gynecological pathology contributes particularly to the evaluation of complicated features associated with neoplasms. Technical advances have been made in immunohistochemistry with respect to gynecological tumors. These important advances and their usefulness for the diagnostic pathology of certain gynecological tumors receive due consideration in this volume.

In addition, remarkable recent progress in the fields of basic science, especially in molecular biology, has greatly contributed to the elucidation of pathologic processes involved in a variety of human disorders, and particularly the molecular basis of human neoplasia. These state of the art techniques are now being introduced into clinical medicine and pathology, including gynecological oncology and pathology. They may not change the practice of gynecology and/or pathology in the immediate future but will certainly become the techniques of the 1990s within oncology. Therefore, it is becoming increasingly important for gynecological pathologists and oncologists to have a grasp of basic ideas concerning molecular pathology. Recent advances in molecular pathology are discussed in several chapters in this volume, covering a variety of gynecological neoplasms. Three chapters are devoted exclusively to the application of new molecular and/or biology techniques to gynecological neoplasms; these chapters deal with (a) human papillomavirus with relation to cervical neo-plasms, (b) flow cytometry, and (c) oncogenes.

It should be emphasized that great advances have recently been made in the field of gynecological pathology by the detailed analysis of morphologic findings corroborated by clinicopathologic study. The significance of such study is sometimes overlooked by the scientific community. One should not forget, however, that these new histopathologic findings may have a broad and pronounced impact on the routine diagnosis and management of patients with gynecological neoplasms. Therefore, new developments in the histopathology of gynecological neoplasia are also covered within this volume. Some excellent and valuable contributions in the field of gynecological oncology have been made by those interested in surgical pathology. As regards the surgical pathology of neoplasms, follow-up is absolutely essential in evaluating certain histologic findings suggestive of malignancy. Treatment of the patient for a gynecological tumor may have a marked effect not only on the results of follow-up study but also on the morphologic features of subsequent biopsies. Therefore, gynecological pathologists are required to have a thorough knowledge of the various treatments of gynecological tumors. Several chapters in this volume have been written by gynecological oncologists who have been trained in anatomic pathology and who currently practice cytologic and/or histopathologic diagnosis of gynecological disorders. Consequently, while this volume is primarily intended for practicing surgical pathologists, the editor believes that it will also be of value to gynecological oncologists who depend on surgical pathologists for the management of patients.

The editor has much pleasure in acknowledging the valuable editorial suggestions of Prof. Steven G. Silverberg, Department of Pathology, The George Washington University Medical Center, and Prof. Akira Yajima, Department of Obstetrics and Gynecology, Tohoku University School of Medicine, both of whom worked with me at the Department of Pathology, Tohoku University of School of Medicine. The generous advice and help received from the staff of Springer-Verlag are also appreciated, as is their patience in waiting for me to assemble the various chapters. Finally, I wish to thank all cuntributors to this volume, who are currently practicing in the USA, Japan, and Germany and have generously given of their precious time in order that this volume may be completed.

Sendai, September 1991 NOBUAKI SASANO

# Contents

# Endometrial Carcinomas

G. DALLENBACH-HELLWEG



## 1 Introduction

As with knowledge of tumors of all tissues of the body, so our knowledge of endometrial tumors is in constant need of revision. On the one hand, such a revision represents the recognition of new tumor types, which usually arise because of changes in the environment, whereas other types of tumor become less common. On the other hand, progress in diagnostic methods has enabled us to define much of the fine structure and histogenesis of tumors. From these developments we are able to draw inferences about prognosis and therapy of

Current Topics in Pathology
Volume 85, Ed. N. Sasano

the tumors. With the purpose of this book in mind, I restrict myself only to new advances in our knowledge of endometrial tumors made during the last 10 years, eschewing a comprehensive review of endometrial tumors in general.

The endometrium differs from other tissues of the body in many ways: as the main target organ for the female sex hormones, its growth and regression are entirely under hormonal control. The speed of growth stimulated by estrogens exceeds by far that known for other regenerating tissues. Prolonged unopposed estrogen stimulation will result in either diffuse or focal hyperplasia, often with the formation of polyps, which are comparable to benign tumors elsewhere. For this reason, benign epithelial growths of the endometrium are generally considered as focal hyperplasias, which under longstanding appropriate stimulation and mutational change may progress to malignancy.

The incidence of endometrial carcinoma has increased remarkably over the past 50 years; it is now considered to be the most common invasive neoplasm of the female genital tract in the United States (WALKER and JICK 1979; KURMAN and NORRIS 1987). Because this increase can be measured in almost like extent outside the United States, with a few geographic exceptions, the disease, and its possible prevention, has become a major concern worldwide.

## 2 Etiology

For the great majority of endometrial carcinomas, a close relationship between endogenous or exogenous hyperestrogenism and carcinogenesis can be confirmed (for review of the literature: DALLENBACH-HELLWEG 1987; KURMAN and NORRIS 1987). This relationship appears plausible in view of the excessive growth stimulation of the endometrial glands induced by unopposed estrogens. The causes of endogenous hyper-estrogenism are manifold, ranging from overproduction of estrogen by the ovaries, to liver damage with failure to metabolize estrogens, or to enhanced conversion of androstenedione to estrogen in fat cells in obese women. In addition, the rise in frequency of endometrial carcinoma parallels the rise in the use of substitutional exogenous estrogens during the climacteric period. After it was learned that exogenous estrogens are associated with endometrial carcinoma, their use decreased, and in the following decade the incidence of endometrial carcinoma also declined in that age group (WALKER and JICK 1980). On the other hand in women over 60 years of age the endometrial cancer rates are continuously rising. This can be explained by the assumption that an additional carcinogenic mechanism may be involved in old age, and that there may be two different forms of endometrial cancer (BOKHMAN 1983; HACHISUGA 1986). This assumption is supported by the observation that poorly differentiated carcinomas originating from pluripotent müllerian epithelium predominate in old age, whereas patients in the early postmenopause usually develop well-differentiated adenocarcinomas of the endometrial type. Recent observations of increased incidences of endometrial carcinoma in patients with breast carcinoma under adjuvant tamoxifen treatment (KILLAKEY et al. 1985; FORNANDER et al. 1989; NUOVO et al. 1989) suggest a stimulatory effect of estrogen antagonists on metaplastic müllerian target cells in the endometrium (see below). A similar effect may be observed with prolonged use of synthetic gestagens which are now routinely added to the pre- and postmenopausal estrogen substitution therapy. The increase of the mucinous type of endometrial adenocarcinoma recently observed may be closely related to that change in hormone substitution (DALLENBACH-HELLWEG et al. 1991).

## 3 Precursors

### 3.1 Morphology

As might be expected from the causal relationship of unopposed hyperestrogenism to the development of endometrial carcinoma, various stages of endometrial hyperplasia developing under elevated estrogen levels have to be considered as potential precursors of adenocarcinomas with endometrial differentiation, the most frequent type of endometrial carcinoma. Estrogen-stimulated endometrial hyperproliferation results in a continuum of hyperplastic changes of various degrees of severity and malignant potential.

*Glandular-cystic (simple) hyperplasia* is characterized by hyperproliferation of glands and stroma, usually without new gland formation and often resulting in cystic dilatation of the proliferating glands. New gland formation and glandular crowding with gradual loss of intervening stroma lead to *adenomatous (complex) hyperplasia*. The adenomatous growth may be only focal (*mild* adenomatous hyperplasia) or diffuse (*moderate* adenomatous hyperplasia), whereby structural alterations are observed without cytologic atypias. In severe adenomatous (atypical) hyperplasia, the structural alterations are accompanied by cytologic atypias. The relative risk of developing a carcinoma increases with the grade of severity of the hyperplasia. According to follow-up studies, cytologic atypia was a discriminating factor. The progression rate of hyperplasia without atypia was only 1%–8%, as compared to 29% in hyperplasias with atypia (severe adenomatous hyperplasia; KURMAN et al. 1985). The individual pattern of hyperplastic growth is maintained during all stages of carcinogenesis: adenomatous hyperplasia with foci of squamous metaplasia or morules will progress to adenocarcinoma with metaplasia (adenoacanthoma). When the preceding adenomatous hyperplasia has contained glands lined by ciliated cells, such cells will also be seen in the carcinoma developing from it.

For the second form of endometrial carcinoma with müllerian differentiation corresponding types of metaplasia are suggested as possible cells of origin. Whereas squamous metaplasia and ciliated cell changes in the endometrium have been shown to develop under estrogen stimulation (HENDRICKSON and KEMPSON 1980b; THOM et al. 1981) and are consequently found in hyperplastic endometria, other types of metaplasia, such as mucinous and serous papillary metaplasia, and clear cell and eosinophilic cell changes generally are not related to hyperestrogenism and may even be seen in atrophic endometria (Fig. 1). Some of these other types of metaplasia may, however, be associated with tamoxifen therapy or high doses of exogenous gestagens that also cause hyperproliferation of endocervical glands with microglandular hyperplasia. It is interesting that the endometrial carcinomas developing after tamoxifen therapy (personal observation, and see p. 30) are often of the endocervical or mixed müllerian type. A patient recently seen in consultation developed an endocervical type mucinous adenocarcinoma of the endometrium following high dosages of gestagens given for severe adenomatous hyperplasia. Her endometrium showed regressive changes with atrophic endometrial glands and decidualization of endometrial stroma, foci of mucinous metaplasia, and clear cell changes in the regions about the carcinoma (Fig. 2). These observations suggest that various types of metaplasia developing under excessive stimulation with antiestrogens or exogenous gestagens may be causally related to some of the "nonendometrial" types of endometrial carcinoma with müllerian differentiation, which usually are associated with endometrial atrophy and predominate in the late postmenopause (Table 1).

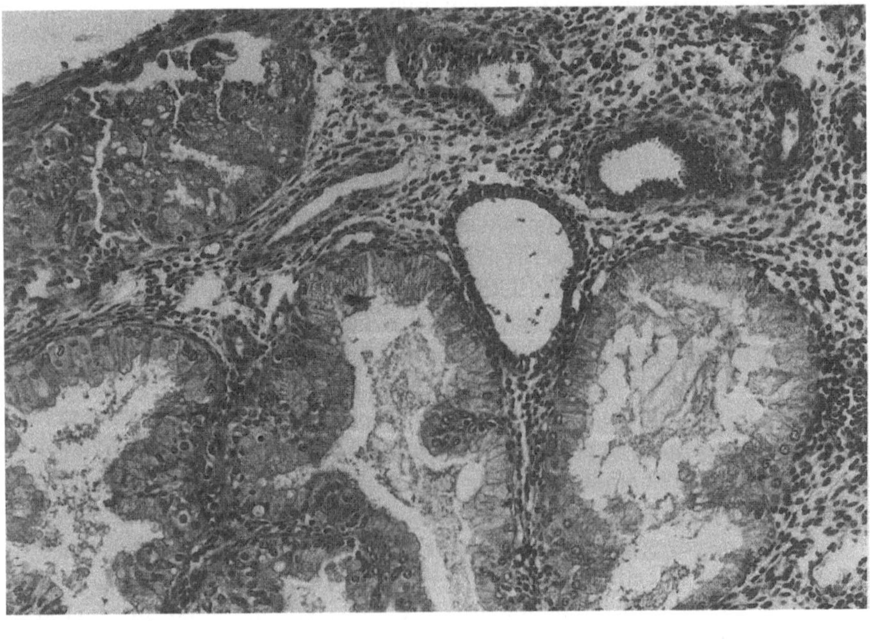

**Fig. 1.** Mucinous metaplasia in atrophic endometrium after therapy with tamoxifen. H&E, × 140

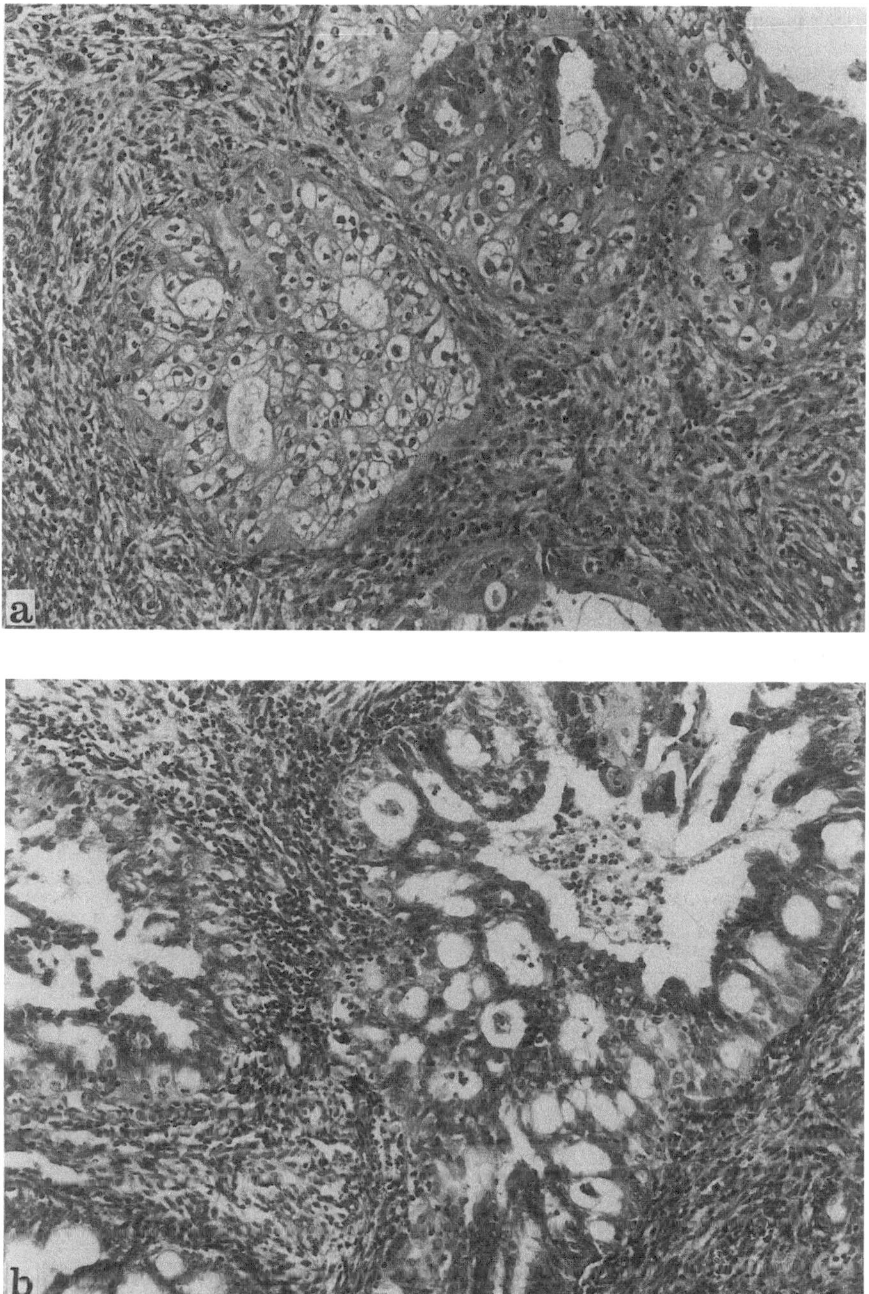


**Fig. 2.** Clear cell changes (**a**) adjacent to early mucinous adenocarcinoma and (**b**) following gestagen therapy for juvenile adenomatous hyperplasia. H&E, × 140

**Table 1.** Possible origin of different types of endometrial carcinoma from various metaplastic states. (DALLENBACH-HELLWEG 1987)

| | |
|---|---|
| Adenomatous hyperplasia → | Adenocarcinoma, endometrial type |
| With ciliated cells → | Adenocarcinoma, ciliated cell type |
| With squamous metaplasia and morules → | Adenoacanthoma<br>Adenosquamous carcinoma<br>Squamous cell carcinoma |
| Mucinous metaplasia → | Mucinous adenocarcinoma<br>Mucoepidermoid adenocarcinoma |
| Clear cell metaplasia → | Clear cell carcinoma |
| Papillary metaplasia → | Serous papillary carcinoma |

## 3.2 Differential Diagnosis

The distinction of adenomatous hyperplasia from a well-differentiated carcinoma may be difficult because of their morphologic similarities, such as back-to-back positioning of glands, epithelial stratification, and nuclear atypia (WELCH and SCULLY 1977; TAVASSOLI and KRAUS 1978; HENDRICKSON and KEMPSON 1980a). The most important and reliable criterion of the beginning of carcinomatous growth appears to be stromal invasion. Early carcinoma can be

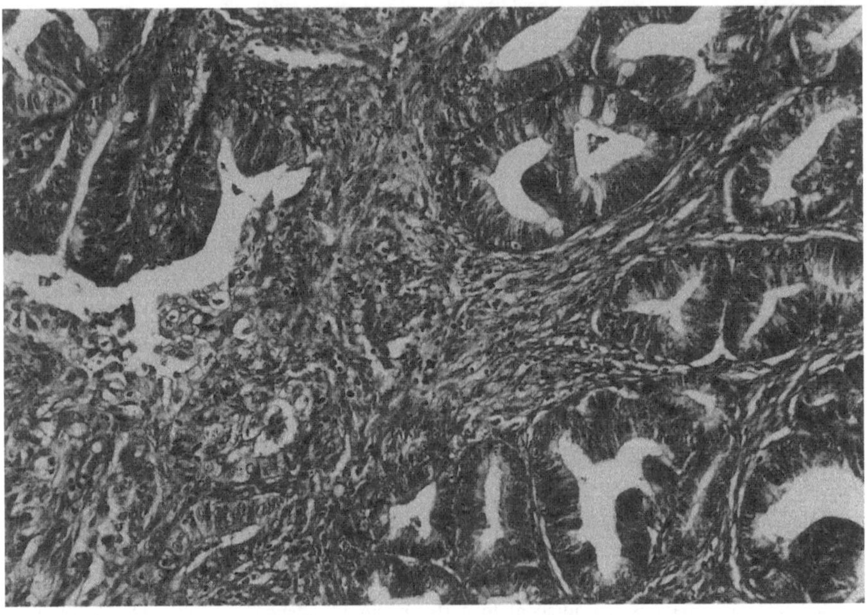

**Fig. 3.** Desmoplastic stromal reaction consisting of proliferating fibroblasts and sparse lymphocytic infiltrates around invading carcinomatous glands. (DALLENBACH-HELLWEG 1987) H&E, × 140

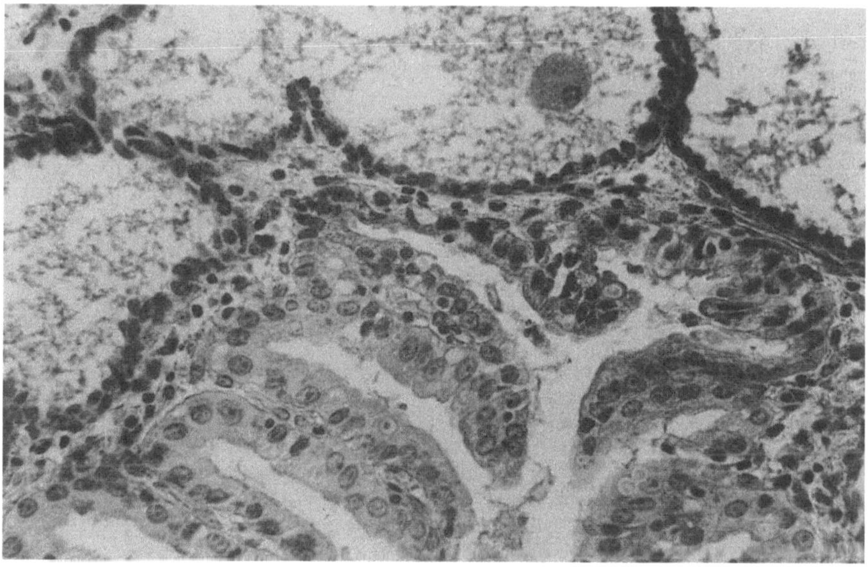

**Fig. 4.** Eosinophilic metaplasia in cystic–atrophic endometrium. (DALLENBACH-HELLWEG 1987) H&E, × 330

recognized by an altered fibroblastic (desmoplastic) stromal reaction around the invading atypical glands, by a confluent glandular pattern with microalveolar or cribriform proliferation, by replacement of stroma, by an extensive papillary pattern, and by large areas of squamous metaplasia. One of these criteria, if it occupies an area 4.2 mm in diameter, equaling one-half of a low-power field, is sufficient for a diagnosis of stromal invasion (KURMAN and NORRIS 1982; NORRIS et al. 1983). A desmoplastic stromal reaction can be distinguished by the densely packed spindle-shaped fibroblasts with elongated nuclei around the invading glands (Fig. 3). The various glandular patterns diagnostic of stromal invasion need not include cytologic atypias. On the other hand, cells with a high grade of nuclear atypia are, regardless of the area they occupy, highly suspicious of stromal invasion elsewhere in the endometrial specimen. Such atypical cytologic changes are immediate precursors of early carcinoma, which may develop either focally or multicentrically within an adenomatous hyperplasia. The early carcinomatous foci have compressed borders and may be surrounded by lymphocytic infiltrates about the desmoplastic stromal reaction (Fig. 2b).

Areas with cytologic atypias in severe adenomatous hyperplasia must, on the other hand, be distinguished from foci of müllerian metaplasia, which may show similar cytoplasmic changes such as eosinophilia. Benign metaplastic cells can best be recognized by their regular, euploid nuclei (Fig. 4) as compared to the atypical nuclei in pleomorphic cells seen focally in severe adenomatous hyperplasia.

**Table 2.** Carcinomas of the endometrium

| Histogenesis | Structure | Grading | Survival rate (%) | Relative frequency (%) [a] |
|---|---|---|---|---|
| Endometrial | Adenocarcinoma | | | 39.6 |
| | Glandular or | Grade 1 | 93 | |
| | Glandular–papillary | Grade 2 | 76 | |
| | Solid | Grade 3 | 61 | |
| | Secretory | Grade 1 | 87 | |
| | Ciliated cell | Grade 1 | | |
| | Adenocarcinoma with squamous metaplasia | | | |
| | Adenoacanthoma | Grade 1 | 87 | 21.7 |
| | Adenosquamous carcinoma | Grades 2+3 | 47 | 6.9 |
| Endocervical | Mucinous adenocarcinoma | Grades 1+2 | | 18 |
| | Mucoepidermoid adenocarcinoma | Grades 2+3 | 47 | |
| | Clear cell carcinoma | | | 4 |
| | Glandular or papillary | Grade 2 | 35 | |
| | Solid | Grade 3 | | |
| Serous | Serous papillary carcinoma | Grades 1+2 | 45 | 6 |
| | | Grade 3 | 11 | |
| Ectocervical | Squamous cell carcinoma | Grades 1, 2, or 3 | | |

[a] Approximate: collected and summarized from several studies (CHRISTOPHERSON et al. 1982; CHAMBERS et al. 1982; FANNING et al. 1989; personal studies)

# 4 Histogenetic Classification, Staging, and Grading

## 4.1 Classification

Since virtually all endometrial carcinomas develop from descendants of müllerian epithelium, they can be subdivided histogenetically (Table 2). Such a classification is sensible for several reasons: the etiology of the two major forms of endometrial carcinoma (that with endometrial differentiation and that with müllerian differentiation) differs; both forms are associated with different hormonal stimuli. The survival rates differ considerably and appear to be even more dependent on the cell of origin than on the histologic tumor grade. Identification of various histogenetic subtypes is possible with modern immunohistochemical techniques, even in the poorly differentiated tumors.

In addition to the histogenetic type, other prognostic parameters are important guidelines when deciding upon treatment, such as the tumor stage with depth of myometrial invasion, lymphatic invasion, and the histologic grade (CONNELLY et al. 1982; NG and REAGAN 1970).

## 4.2 Staging

The staging of endometrial carcinomas, according to FIGO, has recently been revised to comply with surgical staging (CREASMAN 1990):

| | | |
|---|---|---|
| Stage 1A | G123: | Tumor limited to endometrium |
| Stage IB | G123: | Invasion to less than one-half the myometrium |
| Stage IC | G123: | Invasion to more than one-half the myometrium |
| Stage IIA | G123: | Endocervical glandular involvement only |
| Stage IIB | G123: | Cervical stromal invasion |
| Stage IIIA | G123: | Tumor invades serosa and/or adnexa, and/or positive peritoneal cytology |
| Stage IIIB | G123 | Vaginal metastases |
| Stage IIIC | G123: | Metastases to pelvic and/or para-aortic lymph nodes |
| Stage IVA | G123: | Tumor invasion of bladder and/or bowel mucosa |
| Stage IVB | : | Distant metastases including intra-abdominal and/or inguinal lymph nodes |

For endocervical or cervical invasion, the surgical staging is more precise. The advantage of a fractionated D and C for predicting cervical involvement lies in the fact that it allows a preoperative staging. The value of that procedure is, however, dependent upon the technique used. Only adequate cervical specimens can be evaluated to prevent false-positive or false-negative results (FRAUENHOFFER et al. 1987; COWLES et al. 1985; Weiner et al. 1980). When the endocervical curettings contain only free-floating fragments of carcinomatous tissue, cervical invasion can never be excluded or proved.

### 4.3 Grading

Every type of endometrial carcinoma should be classified, in addition, for its degree of histologic differentiation. The new grading system, according to FIGO, is like the previous one based on *architectural criteria*:
G1 = 5% or less of a nonsquamous or nonmorular solid growth pattern
G2 = 6%–50% of a nonsquamous or nonmorular solid growth pattern
G3 = more than 50% of a nonsquamous or nonmorular solid growth pattern

With this FIGO classification the 5-year survival rates correspond closely with tumor grade (see Table 2). In general, grade 3 tumors present with deep myometrial invasion and early lymphatic spread, whereas grade 1 tumors are rarely seen in this advanced stage at the time of surgery.

In addition to architectural changes, the degree of *nuclear atypia* is considered to be important for grading (CONNELLY et al. 1982; KURMAN and NORRIS 1987). Evaluation of nuclear atypia seems to be of particular value for clear cell and serous papillary carcinomas, which have a poor prognosis regardless of their histologic grade as defined by FIGO. Both these types of carcinoma may have well-preserved glands or papillae but pronounced nuclear atypias. Since, in addition, some carcinomas vary in their differentiation from one area to another, a combination of grading based on architectural and nuclear criteria might be best, as shown and recommended in a recent comparative study of 164 patients (MITTAL et al. 1988). The nuclear grade should include the mitotic index, or even better, the proliferation rate, as measured with proliferation markers such as KI 67. According to a recent recommendation of the Committee of the International Society of Gynecological Pathologists, notable nuclear atypia, inappropriate for the architectural grade, should raise the grade of a grade 1 or grade 2 tumor by 1.

Measurement of the *steroid receptor content* of the carcinomatous cells is valuable in two respects: First, it identifies the carcinomas with endometrial differentiation that have developed under hormonal stimulation and show a better prognosis: up to 81% of all low-grade carcinomas are receptor-positive, as compared with only 12% of high-grade tumors. Second, since only those patients with receptor-positive carcinomas will profit from adjuvant gestagen therapy, it helps in deciding postoperative treatment.

## 5 Carcinomas with Endometrial Differentiation

Adenocarcinomas with endometrial differentiation constituted approximately 86% (HERTIG and GORE 1960), but recently slightly less (WALKER and JICK 1980) of all endometrial carcinomas. Their peak incidence lies in the early postmenopause, with an average age of around 57 years.

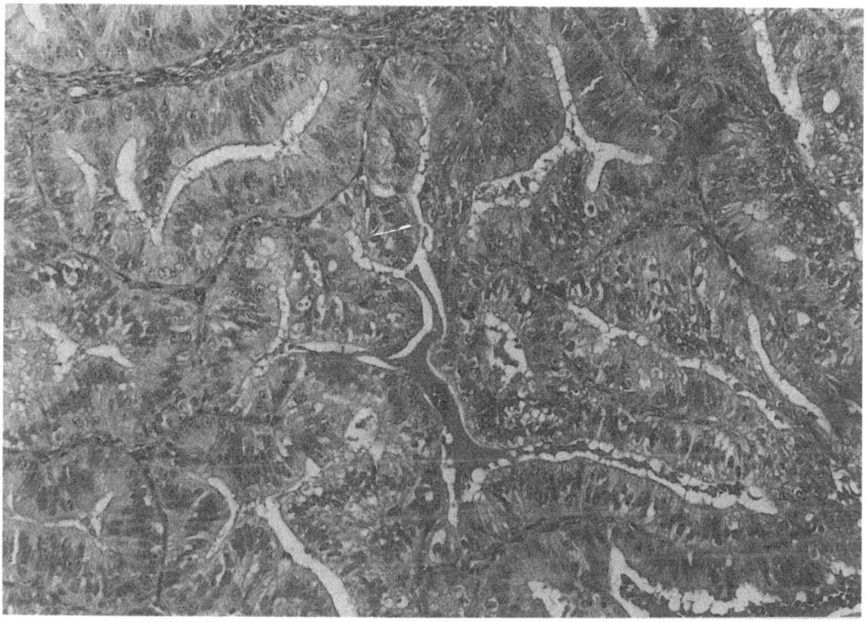

**Fig. 5.** Adenocarcinoma, endometrial type, well differentiated. H&E, × 140

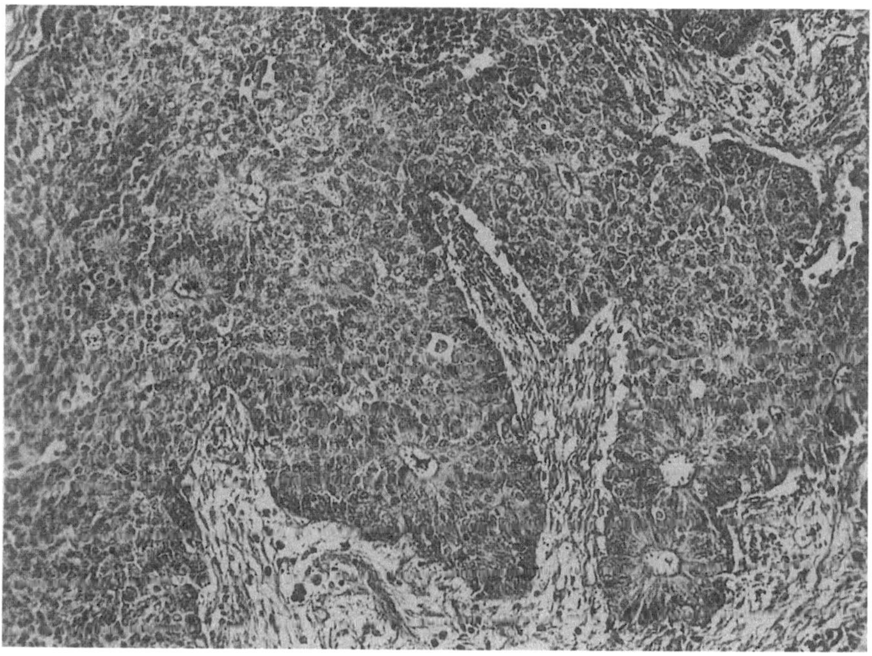

**Fig. 6.** Adenocarcinoma, endometrial type, undifferentiated (solid), with pseudorosette formation. (DALLENBACH-HELLWEG 1987) H&E, × 140

## 5.1 Glandular or Glandular–Papillary Adenocarcinoma

In glandular or glandular–papillary adenocarcinoma, the carcinomatous glands in the well-differentiated type (Fig. 5) resemble those of the preceding adenomatous hyperplasia both light and electron microscopically (THRASHER and RICHART 1972; AYCOCK et al. 1979). Partly undifferentiated carcinomas may contain microglandular areas occasionally separated sharply from the well-differentiated areas. Undifferentiated solid adenocarcinoma consists of solid areas of disorderly arranged carcinomatous cells. The adenomatous nature of the tumor may be detected by finding pseudorosette formations in some parts of the tumor (Fig. 6). These can be used to distinguish solid adenocarcinoma from undifferentiated squamous cell carcinoma. Such pseudorosettes often contain small amounts of mucus in their centers, which may become evident with the PAS stain. If these are lacking, ultrastructural or immunohistochemical studies may help in the differentiation: the undifferentiated carcinomatous cells retain the complex patterns of intermediate filaments shown by their cells of origin (see below).

*Secretory adenocarcinoma* is rare. The secretory changes of well-differentiated carcinomatous glands (Fig. 7) may be the result of previous therapy with high doses of gestagen. In patients without a history of gestagen use, an endogenous source for the progestational effect may be difficult to clarify, since most of these patients are postmenopausal (CHRISTOPHERSON et al. 1982).

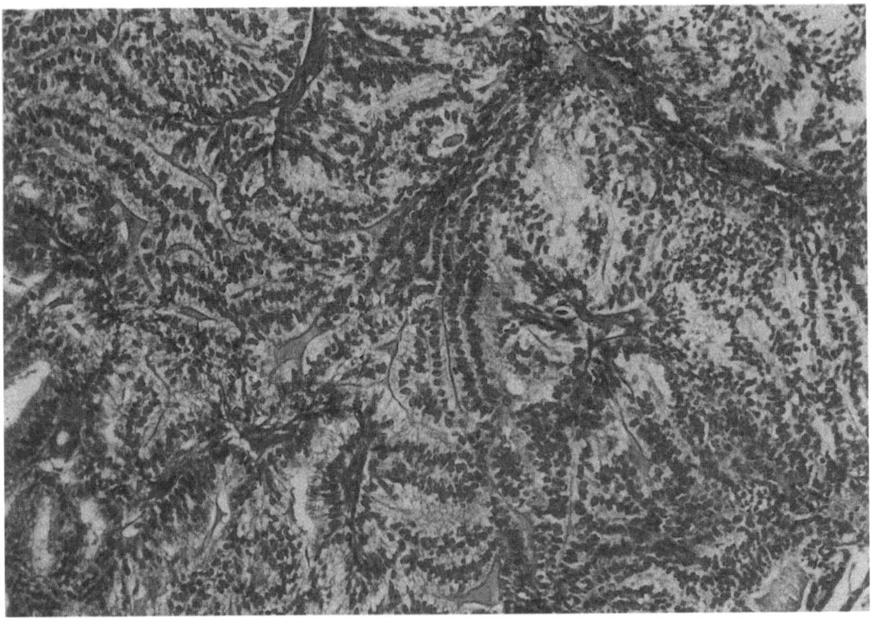

**Fig. 7.** Secretory adenocarcinoma, endometrial type. (DALLENBACH-HELLWEG 1987) H&E, × 140

The rare *ciliated cell type adenocarcinoma* is closely associated with previous exogenous estrogen treatment (HENDRICKSON and KEMPSON 1980b).

## 5.2 Adenocarcinoma with Squamous Metaplasia

Adenocarcinoma with squamous metaplasia is the type most frequently seen in patients who have previously taken estrogens (ROBBOY and BRADLEY 1979). The well-differentiated form, *adenoacanthoma*, is a glandular papillary adenocarcinoma of the endometrial type with nodular regions of squamous metaplasia or morules that mingle with the glandular cells from which the squamous cells apparently arise by metaplasia (Fig. 8). Ultrastructurally, they are usually surrounded by an intact basal lamina. In spite of their regular appearance, these squamous cell nodules are potentially malignant and may be found in the metastases of these carcinomas (CHARLES 1965).

In the poorly differentiated form, *adenosquamous carcinoma*, the glandular and solid-squamous portions are closely mixed but in a disorderly fashion. Some glands may be well-differentiated, whereas others develop aberrantly as small compact acini. Mucus is sparse. The adjacent solid regions consist of immature squamous metaplasia with atypical nuclei, frequent mitoses, and variably abundant acidophilic cytoplasm (Fig. 9). Ultrastructurally, both cellular components can be clearly distinguished, but cells intermediate between

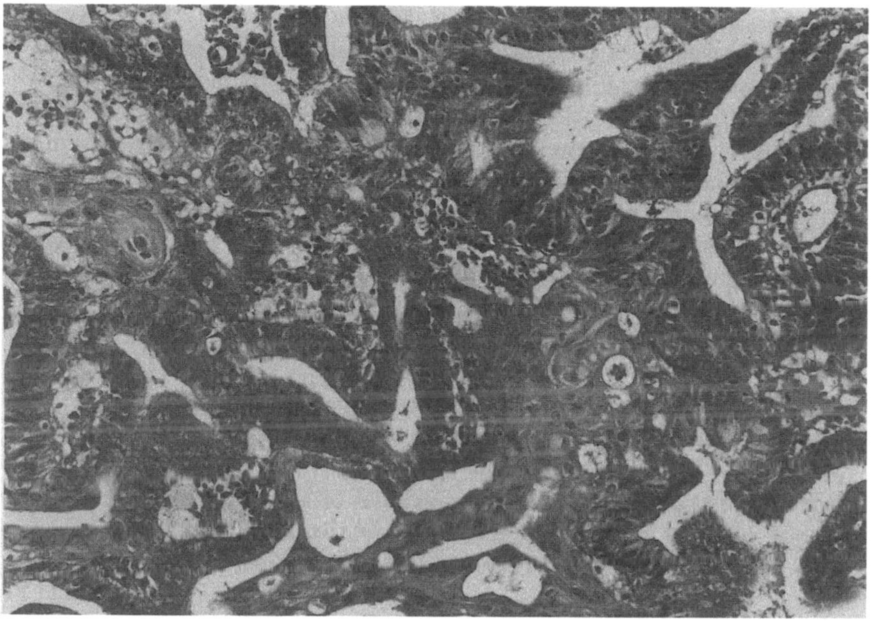

**Fig. 8.** Adenoacanthoma,well differentiated. H&E, × 140

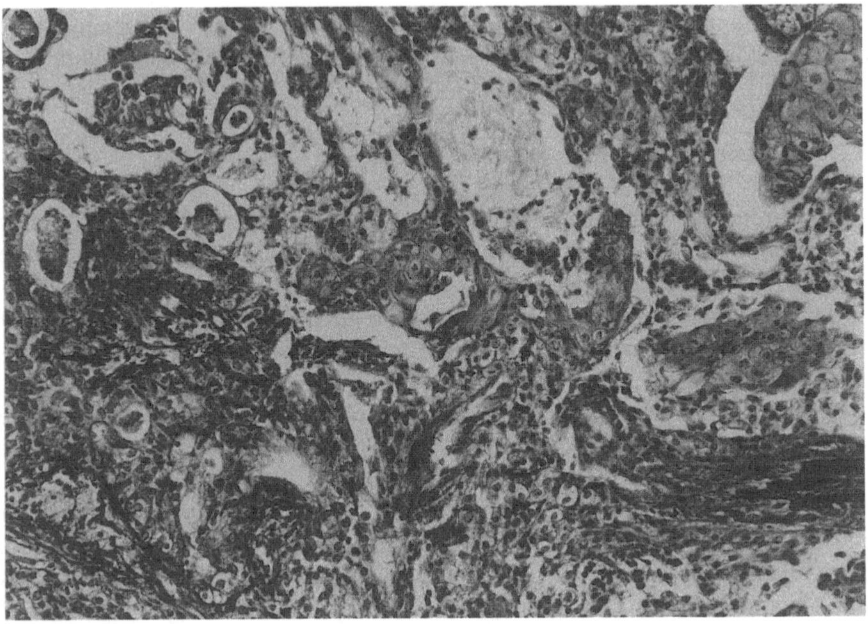

**Fig. 9.** Adenosquamous carcinoma, poorly differentiated. H&E, × 140

glandular and squamous elements may be seen, suggesting that the two cell types differentiate from the same stem cell (FU et al. 1979). In this type of carcinoma, irrespective of the stage of differentiation of the glandular elements, the squamous component with aneuploid nuclei is usually responsible for early deep myometrial invasion (DEMOPOULOS et al. 1986).

Because of their differences in prognosis, it is important to distinguish the well-differentiated adenoacanthoma with a 5-year survival rate of 87% from the poorly differentiated adenosquamous carcinoma with a 5-year survival rate of 47% (ALBERHASKY et al. 1982; CONNELLY et al. 1982). The endometrial type of adenosquamous carcinoma can be distinguished from the endocervical type by immunohistochemistry, especially with antibodies to carcinoembryonic antigen (CEA) and vimentin (see below).

## 5.3 Adenocarcinoma in Young Women

In women under 40 years of age the diagnosis of a well-differentiated adenocarcinoma with or without squamous metaplasia must be made with great caution. Clinical experience has shown that even extensive adenomatous proliferation with adenoacanthosis is reversible in young women and should be diagnosed as adenomatous hyperplasia (DALLENBACH-HELLWEG et al. 1971; FECHNER and KAUFMAN 1974; MOUKHTAR et al. 1977; NORRIS et al. 1983; LEE and

SCULLY 1989). Invasive adenocarcinoma in young women is extremely rare and should be diagnosed only when unequivocal signs of invasion such as a desmoplastic stromal response or confluence of adenomatous proliferation and nuclear atypicality are present.

# 6 Carcinomas with Müllerian Differentiation

Unlike the carcinomas with endometrial differentiation, this group of endometrial carcinomas originates from pluripotent müllerian epithelium and may develop in endometria with low or even absent proliferative activity independent of estrogenic hyperstimulation. Their peak incidence usually lies in the late postmenopause.

## 6.1 Mucinous Adenocarcinoma

Mucinous adenocarcinoma structurally and histochemically closely resembles the mucinous type of endocervical adenocarcinoma (Fig. 10). Microglandular or solid areas may be found between well-differentiated cystic glands filled with

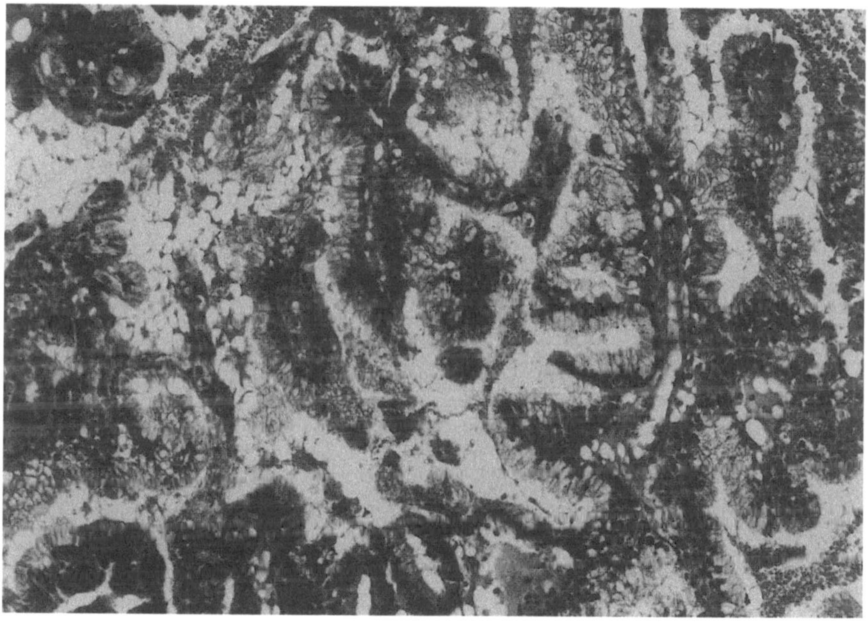

**Fig. 10.** Mucinous adenocarcinoma. H&E, × 140

mucus. At the margins of the carcinoma remnants of endocervical metaplasia can often be seen. The patients with these tumors have frequently had previous therapy with antiestrogens (tamoxifen) or synthetic gestagens. Consequently their endocervical mucosa may be equally stimulated, showing adenomatous or microglandular proliferation. In such instances, the hormonal stimulus that causes hyperproliferation of endocervical glands apparently leads to endocervical metaplasia of the endometrium, which then undergoes malignant change. Since the adjuvant treatment for this type of carcinoma will undoubtedly prove to be quite different from that for the adenocarcinoma of endometrial differentiation, it is very important to distinguish between the two types. That distinction is readily made by recalling the structural differences between endometrial and endocervical differentiation, and by noting how the cytoskeletons of the carcinomatous cells stain: at least some of the mucin-secreting carcinomatous glands with endocervical differentiation are positive with anti-CEA (see p. 23), and their reaction with anti-vimentin is consistently negative. On the other hand, to distinguish mucinous adenocarcinoma of the endometrium, which has a fairly good prognosis (MELHEM and TOBON 1987), from that of the endocervix with an unfavorable prognosis is impossible histologically and can be achieved only topographically, since both carcinomas produce almost identical acid mucopolysaccharides (CZERNOBILSKY et al. 1980; TILTMAN 1980; ROSS et al. 1983) and have a similar composition of intermediate filaments (WAHLSTRÖM et al. 1979)

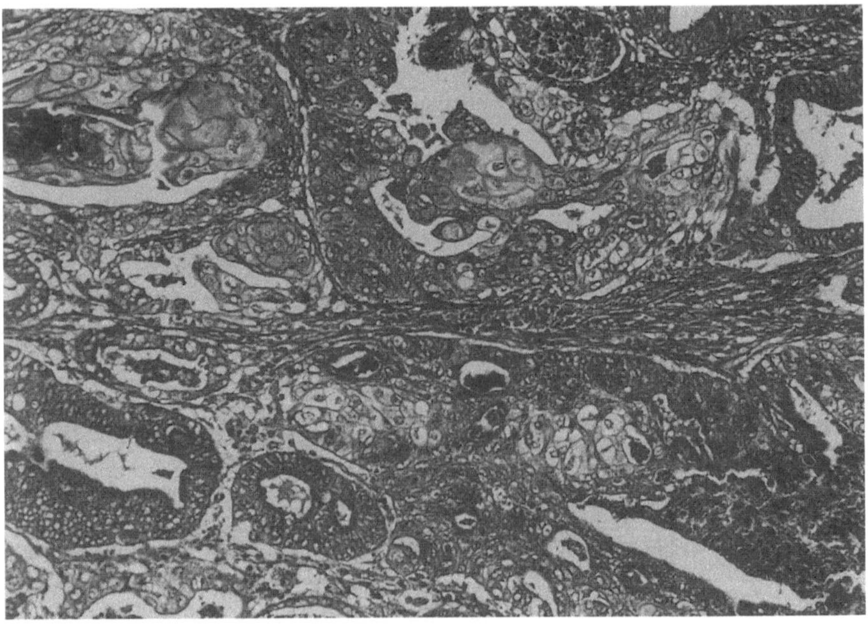

**Fig. 11.** Mucoepidermoid adenocarcinoma. PAS, × 140

## 6.2 Mucoepidermoid Adenocarcinoma

Mucoepidermoid adenocarcinoma consists mainly of poorly differentiated strands of epidermoid cells with monocellular keratinization or mucin formation, intermingled with mucinous glands (Fig. 11). These carcinomas, too, usually arise from endocervical metaplasias in the endometrium, in which the bipotential metaplastic cells may produce either keratin or mucin (DALLENBACH-HELLWEG et al. 1988). They are more aggressive than mucinous adenocarcinomas without squamous differentiation. To distinguish them from a primary mucoepidermoid adenocarcinoma of the endocervix is possible only topographically. The age of the patient, however, is important: the average age of patients with a mucoepidermoid adenocarcinoma of the endometrium is 69 years (DALLENBACH-HELLWEG et al. 1988), whereas that of patients whose carcinomas arise in the endocervix is 39 years (DALLENBACH-HELLWEG 1984).

## 6.3 Clear Cell Carcinoma

Clear cell carcinoma, too, develops in the senile patient. It closely resembles clear cell carcinoma of the ovary, cervix, and vagina, both light and electron microscopically (KURMAN and SCULLY 1976; HORIE et al. 1977). Although their structural identity is incomplete (EASTWOOD 1978), clear cell carcinomas most

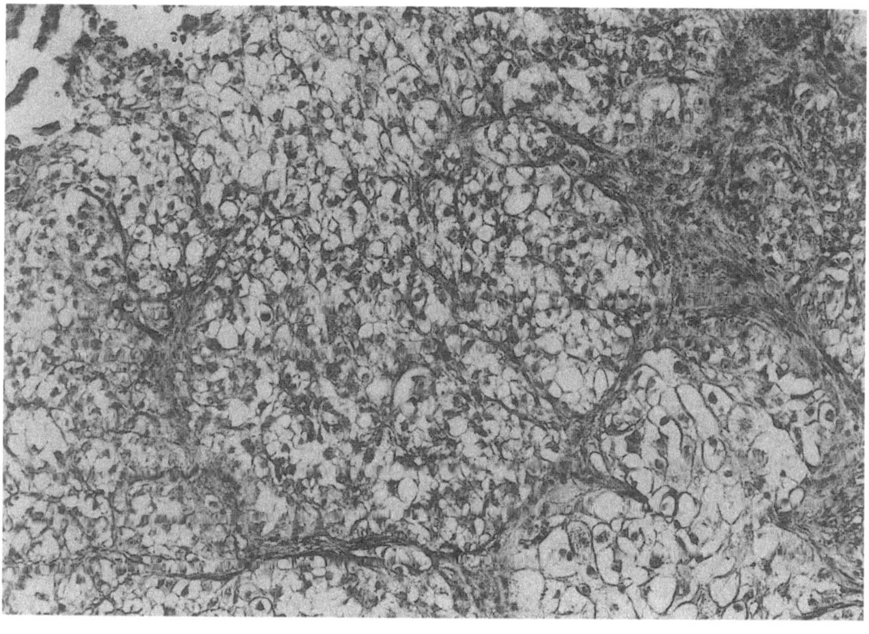

**Fig. 12.** Clear cell carcinoma, solid. H&E, × 140

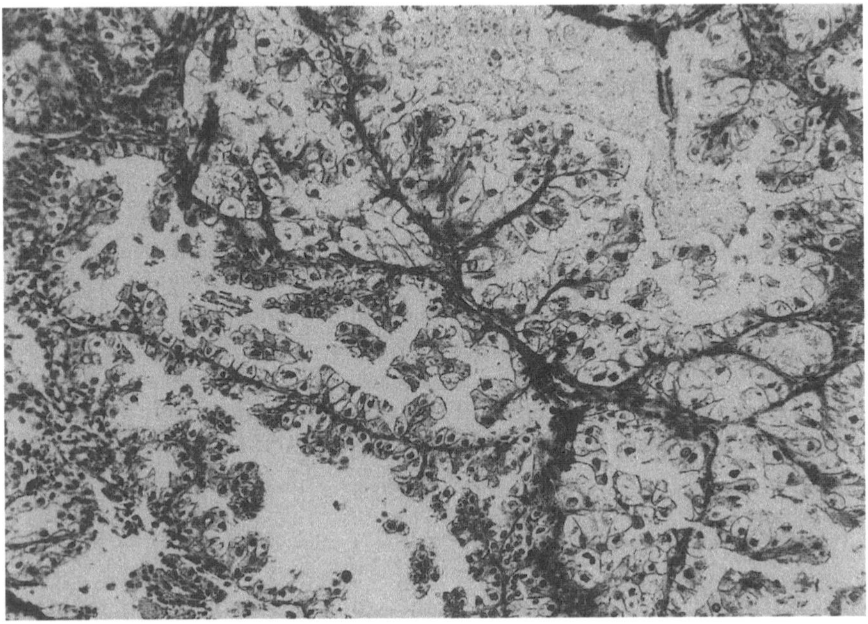

**Fig. 13.** Arias–Stella reaction of hypersecreting endometrial glands. (DALLENBACH-HELLWEG 1987) H&E, × 140

likely arise from disturbed metaplasia of endocervical reserve cells in the endometrium, whereby the reserve cells, presumably through faulty differentiation, remain at an intermediary stage of development between incomplete keratinization and the secretion of mucus (DALLENBACH-HELLWEG and LANG 1991). The clear cells are either arranged in solid nests or form glands, cysts, or papillae, often with nuclei in a hobnail position (Fig. 12). Nuclear atypia is marked, and mitoses are frequent. The clear cell cytoplasm may contain glycogen or diastase-resistant hyaline inclusions. The 5-year survival rate of all grades of this highly malignant neoplasm is only 35% (CHRISTOPHERSON et al. 1982). The microscopic distinction from a clear cell carcinoma of the endocervix may be impossible. On the other hand, it is easy to distinguish it from a secretory adenocarcinoma, the cells of which may also have clear cytoplasm, since the latter lacks nuclear and cellular pleomorphism. The glandular type of clear cell carcinoma may occasionally be confused with a very pronounced Arias–Stella reaction of hypersecreting endometrial glands during pregnancy (Fig. 13). This can be avoided when the entire endometrial specimen is examined and correlated with the clinical history.

## 6.4 Serous Papillary Carcinoma

Serous papillary carcinoma almost exclusively develops in the senile patient with an average age between 66 (HENDRICKSON et al. 1982) and 73 years (LIU

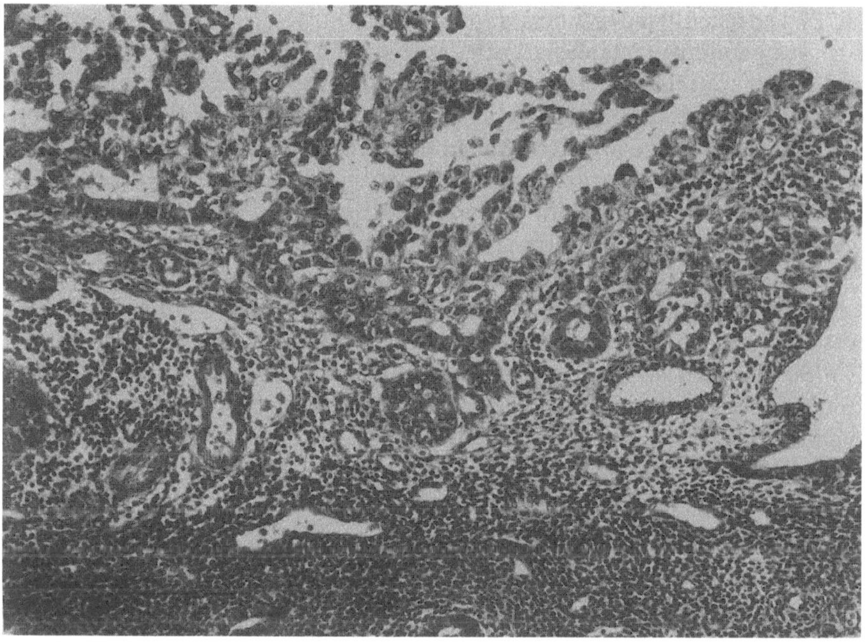

**Fig. 14.** Serous papillary metaplasia of endometrial surface epithelium. (DALLENBACH-HELLWEG 1987) H&E, × 140

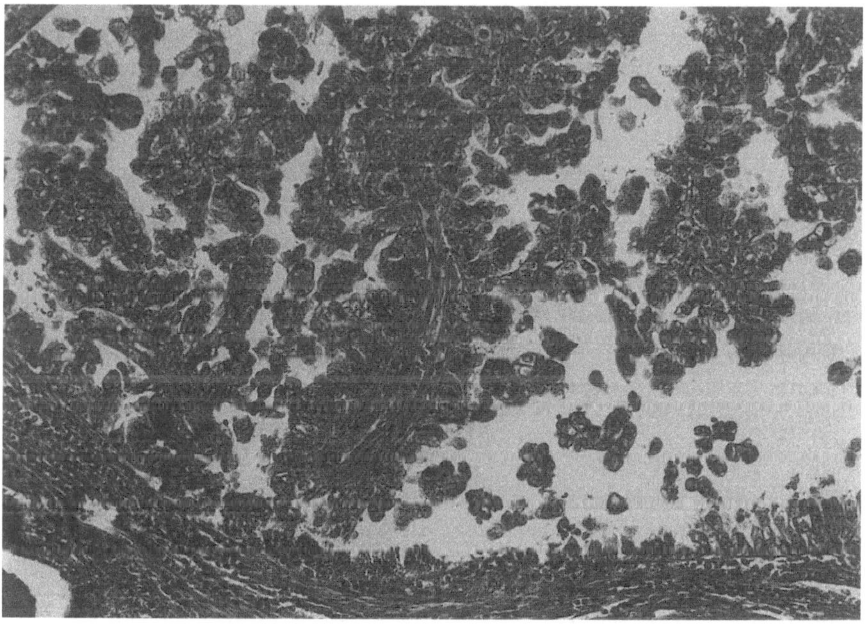

**Fig. 15.** Serous papillary carcinoma. H&E, × 140

1972), and usually independent of previous hormone therapy. It originates from a serous papillary metaplasia in the endometrial surface epithelium (Fig. 14) and fills the uterine cavity with an exophytic growth grossly resembling placental tissue but surrounded by an atrophic uterus. By the time the tumor is detected it may have already invaded the myometrium and spread beyond the uterus. Its histologic structure is almost identical to that of serous papillary carcinoma of the ovary with its complex branching epithelial papillae and marked nuclear pleomorphism (Fig. 15). Ultrastructurally, paranuclear microfilaments and tonofilaments are more prominent than in endometrial type adenocarcinoma (SATO et al. 1984). The 5-year survival rate in a recent study was found to be only 45% for stages 1 and 2, and 11% for stages 3 and 4 (CHAMBERS et al. 1987). It is important of distinguish this serous papillary carcinoma from papillary structures of a well-differentiated edenocarcinoma of endometrial type, which are broader and usually have stratified columnar, more regular carcinomatous cells, because the latter has a much more favorable prognosis (see Table 2).

### 6.5 Squamous Cell Carcinoma

Squamous cell carcinoma of the endometrium is extremely rare (MELIN et al. 1979). It may develop in the late postmenopause from a generalized squamous metaplasia or an ichthyosis uteri (BERSCH et al. 1984). Only two cases have been reported before the menopause (YAMASHINA and KOBARA 1986). The prognosis is poor (SIMON et al. 1988). More often what seems to be a squamous cell carcinoma of the endometrium represents a squamous cell carcinoma of the cervix that has grown up into the uterine cavity (KANBOUR and STOCK 1978). Consequently, a primary squamous cell carcinoma of the endometrium can only be diagnosed in a uterus with a normal ecto- and endocervix, and in the absence of endometrial adenocarcinoma.

## 7 Undifferentiated Carcinomas

Undifferentiated carcinomas may be unclassifiable of light microscopy. Electron microscopy and immunohistochemistry can be helpful in the differential diagnosis (see below). They may be large or small celled. Some of the small cell variety may show neuroendocrine differentiation and contain argyrophilic cells (UEDA et al. 1977; OLSON et al. 1982; see chapter by Ueda).

## 8 Metastatic Carcinomas

Carcinomas may involve the endometrium and the ovary simultaneously, making it difficult to distinguish between two primary tumors and/or metastases to either site. The distinction is nonetheless important, because the prognosis and treatment differ. In a series of 34 such simultaneous carcinomas, 12 were classified as two independent carcinomas, 22 as metastases (ULBRIGHT and ROTH 1985). Since well-differentiated endometrial adenocarcinomas seldom metastasize, an ovarian carcinoma found at the same time usually represents a second primary tumor. On the other hand, endometrial carcinomas with müllerian differentiation, like serous papillary carcinomas, tend to metastasize early to the ovaries (EIFEL et al. 1982). Metastases from extragenital primary carcinomas are rare and most often poorly differentiated. In these instances the primary carcinoma is most often located in the breast (47%) or gastrointestinal tract (35%), rarely in the kidney (3%) (KUMAR and HART 1982).

## 9 Immunohistochemistry

The subdivision of invasive endometrial carcinomas made possible by their structural differences can be substantiated by their individual and specific immunohistochemical reactions. All the types of carcinoma mentioned retain the complex pattern of intermediate filaments shown by their cells of origin. Hence, tumors derived from the different types of epithelial cell originating from the müllerian duct can be distinguished by their specific cytokeratin polypeptide patterns. The carcinomatous cells derived from metaplastic endocervical epithelium in addition acquire a more or less distinctly positive reaction with anti-CEA, which indicates malignant transformation.

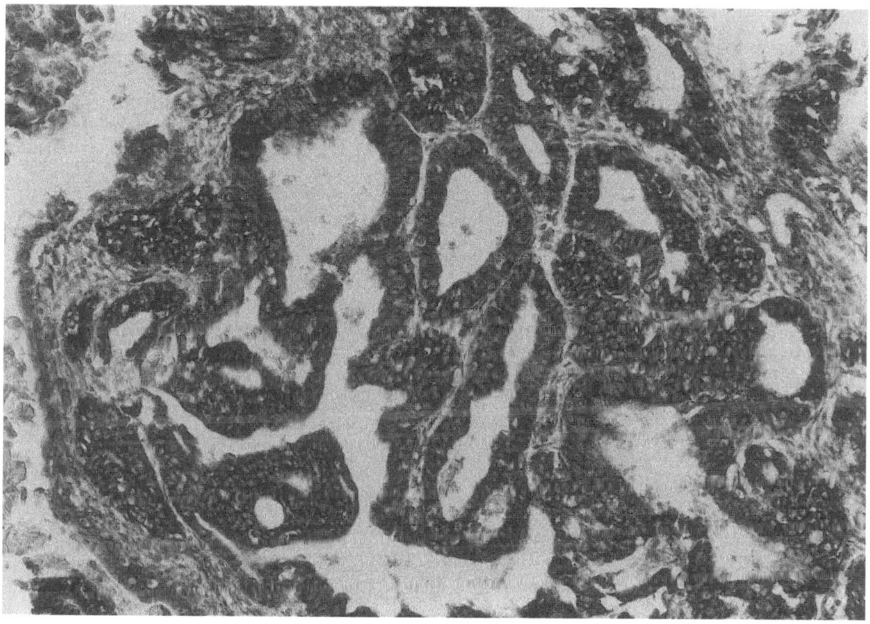

**Fig. 16.** Adenocarcinoma with endometrial differentiation. Positive reaction of carcinomatous glands with antivimentin. × 140

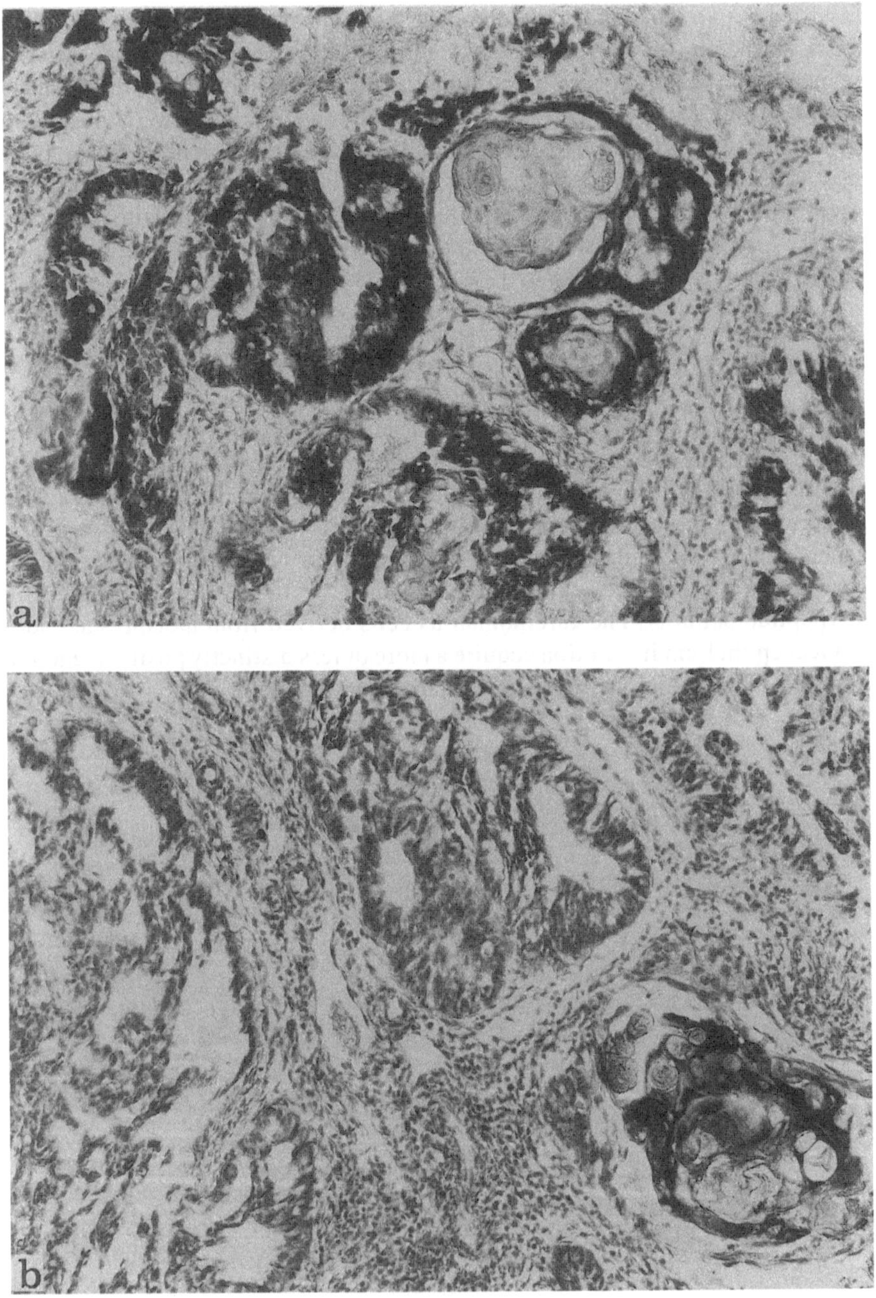

Fig. 17 a, b. Adenoacanthoma. Carcinomatous glands react positively with anticytokeratin 8 (a), whereas foci of squamous metaplasia are positive with anticytokeratin 13 (b). × 140

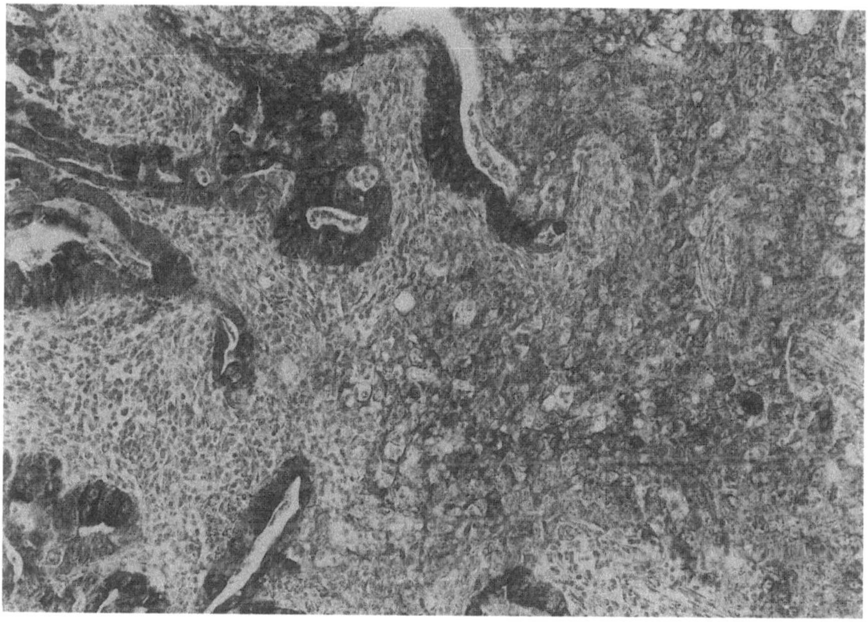

**Fig. 18.** Adenosquamous carcinoma. Carcinomatous glands are positive and solid carcinomatous areas negative with anticytokeratin 8, indicating incomplete squamous differentiation. × 140

## 9.1 Adenocarcinomas with Endometrial Differentiation

Adenocarcinomas with endometrial differentiation show, like normal endometrial glands, a distinctly positive reaction for cytokeratins 7, 8, 18, and 19 (MOLL et al. 1983; CZERNOBILSKY et al. 1984). The reactions with anticytokeratins typical of complex epithelial cells are negative. In addition, the majority of carcinoma cells of endometrial differentiation stain for vimentin (Fig. 16) just as proliferative normal endometrial glandular cells do, whereas secreting glandular epithelial cells are only weakly positive or even negative with antivimentin. When we studied only carcinomas with unequivocal endometrial differentiation, nearly all of our cases showed a coexpression of vimentin and cytokeratin. Similar results were reported by McNUTT et al. (1985) and PUTS et al. (1987). DABBS et al. (1986) found a positive vimentin reaction in 65% of all endometrial adenocarcinomas (including some of müllerian differentiation). The reaction for CEA is negative (see also WAHLSTRÖM et al. 1979; UEDA et al. 1983). The variable results with the reaction for CEA on endometrial adenocarcinomas published by other authors (MAES et al. 1988; and previous references cited there) can be explained in part by the areas of endocervical differentiation within an otherwise endometrial type adenocarcinoma. In addition, some endometrial carcinomas may react positively with anti-CEA at the small luminal rim of the carcinomatous glandular epithelial cells, where acid mucopolysaccharides at the apical end of the glandular cells are located in 80% of well-differentiated endometrial adenocarcinomas (SORVARI 1969). Such a reaction should be disregarded, since it lies outside the cytoplasm.

Adenocarcinomas with squamous metaplasia, regardless of their degree of differentiation, give identical immunohistochemical reactions in their adenomatous regions, whereas the foci of squamous metaplasia are positive with anticytokeratins 5 and 13, but negative with anticytokeratins 7, 8, 18, and 19 and with antivimentin (Fig. 17). By these reactions poorly differentiated areas of adenosquamous carcinoma can be recognized either as adenomatous or as squamous (Fig. 18).

## 9.2 Carcinomas with Müllerian Differentiation

Carcinomas with müllerian differentiation show, independent of their histologic grade, focally different coexpressions of intermediate filaments that correspond to their differences in cellular structure. Mucinous adenocarcinomas and well-differentiated mucinous areas in müllerian mixed carcinomas, like mucoepidermoid adenocarcinomas, are positive for cytokeratins 7, 8, 18 and 19, but negative for cytokeratins 5 and 13 and for vimentin. The reaction for CEA is inconsistently positive, varying in intensity from area to area (Fig. 19). The

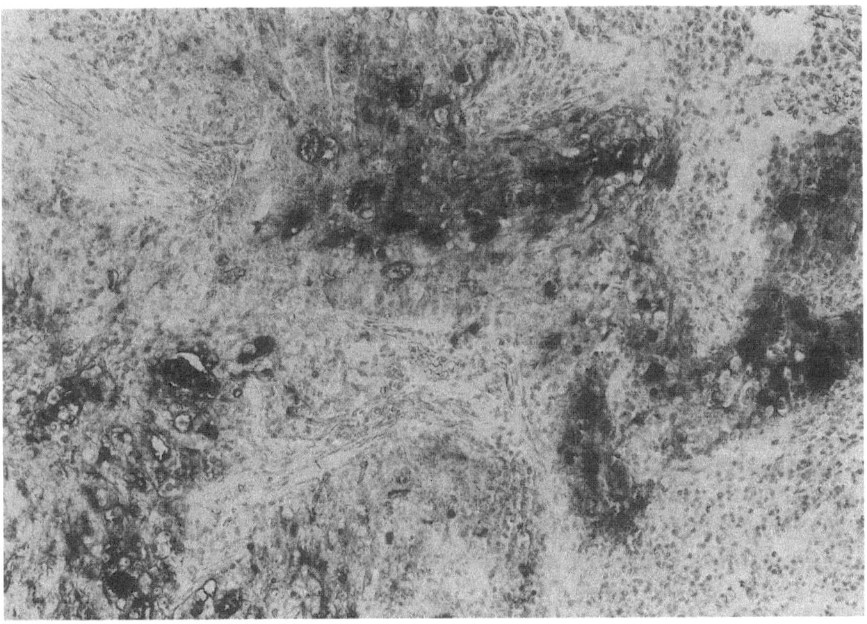

**Fig. 19.** Mucinous adenocarcinoma, poorly differentiated. Reaction with anti-CEA focally positive. × 140

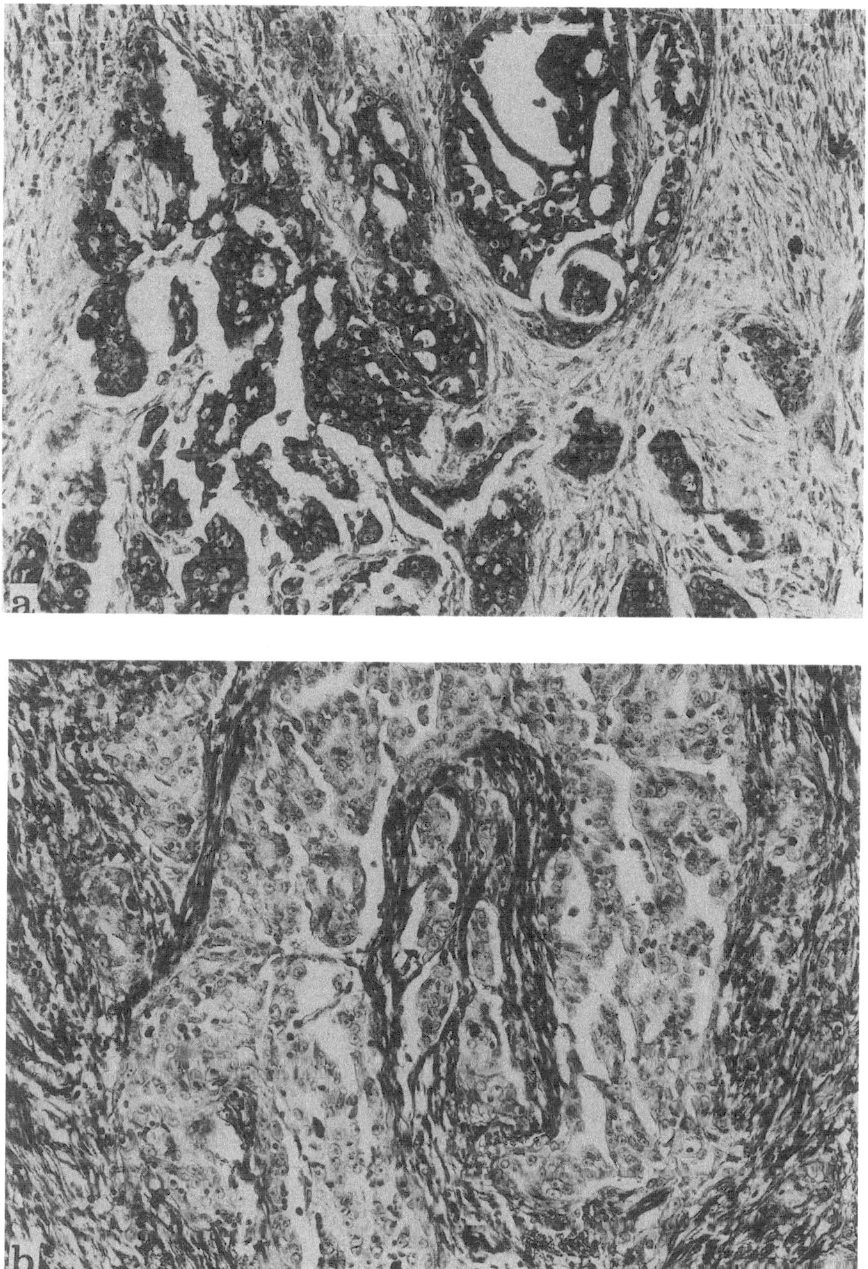

**Fig. 20 a, b.** Serous papillary carcinoma. Positive reaction with anticytokeration 8 (**a**), whereas most carcinomatous cells react negatively with antivimentin (**b**). × 140

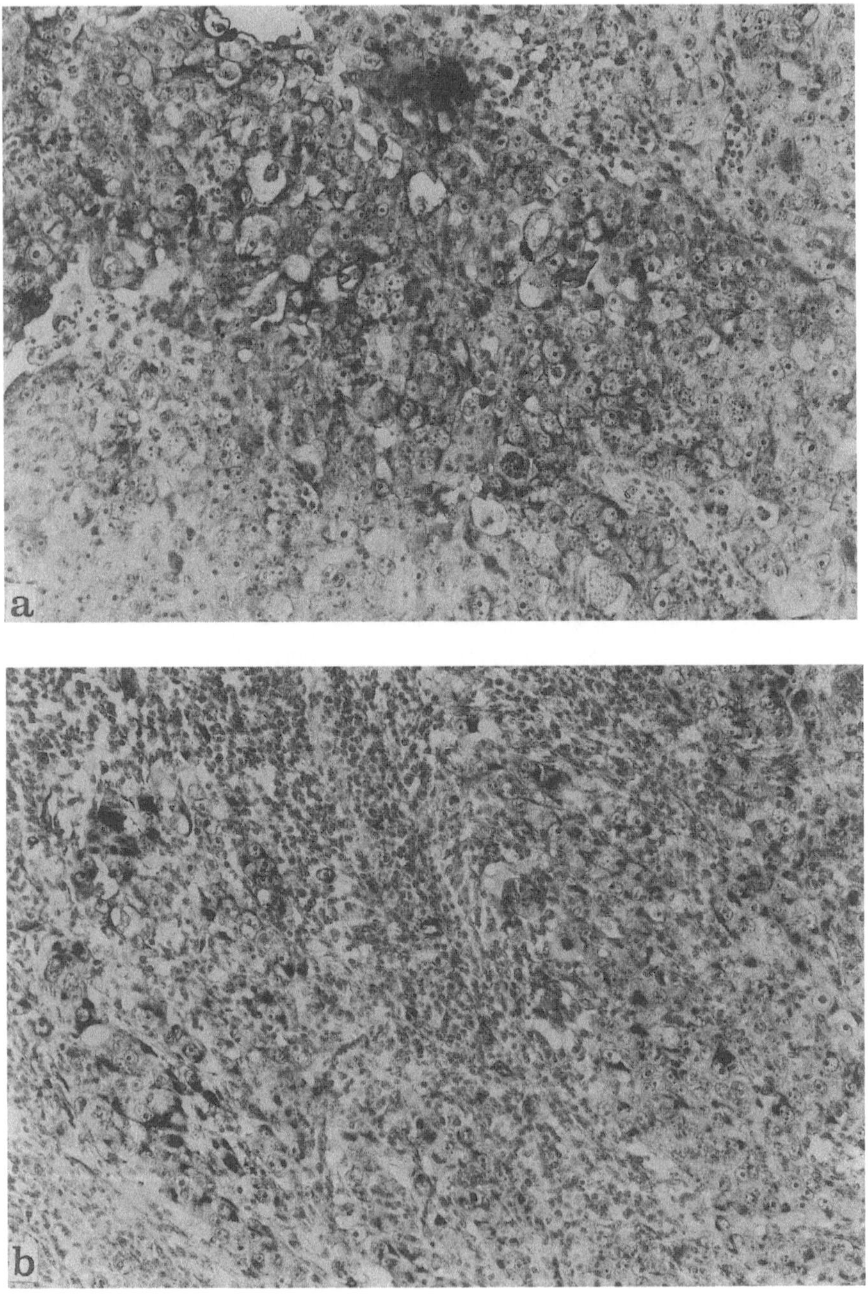

**Fig. 21 a, b.** Undifferentiated carcinoma. Coexpression of **(a)** cytokeratin 8 and **(b)** vimentin in several foci. × 140

areas with squamous differentiation in mucoepidermoid adenocarcinomas coexpress cytokeratins 5 and 13 but are CEA-negative. Clear cell carcinomas, because of their clear cytoplasm, generally have reduced numbers of intermediate filaments. Consequently, no extensive reactions can be expected. They show a weak coexpression of cytokeratins 5, 13, 7, 8, 18, and 19, but are negative for vimentin and usually negative for CEA, although the reaction with anti-CEA may occasionally be weakly positive. Serous papillary carcinomas are negative for cytokeratins 5 and 13, but positive for cytokeratins 7, 8, 18, and 19 (Fig. 20a). Their reaction with antivimentin varies: it is positive in some of the carcinomatous cells, but negative in others (Fig. 20b). Their reaction for CEA is negative (Sasano et al. 1990).

## 9.3 Undifferentiated Carcinomas

In undifferentiated carcinomas the cells of origin can often be identified by their coexpression of intermediate filaments (Fig. 21). In addition argyrophilic cells can be detected in 26% (Aquirre et al. 1984) to 68% (Bannatyne et al. 1983) of these endometrial carcinomas, some of which also reveal neurosecretory granules ultrastructurally and react with antibodies against neuroectoderm (Ueda et al. 1986). Since patients with these carcinomas manifest no hormonal aberrations (Scully et al. 1984) these argyrophil cells may merely be an incidental finding.

## 9.4 Differential Diagnosis

Histogenetic differentiation between the various types of endometrial carcinoma is clinically important to avoid treatment failures (Burke et al. 1990), since these carcinomas vary in their prognosis and response to therapy (Table 3). The differentiation cannot always be made on H&E slides alone, particularly when the carcinoma under study is poorly differentiated throughout. Equally important is the differentiation between carcinomas originating in the endometrium and those originating in the endocervix. Since the mucopolysaccharides of endometrial glands differ histochemically in quality and quantity from those of endocervical glands, the adenocarcinomas arising from these two types of gland can usually be readily distinguished with appropriate immunohistochemical methods, such as mucus-associated antigens (Maes et al. 1988). In addition, if staining for vimentin is positive that excludes the endocervix as the primary site for the carcinoma (Dabbs et al. 1986).

On the other hand, the differentiation between endocervical and endometrial carcinomas of either mucinous or mucoepidermoid or clear cell origin may prove to be very difficult, because of the common histogenetic derivation and their nearly identical contents of sulfated and nonsulfated acid mucopolysaccharides (Czernobilsky et al. 1980; Tiltman 1980). As already pointed out, that distinction can only be made topographically.

**Table 3.** Coexpression of intermediate filaments in the various types of endometrial carcinoma

| | Cytokeratins 5, 13 | Cytokeratins 7, 8, 18, 19 | Vimentin | CEA |
|---|---|---|---|---|
| Normal endometrium | | | | |
| Secretory | – | + | (+) | – |
| Proliferative | – | + | + | – |
| Hyperplasia | – | + | + | – |
| Adenocarcinoma, endometrial | – | + | + | – |
| Adenocarcinoma with squamous metaplasia: | | | | |
| Adenomatous area | – | + | + | – |
| Squamous area | + | – | – | +/(+) |
| Mucinous adenocarcinoma | – | + | – | –/(+) |
| Clear cell carcinoma | (+) | (+) | – | – |
| Serous papillary carcinoma | – | + | –/+ | – |

Various other methods have been tested and found of little value for purposes of differential diagnosis or predicting prognosis. For example, the results of an immunohistochemical localization of CA 125 in 44 endometrial adenocarcinomas suggested that high CA 125 expression may be associated with increased metastatic potential (BERCHUCK et al. 1989).

## 9.5 Steroid Receptors

*Estrogen receptors* in the nuclei of endometrial carcinoma cells can be visualized immunohistochemically with monoclonal antibodies against estrophilin (ER-ICA assay) or with a monoclonal antihuman estrogen receptor antibody (H 222spγ). Whereas well-differentiated adenocarcinomas of endometrial differentiation show intense nuclear positivity (Fig. 22), poorly differentiated carcinomas react heterogeneously, and solid adenocarcinomas may be entirely receptor-negative (CHARPIN et al. 1986; PERTSCHUCK et al. 1986; LANG et al. 1989). As compared with the biochemical analysis of estrogen receptors (MUTCH et al. 1987), the immunohistochemical detection in general is more sensitive and specific.

The immunohistochemical distribution of the *progesterone receptors*, as measured with antireceptor antibodies (PR-ICA or JZB 39), corresponds to that

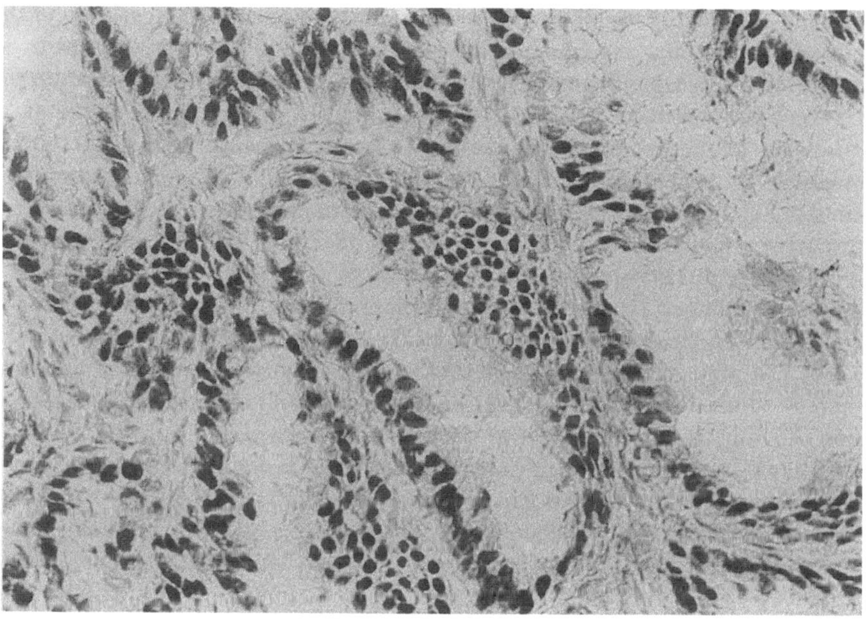

**Fig. 22.** Well-differentiated adenocarcinoma, endometrial type. High content of intranuclear estrogen receptor, as demonstrated with the ER-ICA assay. × 350

of the estrogen receptors (SEGRETI et al. 1989) and is equivalent to the biochemical assays (EHRLICH et al. 1981; UTAAKER et al. 1987). This can be explained by the fact that the production of progesterone receptors depends on the presence of estrogen receptors. Hence the number and intensity of both types of hormone receptor are fairly reliable parameters for the degree of differentiation of endometrial carcinomas and also for their response to adjuvant hormone therapy.

## 10 Gestagen Therapy

Since hormonal action is dependent on the presence of equivalent receptors in target cells, only well-differentiated receptor-positive carcinoma cells will be susceptible to hormone therapy. As histophotometric measurements of carcinomatous tissue cultured in vitro have shown, gestagen therapy decreases the synthesis of DNA and RNA (NORDQVIST 1970; HUSTIN 1975; SIMON and HÖLZEL 1979). At the same time, gestagens may exert and antiestrogenic effect by preventing estrogen from binding to its receptor. In well-differentiated endometrial carcinomas the histologic changes produced by gestagen therapy resemble those that develop in the endometrium during a normal secretory phase. After 3 days of treatment, secretory vacuoles appear in the carcinomatous cells, and the number of mitoses decreases. As therapy continues, the production of glycogen and mucus by the carcinomatous glands increases, and the stroma becomes decidualized. Many follow-up studies have shown a regression of the primary carcinoma, and its metastases in only about 30% of the patients who had received gestagen therapy (PIVER et al. 1980; for review of the literature see DALLENBACH-HELLWEG 1987). In contrast, poorly differentiated carcinomas often fail to regress following gestagen therapy, because their progesterone receptors are decreased or lacking (YOUNG et al. 1976). Since most carcinomas contain heterogeneous cells, some of which contain hormone receptors and are responsive to gestagens, while others lack receptors and are unresponsive, receptor analysis may provide the best criterion for selecting therapy. Prolonged treatment with gestagens may eventually suppress the formation of the estrogen and progesterone receptors (BJERSING 1977; RODRIQUEZ et al. 1979; VIHKO et al. 1980). To prevent that suppression, tamoxifen may be added to the gestagen therapy, since it blocks estrogen-promoted growth and increases the concentration of progesterone receptors at the same time. This may, however, lead to gestagenic overstimulation of endometrial glandular cells, provoking an endocervical metaplasia with excessive cellular proliferation paralleling microglandular hyperplasia of the endocervix. As already noted, in some instances endometrial carcinomas with endocervical differentiation have developed in patients treated with tamoxifen for their breast carcinoma (see p. 4), and after prolonged gestagen therapy as well. For this reason, adjuvant therapy with gestagens is contraindicated in endometrial adenocarcinomas with endocervical differentiation like mucinous carcinomas.

## 11 Radiation Therapy

In contrast to their response to gestagen therapy, well-differentiated adenocarcinomas are usually resistant to radiation therapy whereas the poorly differentiated or undifferentiated types respond to it fairly well and independently of their histogenetic origin. Carcinomas vary in their radiosensitivity mainly because of differences in their mitotic activity, for cells in mitosis are most susceptible to irradiation (Tubiana 1971).

The morphologic changes seen after radiation therapy can be manifold. In general, preexisting glandular patterns become distorted; the nuclei of the carcinoma cells appear pleomorphic and can be greatly enlarged and hyperchromatic due to replication of DNA without cell division. In the cytoplasm, damage to various organelles and destruction of lysosomal membranes may result in vacuolation. Despite these cytologic changes, some of the damaged tumor cells may still be viable and capable of replication.

## References


Aguirre P, Scully RE, Wolfe HJ, De Lellis RA (1984) Endometrial carcinoma with argyrophil cells: a histochemical and immunohistochemical analysis. Hum Pathol 15:210–217

Alberhasky RC, Connelly PJ, Christopherson WM (1982) Carcinoma of the endometrium. IV. Mixed adenosquamous carcinoma. A clinical-pathological study of 68 cases with long-term follow-up. Am J Clin Pathol 77:655–664

Aycock NR, Jollie WP, Dunn LJ (1979) An ultrastructural comparison of human endometrial adenocarcinoma with normal postmenopausal endometrium. Obstet Gynecol 53:565–571

Bannatyne P, Russell P, Wills EJ (1983) Argyrophilia and endometrial carcinoma. Int J Gynecol Pathol 2:235–254

Berchuck A, Soisson AP, Clarke-Pearson DL et al. (1989) Immunohistochemical expression of CA 125 in endometrial adenocarcinoma: correlation of antigen expression with metastatic potential. Cancer Res 49:2091–2095

Bersch W, Wolfmüller H, Raufelder W (1984) Beitrag zur Ichthyosis uteri mit und ohne maligne Neoplasie. Pathologe 5:148–152

Bjersing L (1977) Endometrial hyperplasia and carcinoma: histopathology and hormonal factors. Acta Obstet Gynecol Scand 65:83–88

Bokhman JV (1983) Two pathogenetic types of endometrial carcinoma. Gynecol Oncol 15:10–17

Burke TW, Heller PB, Woodward JE, Davidson SA, Hoskins WJ, Park RC (1990) Treatment failure in endometrial carcinoma. Obstet Gynecol 75:96–101

Chambers JT, Merino M, Kohorn ET et al. (1987) Uterine papillary serous carcinoma. Obstet Gynecol 69:109–113

Charles D (1965) Endometrial adenoacanthoma. Cancer 18:737–750

Charpin C, Martin PA, Lavaut MN et al. (1986) Estrogen receptor immunocytochemical assay (ER-ICA) in human endometrium. Int J Gynecol Pathol 5:119–131

Christopherson WM, Alberhasky RC, Connelly PJ (1982) Carcinoma of the endometrium: I. A clinicopathologic study of clear-cell carcinoma and secretory carcinoma. Cancer 49:1511–1523

Connelly PJ, Alberhasky RC, Christopherson WM (1982) Carcinoma of the endometrium. III. Analysis of 865 cases of adenocarcinoma and adenoacanthoma. Obstet Gynecol 59:569–575

Cowles TA, Magrina JF, Masterson BJ, Capen CV (1985) Comparison of clinical and surgical staging in patients with endometrial carcinoma. Obstet Gynecol 66:413–416

Creasmen WT (1990) Gradutate education. New gynecologic cancer staging. Obstet Gynecol 75:287–288

Czernobilsky B, Katz Z, Lancet M, Gaton E (1980) Endocervical-type epithelium in endometrial carcinoma. Am J Surg Pathol 4:481–489

Czernobilsky B, Moll R, Franke WW, Dallenbach-Hellweg G, Hohlweg-Majert P (1984) Intermediate filaments of normal and neoplastic tissues of the female genital tract with emphasis on problems of differential tumor diagnosis. Pathol Res Pract 179:31–37

Dabbs DJ, Geisinger KR, Norris HT (1986) Intermediate filaments in endocervical carcinomas: the diagnostic utility of vimentin patterns. Am J Surg Pathol 10:568–576

Dallenbach-Hellweg G (1984) On the origin and histological structure of adenocarcinoma of the endocervix in women under 50 years of age. Pathol Res Pract 179:38–50

Dallenbach-Hellweg G (1987) Histopathology of the endometrium. Springer, Berlin Heidelberg New York

Dallenbach-Hellweg G, Lang-Avérous G, Hahn U (1991) The value of immunohistochemistry in the differential diagnosis of endometrial carcinomas. APMISF 99:91–99

Dallenbach-Hellweg G, Lang G (1991) Immunohistochemical studies on uterine tumors: invasive adeno-carcinomas of the endocervix and their precursors. Pathol Res Pract 187:36–43

Dallenbach-Hellweg G, Weber J, Stoll P, Velten CH (1971) Zur Differentialdiagnose adenomatöser Endometriumhyperplasien junger Frauen. Arch Gynäkol 210:303–320

Dallenbach-Hellweg G, Dallenbach C, Lang G (1988) Zur Histogenese und Morphologie der Mukoepidermoiden Adenokarzinome des Corpusendometrium. Pathologe 9:351–357

Demopoulos RI, Dubin N, Noumoff J et al. (1986) Prognostic significance of squamous differentiation in stage 1 endometrial adenocarcinoma. Obstet Gynec 68:245–250

Eastwood J (1978) Mesonephroid (clear cell) carcinoma of the ovary and endometrium. A comparative prospective clinico-pathological study and review of literature. Cancer 41:1911–1928

Ehrlich CE, Young PCM, Cleary RE (1981) Cytoplasmic progesterone and estradiol receptors in normal, hyperplastic, and carcinomatous endometria: therapeutic implications. Am J Obstet Gynecol 141:539–546

Eifel P, Hendrickson M, Ross J et al. (1982) Simulataneous presentation of carcinoma involving the ovary and the uterine corpus. Cancer 50:163–170

Fanning J, Erang MC, Peters AJ, Samuel M, Harmon ER, Bates JS (1989) Endometrial adenocarcinoma histologic subtypes: clinical and pathologic profile. Gynecol Oncol 32:288–291

Fechner RE, Kaufman RH (1974) Endometrial adenocarcinoma in Stein–Leventhal syndrome. Cancer 34:444–452

Fornander T, Cedermark B, Mattsson A et al. (1989) Adjuvant tamoxifen in early breast cancer: occurrence of new primary cancers., Lancet I:117–120

Frauenhoffer EF, Zaino RJ, Wolff TV, Whitney CH (1987) Value of Endocervical curettage in the staging of endometrial carcinoma. Int J Gynecol Pathol 6:195–202

Fu YS, Parks PJ, Reagen JW, Wentz WB, Storaasli JP (1979) The ultrastructure and factors relating to survival of endometrial cancers. Am J Diag Gynecol Obstet 1:55–

Hachisuga T (1986) Endometrial carcinoma. A histopathologic analysis of 155 cases with special reference to prognostic factors and background lesions. Fukuoka Igaku Zasshi 77:314–332

Hendrickson MR, Kempson RL (1980a) The differential diagnosis of endometrial adenocarcinoma. Some viewpoints concerning a diagnostic problem. Pathology 32:35–61

Hendrickson MR, Kempson RL (1980b) Endometrial epithelial metaplasias—proliferations frequently misdiagnosed as adenocarcinoma: report of 89 cases and proposed classification. Am J Surg Pathol 4:525–542

Hendrickson MR, Ross J, Eifel P et al. (1982) Uterine papillary serous carcinoma. Am J Surg Pathol 6:93–108

Hertig AT, Gore H (1960) Tumors of the female sex organs, part 2. In: Atlas of tumor pathology, Sect. IX, fasc. 33. Armed Forces Institute of Pathology, Washington DC

Horie A, Yasumoto K, Ueda H et al. (1977) Clear cell adenocarcinoma of the uterus—ultrastructural and hormonal study. Acta Pathol Jpn 27:907–915

Hustin J (1975) Effect of protein hormones and steroids on tissue cultures of endometrial carcinoma. Br J Obstet Gynaecol 82:493–500

Kanbour A, Stock J (1978) Squamous cell carcinoma in situ of the endometrium and fallopian tube as superficial extension of invasive cervical carcinoma. Cancer 42:570–580

Killakey MA, Hakes TB, Pierce VK (1985) Endometrial adenocarcinoma in breast cancer patients receiving antiestrogens. Cancer Treat Rep 69:237–238

Kumar NB, Hart WR (1982) Metastases to the uterine corpus from extragenital cancers—a clinicopathologic study of 63 cases. Cancer 50:2163–2169
Kurman RJ, Norris HJ (1982) Evaluation of criteria for distinguishing atypical endometrial hyperplasia from well-differentiated carcinoma. Cancer 49:2547–2559
Kurman RJ, Norris HJ (1987) Endometrial carcinoma. In: Kurman RJ (ed) Blaustein's pathology of the female genital tract. Springer, New York Berlin Heidelberg
Kurman RJ, Scully RE (1976) Clear cell carcinoma of the endometrium. An analysis of 21 cases. Cancer 37:872–882
Kurman RJ, Kaminski PF, Norris HJ (1985) The behavior of endometrial hyperplasia. A long-term study of "untreated" hyperplasia in 170 patients. Cancer 56:403–412
Lang G, Lang M, Dallenbach-Hellweg G (1989) Immunhistochemische Rezeptorbefunde im Endometrium und therapeutische Konsequenzen bei endogenen und exogenen Funktionsstörungen und im Karzinom. Geburtshilfe Frauenheilkd 49:1025–1100
Lee KR, Scully RE (1989) Complex endometrial hyperplasia and carcinoma in adolescents and young women 15 to 20 years of age: a report of 10 cases. Int J Gynecol Pathol 8:201–219
Liu CT (1972) A study of endometrial adenocarcinoma with emphasis on morphologically variant types. Am J Clin Pathol 57:562–573
Maes G, Fleuren GJ, Bara J, Nap M (1988) The distribution of mucins, carcinoembryonic antigen, and mucus-associated antigens in endocervical and endometrial adenocarcinomas. Int J Gynecol Pathol 7:112–122
McNutt MA, Bolen JW, Gown AM et al. (1985) Coexpression of intermediate filaments in human epithelial neoplasms. Ultrastruct Pathol 9:31–43
Melhem MF, Tobon H (1987) Mucinous adeno-carcinoma of the endometrium. a clinico-pathological review of 18 cases. Int J Gynecol Pathol 6:347–355
Melin JR, Wanner L, Schulz DM, Cassel EE (1979) Primary squamous cell carcinoma of the endometrium. Obstet Gynecol 53:115–119
Mittal KR, Schwartz PE, Barwick KW (1988) Architectural (FIGO) grading, Nuclear grading, and other prognostic indicators in stage I endometrial adenocarcinoma with identification of high-risk and low-risk groups. Cancer 61:538–545
Moll R, Levy R, Czernobilsky B et al. (1983) Cytokeratins of normal epithelia and some neoplasms of the female genital tract. Lab Invest 49:559–609
Moukhtar M, Aleem FA, Hung HC et al. (1977) The reversible behavior of locally invasive endometrial carcinoma in a chromosomally mosaic (45, X/46, Xr (X)) young woman treated with Clomid. Cancer 40:2957–2966
Mutch DG, Soper JT, Budwit-Novotny DA et al. (1987) Endometrial adenocarcinoma estrogen receptor content: association of clinicopathologic features with immunohistochemical analysis compared with standard biochemical methods. Am J Obstet Gynecol 157:924–931
Ng ABP, Reagan JW (1970) Incidence and prognosis of endometrial carcinoma by histologic grade and extent. Obstet Gynecol 35:437–443
Nordqvist S (1970) The synthesis of DNA and RNA in human carcinomatous endometrium in short-term incubation in vitro and its response to oestradiol and progesterone. J Endocrinol 48:29–38
Norris HJ, Tavassoli FA, Kurman RJ (1983) Endometrial hyperplasia and carcinoma. Am J Surg Pathol 7:839–847
Nuovo MA, Nuovo GJ, McCaffrey M et al. (1989) Endometrial polyps in postmenopausal patients receiving tamoxifen. Int J Gynecol Pathol 8:125–131
Olson N, Twiggs L, Sibley R (1982) Small-cell carcinoma of the endometrium: light microscopic and ultrastructural study of a case. Cancer 50:760–765
Pertschuk LP, Beddoe AM, Gorelic LS, Shain SA (1986) Immunocytochemical assay of estrogen receptors in endometrial carcinoma with monoclonal antibodies. Cancer 57:1000–1004
Piver MS, Barlow JJ, Lurrain JR, Blumenson LE (1980) Medroxyprogesterone acetate (Depo Provera) vs hydroxyprogesterone caproate (Delalutin) in women with metastatic endometrial adenocarcinoma. Cancer 45:268–272
Puts JJG, Moesker O, Aldeweireldt J (1987) Application of antibodies to intermediate filament proteins in simple and complex tumors of the female genital tract. Int J Gyn Pathol 6:257–274
Robboy SJ, Bradley R (1979) Changing trends and prognostic features in endometrial cancer associated with exogenous estrogen therapy. Obstet Gynecol 54:269–277
Rodriquez J, Sen KK, Seski JC et al. (1979) Progesterone binding by human endometrial tissue during the proliferative and secretory phases of menstrual cycle and by hyperplastic and carcinomatous endometrium. Am J Obstet Gynecol 133:660–665

Ross JC, Eifel PJ, Cox RS et al. (1983) Primary mucinous adenocarcinoma of the endometrium. Am J Surg Pathol 7:715–729
Sasano H, Comerfor J, Wilkinson DS et al. (1990) Serous papillary adenocarcinoma of the endometrium. Cancer 65:1545–1551
Sato N, Mori T, Orenstein JM, Silverberg SG (1984) Ultrastructure of papillary serous carcinoma of the endometrium. Int J Gynecol Pathol 2:337–348
Scully RE, Aguirre P, De Lellis RA (1984) Argyrophilla, serotonin, and peptide hormones in the female genital tract and its tumors. Int J Gynecol Pathol 3:51–70
Segreti EM, Novotny DB, Soper JT et al. (1989) Endometrial cancer: histologic correlates of immunohistochemical localization of progesterone receptor and estrogen receptor. Obstet Gynecol 73:780–785
Simon A, Kopolovic J, Beyth Y (1988) Primary squamous cell carcinoma of the endometrium. Gynecol Oncol 31:454–461
Simon WE, Hölzel F (1979) Hormone sensitivity of gynecological tumor cells in tissue culture. J Cancer Res Clin Oncol 94:307–323
Sorvari TE (1969) A histochemical study of epithelial mucosubstances in endometrial and cervical adenocarcinomas with reference to normal endometrium and cervical mucosa. Acta Pathol Microbiol Scand [Suppl] 207:1–85
Tavassoli F, Kraus FT (1978) Endometrial lesions in uteri resected for atypical endometrial hyperplasia. Am J Clin Pathol 70:770–779
Thom MH, Davies KJ, Senkus RJ et al. (1981) Scanning electron microscopy of the endometrial cell surface in postmenopausal women receiving oestrogen therapy. Br J Obstet Gynaecol 88:904–913
Thrasher TV, Richart RM (1972) An ultrastructural comparison of endometrial adenocarcinoma and normal endometrium. Cancer 29:1713–1723
Tiltman AJ (1980) Mucinous carcinoma of the endometrium. Obstet Gynecol 55:244–
Tubiana M (1971) The kinetics of tumour cell proliferation and radiotherapy. Br J Radiol 44:325–000
Ueda G, Sato Y, Yamasaki M et al. (1977) Argyrophil cell adenocarcinoma of the endometrium. Acta Obstet Gynecol Jpn 29:1167–1168
Ueda S, Tsubura A, Izumi H et al. (1983) Immunohistochemical studies on carcinoembryonic antigen in adenocarcinomas of the uterus. Acta Pathol Jpn 33:59–69
Ueda G, Yamasaki M, Inoue M et al. (1986) Immonohistochemical demonstration of HNK-1-defined antigen in gynecologic tumors with argyrophilia. Int J Gynecol Pathol 5:143–150
Ulbright TM, Roth IM (1985) Metastatic and independent cancers of the endometrium and ovary: a clinico-pathologic study of 34 cases. Hum Pathol 16:28–34
Utaaker E, Iversen OE, Skaarland E (1987) The distribution and prognostic implications of steroid receptors in endometrial carcinomas. Gynecol Oncol 28:89–100
Vihko R, Jänne O, Kauppila A (1980) Steroid receptors in normal, hyperplastic and malignant human endometria. Ann Clin Res 12:208–215
Wahlström T, Korhonen M, Lindgren J, Markku S (1979) Distinction between endocervical and endometrial adenocarcinoma with immunoperoxidase staining of carcinoembryonic antigen in routine histologic tissue sections. Lancet II:1159–1160
Walker AM, Jick H (1979) Cancer of the corpus uteri: increasing incidence in the United States. Am J Epidemiol 110:47–51
Walker AM, Jick H (1980) Declining rates of endometrial cancer. Obstet Gynecol 56:733–736
Weiner J, Bigelow B, Demopoulos RI et al. (1980) The value of endocervical sampling in the staging of endometrial carcinoma. Diagn Gynecol Obstet 2:265–268
Welch WR, Scully RE (1977) Precancerous lesions of the endometrium. Hum Pathol 8:503–512
Yamashina M, Kobara TY (1986) Primary squamous cell carcinoma with its spindle cell variant in the endometrium. Cancer 57:340–345
Young PCM, Ehrlich CE, Cleary RE (1976) Progesterone binding in human endometrial carcinomas. Am J Obstet Gynecol 125:353–360

# Mixed Müllerian Tumors

S.G. Silverberg



## 1 Introduction

Mixed müllerian tumors constitute one of the rarer groups of uterine tumors, but have always inspired the interest of clinicians, basic scientists, and pathologists out of proportion to their clinical frequency. They are by definition all composed of an intimate admixture of epithelial and nonepithelial elements, and thus have raised particular questions concerning their histogenesis and pathway of differentiation, as well as the relative contributions of the different elements in determining the natural history, prognosis, and ultimately the treatment of each tumor. The present review will attempt to introduce the major clinical and pathologic features of these lesions, as well as to summarize recent studies related to the questions raised above.

Current Topics in Pathology
Volume 85, Ed. N. Sasano

**Table 1.** International Society of Gynecological Pathologists classification of uterine mixed epithelial–nonepithelial tumors

| |
|---|
| Benign |
| Adenofibroma |
| Adenomyoma |
| Variant—atypical polypoid adenomyoma |
| Malignant |
| Adenosarcoma |
| Homologous |
| Heterologous |
| Carcinosarcoma (malignant mixed mesodermal tumor; malignant mixed müllerian tumor) |
| Homologous |
| Heterologous |
| Carcinofibroma |

## 2 International Society of Gynecological Pathologists Classification

The most recent (1989) classification schema of the International Society of Gynecological Pathologists is reproduced in Table 1. The nomenclature presented provides a prefix ("adeno" or "carcino") which conveys the benign or malignant appearance of the epithelial component, and a suffix ("fibroma," "myoma," or "sarcoma") which indicates the benign or malignant appearance of the nonepithelial component. By definition, any lesion placed in this category must contain separate epithelial and nonepithelial components, both of which are integral parts of the lesion. Thus, endometrial lesions which bear some resemblance to mixed müllerian tumors but which are excluded from this category include: (a) polyps, which are considered to be nonneoplastic; (b) carcinomas with spindle cell (sarcomatoid) metaplasia which are identifiable as such at the light microscopic level with routine (i.e., other than immunohistochemical) staining; (c) pure endometrial stromal tumors (usually benign stromal nodules or low grade endometrial stromal sarcomas) in which the stromal cells focally differentiate into tubular, glandlike, or sex cordlike structures; and (d) pure sex cordlike tumors of the uterus, in which the appearance of epithelial and nonepithelial elements may also be present. Also outside the group of mixed müllerian tumors are the extremely rare teratomas of the uterus, in which neoplastic elements derived from all three germ cell layers are characteristically present, rather than the pure mesodermally derived elements of the mixed müllerian tumors.

It should be noted that, although the discussion in this review will be limited to mixed müllerian tumors of the uterine corpus, these tumors can also be observed in the uterine cervix, the ovary, and elsewhere in the female pelvis. It is assumed that in these situations the neoplasms arise by a process of endometrial metaplasia, and in many cases they can be demonstrated to have arisen in foci of endometriosis (CLEMENT and SCULLY 1978; DELIGDISCH et al. 1988; KAO and NORRIS 1978).

## 3 Carcinosarcoma (Malignant Mixed Mesodermal Tumor)

The preferred nomenclature for this lesion in the new classification is carcinosarcoma, but these tumors are also commonly known as malignant mixed mesodermal tumors or malignant mixed müllerian tumors. Although they are the most common of the neoplasms in the mixed müllerian group, they are nevertheless rare tumors, representing only 2%–3% of all uterine cancers (Spanos et al. 1986). These lesions by definition are composed of epithelial and nonepithelial components which are both histologically malignant. These components must be admixed within the same neoplasm, as opposed to a carcinoma and a sarcoma occurring simultaneously in different portions of the same uterus.

### 3.1 Epidemiologic and Clinical Features

Because these tumors are rare and have usually been studied together with other mixed tumors and pure sarcomas of the uterus, their epidemiologic features are still poorly understood. They are known, however, to share some of the epidemiologic features (nulliparity, obesity, diabetes, etc.) associated more strongly with endometrial carcinoma, and have also been related to a history of prior pelvic radiation (Clement and Scully 1988). A few cases have been reported as occurring on a background of functioning ovarian lesions or exogenous estrogen therapy (Press and Scully 1985).

The great majority of carcinosarcomas occur in elderly postmenopausal women, but well-documented cases have occurred in younger patients, with a single case reported in a 4-year-old girl (Amr et al. 1986).

Like the other tumors in the mixed müllerian group, uterine carcinosarcomas usually present clinically with abnormal vaginal bleeding, and are found to be polypoid, usually solitary masses projecting into the endometrial cavity. Carcinosarcomas are generally large tumors which often fill the uterine cavity and may protrude through the external cervical os. Although the diagnosis of a malignant tumor is generally easily made by endometrial curettage, it is not unusual for only the carcinomatous—or rarely, the sarcomatous—component to be seen prior to hysterectomy. When the initial diagnosis is made on the basis of a cervicovaginal smear, it is also common for only adenocarcinoma to be recognized (Tenti et al. 1989).

### 3.2 Gross and Microscopic Pathologic Features

As mentioned above, uterine carcinosarcomas are usually bulky tumors which project into and may completely fill the endometrial cavity. Compared with endometrial carcinomas, these tumors are generally larger, more often have a smooth surface, and tend to have more fleshy and variegated cut surfaces. They usually invade deeply into the myometrium, and have often spread beyond the uterine corpus at the time of initial surgery.

Microscopically, carcinosarcomas are characterized by an intimate admixture of malignant epithelial and nonepithelial elements (Fig.1). The carcinomatous element is usually an adenocarcinoma of one of the types encountered in pure form in the endometrium—usually endometrioid adenocarcinoma with or without squamous differentiation, but not infrequently serous, clear cell, or another less common type. As a rule, the carcinomatous element tends to be moderately to poorly differentiated, but well-differentiated carcinomas are also observed (SILVERBERG et al. 1990). The carcinomatous component should be distinctly separate from the malignant nonepithelial element to rule out the diagnosis of a metaplastic carcinoma at the light microscopic level (Fig. 2).

The stromal component is usually high-grade sarcoma, but may occasionally be relatively well-differentiated (Fig. 2). Homologous stromal components are usually of endometrial stromal sarcoma (Fig. 3), fibrosarcoma (Fig. 2), or leiomyosarcoma type. About half of all uterine carcinosarcomas are classified as *heterologous*, in that they contain foci of sarcoma differentiating toward elements not normally found in the uterine corpus. The most common type of heterologous sarcoma is rhabdomyosarcoma (Fig. 4), with chondrosarcoma (Fig. 5), osteosarcoma (Fig. 6), and liposarcoma (Fig. 7), in decreasing order of frequency, also encountered. These heterologous elements are usually easily

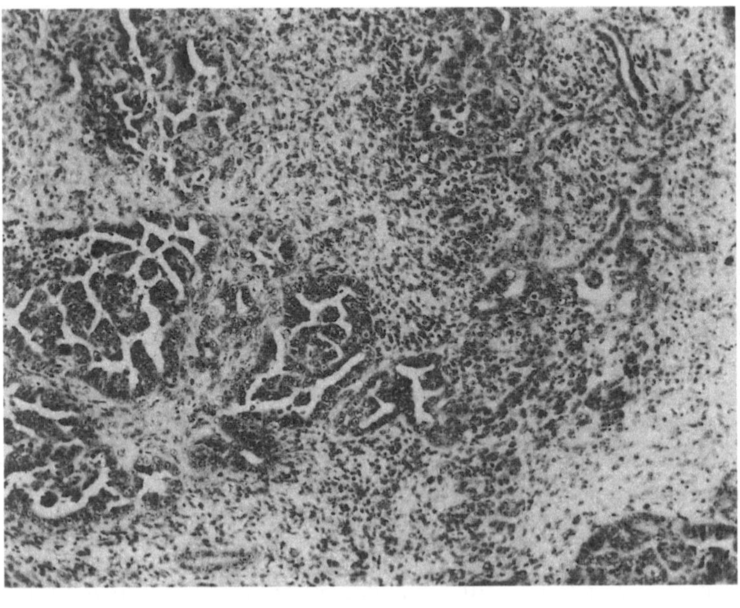

**Fig. 1.** Carcinosarcoma of endometrium, showing intimately admixed malignant glandular and stromal elements. H&E, original magnification. × 100

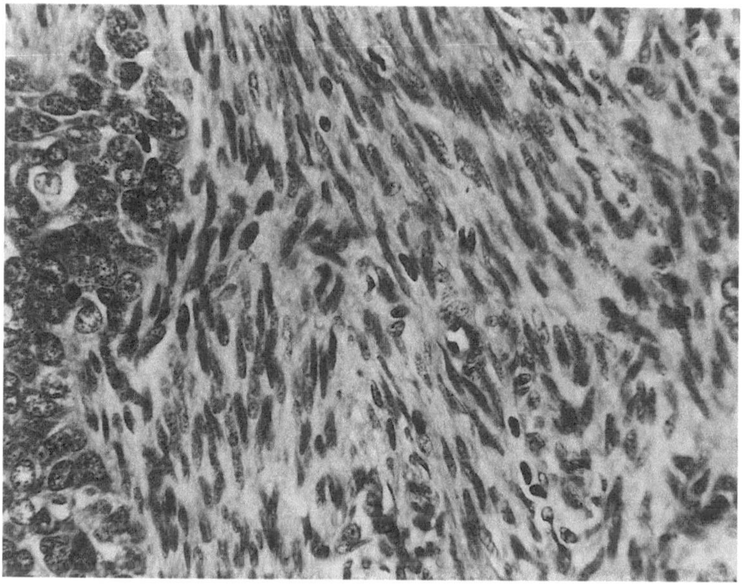

**Fig. 2.** Carcinosarcoma with sharply demarcated malignant glandular and stromal components. The stromal element is a low-grade spindle cell sarcoma resembling fibrosarcoma. H&E, original magnification. × 400

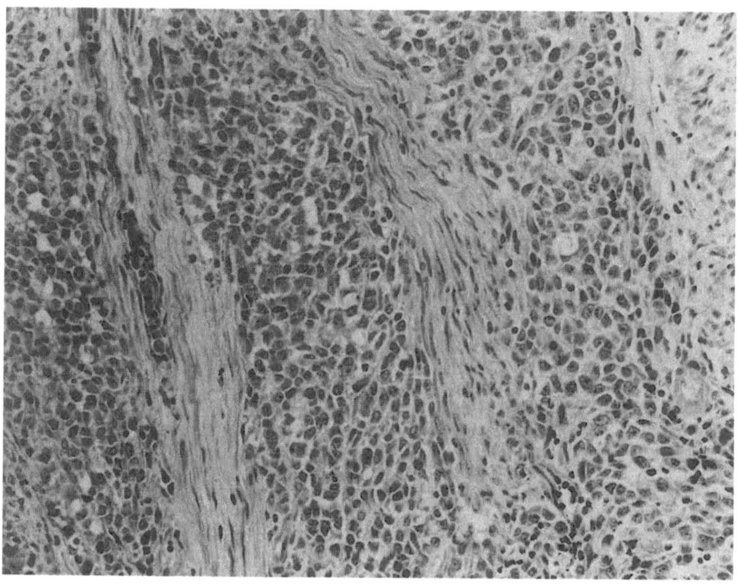

**Fig. 3.** Carcinosarcoma showing infiltrating round cell sarcomatous component. H&E, original magnification. × 200

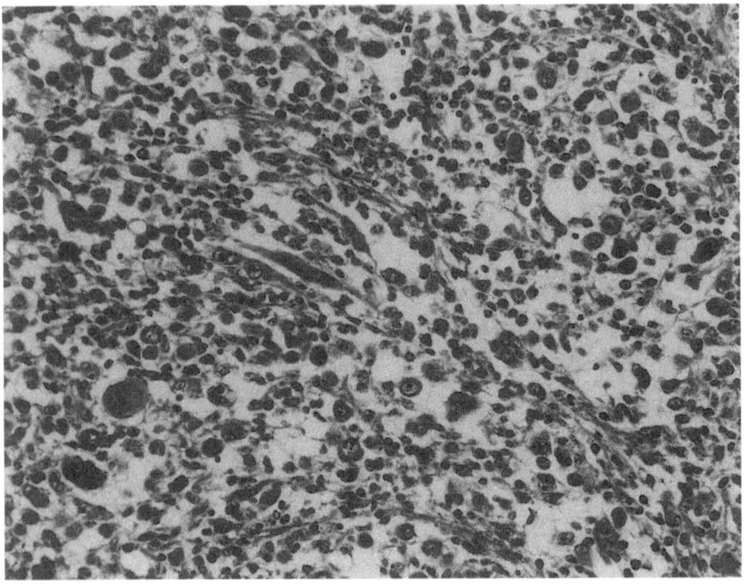

**Fig. 4.** Rhabdomyosarcomatous differentiation in carcinosarcoma, with round and straplike rhabdomyoblasts. H&E, original magnification. ×200

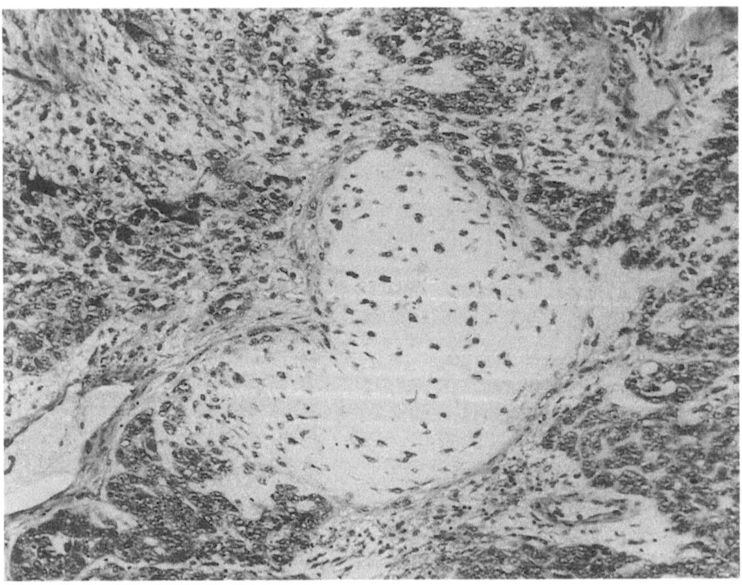

**Fig. 5.** Chondrosarcomatous differentiation in carcinosarcoma. H&E, original magnification. × 100

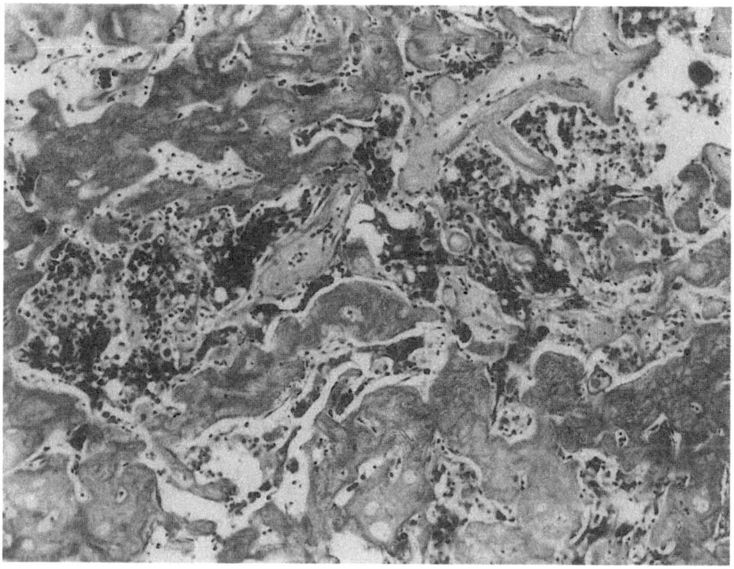

**Fig. 6.** Osteosarcomatous differentiation in carcinosarcoma. H&E, original magnification. × 100

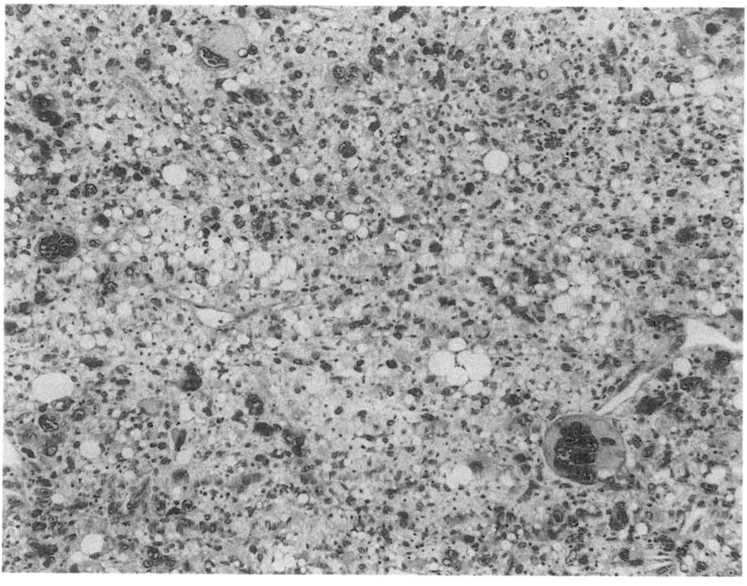

**Fig. 7.** Liposarcomatous differentiation in carcinosarcoma. H&E, original magnification. × 100

diagnosed by conventional light microscopy, but it must be remembered that they are occasionally very focal and must be carefully searched for. In about one-fourth of heterologous carcinosarcomas, more than one heterologous sarcomatous type is present (SILVERBERG et al. 1990). Rarely, foci of neuroectodermal differentiation may be encountered (GERSELL et al. 1989).

### 3.3 Differential Diagnosis

Since carcinosarcomas are usually high-grade malignant tumors, the differential diagnosis from benign entities is rarely a problem. It is not unusual, however, for difficult differential diagnostic problems to arise with other malignant tumors—particularly endometrial carcinoma and adenosarcoma—and the differential diagnosis of homologous from heterologous carcinosarcoma may also be perplexing.

For the differential diagnosis of carcinosarcoma from poorly differentiated endometrial carcinoma with spindle cell metaplasia, it should be remembered that the carcinomatous and sarcomatous elements should be distinct at the light microscopic level for the diagnosis of carcinosarcoma. If the epithelial cells of a poorly differentiated endometrial carcinoma appear to "drop off" into the malignant stromal component (Fig. 8, to be compared with Fig. 2), the diagnosis of poorly differentiated carcinoma should be made. Immunohistochemical and ultrastructural search often reveals epithelial markers in the malignant stromal component of otherwise typical carcinosarcomas (BITTERMAN et al. 1988; DE BRITO et al. unpublished work). Since these techniques are not available in every laboratory of pathology, and since carcinosarcomas in which epithelial markers are demonstrated in the stromal component seem to behave no differently from those in which such markers cannot be demonstrated (DE BRITO et al. unpublished work), we do not recommend the use of these studies for differential diagnosis at the present time.

The differential diagnosis of carcinosarcoma with adenosarcoma is a particularly important one, since adenosarcomas have a considerably more favorable prognosis than carcinosarcomas. Adenosarcoma frequently presents as a smaller tumor in a younger woman than the typical case of carcinosarcoma. At the microscopic level, the epithelial component of adenosarcoma appears histologically benign. The only confusion with carcinosarcoma occurs when the malignant epithelial element of a carcinosarcoma is either sparse in amount—perhaps appearing focally within an otherwise typical adenosarcoma—or unusually well differentiated, or both. By convention, *any* malignant epithelial component within an adenosarcoma changes the diagnosis to carcinosarcoma.

As mentioned above, pure endometrial stromal tumors may contain foci in which the stromal cells differentiate into tubular, glandlike, or sex cordlike structures. The differential diagnosis here is facilitated by the fact that stromal tumors which differentiate in this fashion are almost invariably benign or of

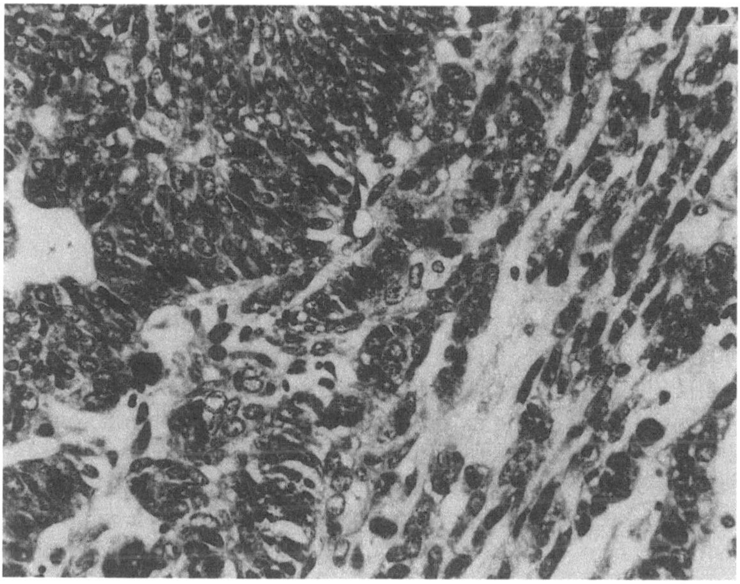

**Fig. 8.** Metaplastic carcinoma of endometrium, showing gradual transition between obvious epithelial component at *left* and spindled component at *right*. H&E, original magnification. ×400

low-grade malignancy (low-grade stromal sarcoma or endolymphatic stromal myosis), and thus do not contain the more poorly differentiated stromal sarcomatous component typical of carcinosarcoma. In addition, the epithelial-appearing component in these pure stromal tumors is generally histologically and cytologically benign as well.

Once the diagnosis of carcinosarcoma is made, differential diagnostic problems arise concerning the present or absence of heterologous elements. For example, eosinophilic hyaline droplets are common in the stroma of both homologous and heterologous carcinosarcomas (Dictor 1982), and should not lead to the confusion of the cells containing them with rhabdomyoblasts. The latter are densely and evenly eosinophilic, may contain cross-striations, and are decorated by an immunostain for myoglobin, in contrast with the globular appearance, variable size, and myoglobin negativity of the stromal hyaline droplets.

We have also found that chondrosarcoma is frequently overdiagnosed within uterine carcinosarcomas, the usual confounder being foci of squamous metaplasia. In contradistinction to squamous metaplasia, the cells of chondrosarcoma show a more glassy cytoplasm, less prominent cell membranes, and a more lacunar appearance, and usually are decorated by an immunostain for S-100 protein. Foci of benign chondroid, osseous, or adipose differentiation may be seen associated with endometrial carcinoma (or even in benign endometria) and do not justify the diagnosis of heterologous carcinosarcoma. At the other extreme, rare pure rhabdomyosarcomas, chondrosarcomas, osteosarcomas, and liposarcomas of the endometrium may be encountered, and should not be diagnosed as carcinosarcoma in the absence of a malignant epithelial component.

### 3.4 Pathogenesis

The pathogenesis and pathway of differentiation of endometrial carcinosarcoma have been of interest to many investigators since these tumors were first recognized. Speculation has centered on whether they represent collision tumors (a mixutre of two histogenetically distinct malignant cell populations), combination tumors (representing an origin of both elements from a common stem cell), or composition tumors (pure carcinomas with reactive atypical but benign stromal elements). These possibilities have been investigated by studies utilizing tissue culture, electron microscopy, heterotransplantation, and immunohistochemistry. Recent tissue culture and heterotransplantation studies (ISHIWATA et al. 1981, 1987; MASUDA et al. 1987) have established that tissue culture lines of human carcinosarcomas can differentiate along both epithelial and nonepithelial lines morphologically, can produce metastases in animals which show both histologic elements, and can demonstrate a change from a carcinomatous to a sarcomatous phenotype. These studies have all been interpreted as supporting the "combination tumor" theory. Ultrastructural studies, on the other hand, have generally emphasized the distinctness of the malignant epithelial and stromal populations (GEISINGER et al. 1987), but our own ultrastructural study (DE BRITO et al. unpublished work), in which by far the largest series of cases was examined, has demonstrated invasion of the stromal component by isolated epithelial cells, as well as occasional hybrid forms between the carcinomatous and sarcomatous phenotypes. These findings were confirmed immunohistochemically in the same cases by DE BRITO et al., and other recent immunohistochemical studies as well have noted that epithelial markers such as cytokeratins and epithelial membrane antigen are frequently displayed by the sarcomatous-appearing cells (AUERBACH et al. 1988; CHUNG et al. 1988; DELIGDISCH et al. 1988; GEISINGER et al. 1987). NOORDUYN and HERMAN (1987) have even suggested that immunohistochemical techniques may demonstrate morphologically unrecognizable heterologous tumor cells within typical ovarian adenocarcinomas.

Additional evidence in favour of the combination theory comes from the recent observations of BITTERMAN et al. (1988) and SILVERBERG et al. (1990) that initial metastases of uterine carcinosarcomas are usually of pure carcinomatous type, less frequently mixed, and only rarely of pure sarcomatous phenotype. In the series of 203 cases reported by SILVERBERG et al. (1990), it was noted that metastates to lymph nodes occurred with approximately the same frequency as in poorly differentiated carcinomas, also suggesting that the carcinomatous element was the driving force—an interpretation supported by the observation that the presence or absence of metastases at initial exploratory laparotomy correlated more closely with the histologic appearance of the carcinomatous element of the primary tumor than that of the sarcomatous element. DELIGDISCH et al. (1988), in a small series of extrauterine carcinosarcomas, noted that metastatic lesions encountered at initial surgery were predominantly epithelial, while subsequent recurrences were composed largely of mesenchymal elements. This observation, if confirmed in larger series and in primary uterine tumors, would also support the hypothesis that a primary malignant stem cell differentiates first into carcinoma and subsequently into the malignant stromal component.

## 3.5 Prognosis and Treatment

As mentioned above, the most important reason for precision in the diagnosis of uterine carcinosarcoma is the extremely unfavorable prognosis of this tumor, with 5-year survival rates in recently reported series ranging between 18% and 39% (DINH et al. 1989; NIELSEN et al. 1988; PODOZASKI et al. 1989). This largely reflects the fact that most cases present with tumor which has already spread to extrauterine sites. The surgical stage and depth of myometrial invasion have been shown to be important prognostic indicators in almost all large published series, although other pathologic factors have been more controversial (SILVERBERG et al. 1990). Early studies suggested that heterologous tumors had a poorer prognosis than homologous ones (NORRIS et al. 1966; NORRIS and TAYLOR 1966), but several more recent studies have shown no significant difference (DINH et al. 1989; NIELSEN et al. 1989; PODOZASKI et al. 1989; SILVERBERG et al. 1990). Rhabdomyosarcoma was also initially considered to be a particularly unfavorable heterologous component (NORRIS et al. 1966), but the recent studies quoted above have also not confirmed this observation.

In the large study of SILVERBERG et al. (1990), certain other features were also related to the frequency of metastases detected at staging laparotomy. A carcinomatous component that was high-grade endometrioid, serous, or clear cell was associated with a higher frequency of metastases, as were deep myometrial invasion, lymphatic or vascular space invasion, and involvement of the isthmus or cervix. On the other hand, features of the stromal component of the primary tumor, including grade, mitotic index, and (as mentioned above) the presence and types of heterologous elements, showed no relation to the presence of metastases at operation. Longer follow-up is required to determine whether these factors may eventually prove to be of some prognostic significance.

DE BRITO et al. (unpublished work) were interested in determining whether epithelial differentiation demonstrated ultrastructurally or immunohistochemically within the "stromal" component was associated with a better or worse prognosis. They were not able to demonstrate any difference between such cases and those in which epithelial markers could not be demonstrated, with the great majority of patients in both groups dead of disease within 2 years. Interestingly, two cases of metaplastic endometrial carcinoma identified by conventional light microscopy were associated with considerable longer survival.

The treatment of uterine carcinosarcoma is predominantly surgical, but adjuvant radiation and chemotherapy are often utilized because of the poor prognosis. Combination chemotherapy has recently been demonstrated to be useful both as adjuvant treatment and for recurrent disease (PETERS et al. 1989).

## 4 Adenofibroma and Adenomyoma

Adenofibroma and adenomyoma are considered together because they represent the benign end of the spectrum of the mixed müllerian tumors. As the diagnostic terms utilized imply, adenofibroma is composed of a benign glandular component and a fibroblastic (or endometrial stromal) element, while adenomyoma comprises a smooth muscle compartment.

### 4.1 Adenofibroma

Adenofibroma was first described in the uterine cervix in 1971 (ABELL 1971), and in the corpus 2 years later (VELLIOS et al. 1973). These tumors have subsequently been reported mostly in association with adenosarcomas, and composite terms for the two tumors have included "benign and low-grade variant of mixed müllerian tumor" (ÖSTÖR and FORTUNE 1980) and "uterine cystosarcoma phyllodes" (VELLIOS 1980). Adenofibroma seems to be considerably rarer than adenosarcoma, since in the large series of CLEMENT and SCULLY (1990b), it comprised only about 5% of tumors in the adenofibroma–adenosarcoma group.

Adenofibromas usually present clinically with abnormal vaginal bleeding in postmenopausal women, although they may be encountered at any age. Like the other tumors in the mixed müllerian group, they present grossly as polypoid masses projecting into the endometrial cavity. Microscopically, the surface of the tumor is usually composed of broad club-shaped papillae (Fig. 9). There is an intimate admixture of epithelial and stromal elements, both of which appear histologically benign (Fig. 10). The epithelial component most commonly resembles proliferative endometrium, but may be flattened or show squamous, mucinous, or other metaplastic changes. The stroma is composed predominantly of cells resembling either benign fibroblasts or endometrial stromal cells or a mixture of these cell types. Stromal cellularity may vary from minimal to marked, but stromal atypia is not noted, cuffs of dense cellular stroma around the glandular component are absent, and mitotic activity is absent or minimal.

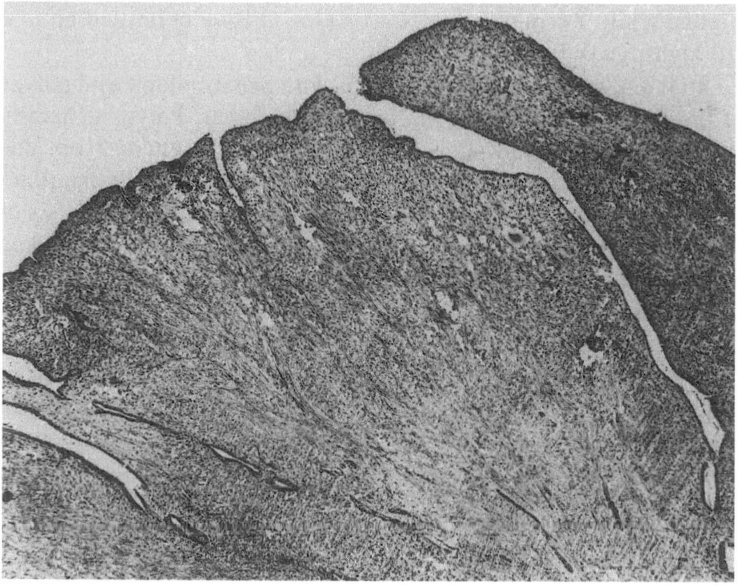

**Fig. 9.** Adenofibroma of endometrium. Note broad club-shaped papillae at surface. H&E, original magnification. × 40

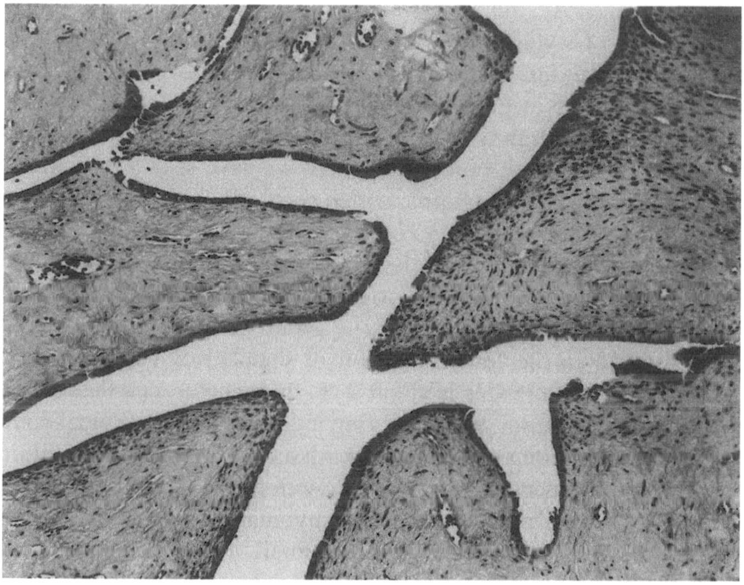

**Fig. 10.** Adenofibroma showing slitlike spaces lined by benign cuboidal glandular epithelium surrounded by paucicellular fibroblastic stroma, H&E, original magnification. × 100

CLEMENT and SCULLY (1990b) have reported fewer than 2 mitotic figures per 10 high-power fields, while ZALOUDEK and NORRIS (1981) have permitted up to 4 mitoses per 10 high-power fields.

The differential diagnosis of adenofibroma is with banal endometrial polyps at one end of the spectrum and adenosarcomas at the other. Polyps generally lack a papillary architecture and show considerable heterogeneity from one microscopic field to the next, whereas adenofibromas are essentially papillary and homogeneous. The distinction from adenosarcoma is made on the basis of the lack of stromal atypia and mitotic activity, as well as the lack of marked stromal hypercellularity and of cuffs of more densely cellular stroma around glands. Borderline lesions should probably be diagnosed as adenosarcoma, since these are many times more common than adenofibromas.

Adenofibromas have thus far been reported as benign lesions, with no cases of distant metastases yet reported. However, three cases have been noted to invade the myometrium, including one which also invaded large myometrial veins (CLEMENT and SCULLY 1990a, b).

## 4.2 Adenomyoma

Adenomyomas are benign polypoid tumors of the uterus in which a benign epithelial component is admixed with a stroma composed largely or exclusively of smooth muscle. In an otherwise unspecified adenomyoma, the glands show no architectural complexity or cytologic atypia. In the more common *atypical polypoid adenomyoma* (APA), the glands exhibit architectural atypia and may show varying degrees of cytologic atypia as well (Fig. 11). Squamous or morular metaplasia, often extensive, is found in most of the cases (Fig. 11), and the smooth muscle stroma is organized in swirling and interlacing fascicles. Mitotic activity in the smooth muscle compartment has been reported as less than 2 mitotic figures per 10 high-power fields, but we have seen a case with a mitotic rate of 9 per 10 high-power fields, which recurred outside the uterus 6 years after hysterectomy (KAKU et al. 1991).

Like the other tumors in the mixed müllerian group, APA is a polypoid tumor which presents clinically with abnormal vaginal bleeding. Unlike the other tumors, however, APA occurs in a younger age group (average age 39 years) and tends to be situated in the lower segment or endocervix (MAZUR 1981; YOUNG et al. 1986). The average size is about 2 cm in diameter, and the tumors are usually well demarcated from the underlying myometrium or cervical wall.

Although adenocarcinoma has been noted both associated with and within APA, malignant behavior has not been reported, with the exception of the one case mentioned above with a mitotically active myomatous stroma. Since the total number of cases thus far reported is still small, further experience is necessary before the natural history of this tumor is completely characterized.

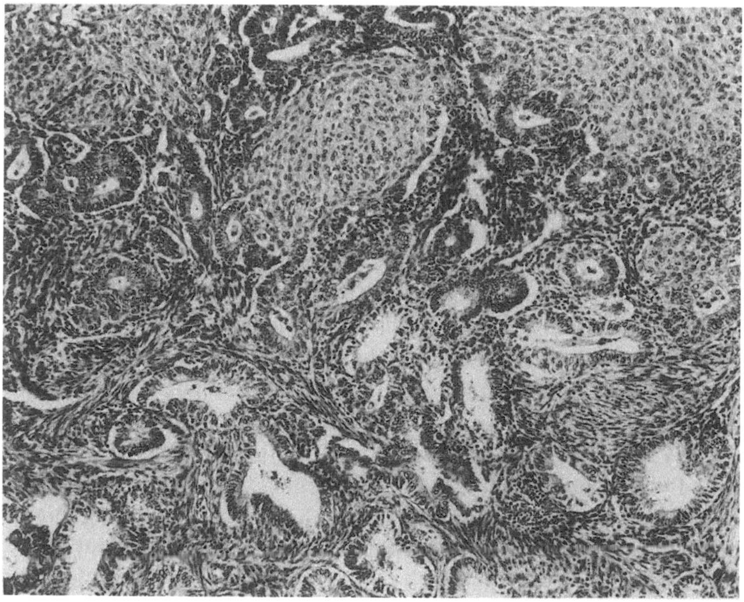

**Fig. 11.** Atypical polypoid adenomyoma. Architecturally atypical glands with extensive morular metaplasia are separated by a stroma composed of whorled fascicles of benign smooth muscle. H&E, original magnification. × 100

## 5 Adenosarcoma

Adenosarcoma was first described in 1974 (Clement and Scully 1974), and by the time of this review several hundred cases have been reported, with the largest series comprising 100 (Clement and Scully 1990b), 31 (Kaku et al. 1991), and 25 (Zaloudek and Norris 1981) cases. Despite the relatively large number of cases in the literature, the recent characterization of the entity still leaves large gaps in our knowledge of its epidemiology, histogenesis, and clinical and pathologic features.

Conceptually, adenosarcoma fills the gap between the completely benign (adenofibroma, adenomyoma) and high-grade malignant (carcinosarcoma) neoplasms in the mixed mullerian group. By definition, it is composed of a benign epithelial and a malignant nonepithelial component. The other tumor in this group with both a benign and a malignant component—*carcinofibroma*—is so rare that only a handful of cases have been reported, and the tumor will not be discussed further in this review.

### 5.1 Clinical and Pathologic Features

Adenosarcomas usually are diagnosed in middle-aged or elderly women, with a mean age between 55 and 60 years, but cases have been seen in younger women and even in children (CLEMENT and SCULLY 1990b; VELLIOS 1980; ZALOUDEK and NORRIS 1981). As already discussed for the other uterine mixed tumors, adenosarcomas usually come to medical attention because of abnormal vaginal bleeding, and are found to be polypoid lesions projecting into the endometrial cavity. Most tumors arise in the uterine fundus, and the average diameter has been reported as about 5 cm (CLEMENT and SCULLY 1990b). The tumor is usually solitary, but multiple, intramyometrial, and extrauterine tumors have all been reported. In several cases, there has been an association with prior pelvic radiation or with exogenous or endogenous hyperestrinism (CLEMENT and SCULLY 1990b).

Microscopically, the diagnosis is made by the finding of benign epithelial elements admixed with a malignant stromal component. This neoplasm shares many features with cystosarcoma phyllodes of the breast, including broad leaflike papillary processes on the surface and deeply situated glands cuffed by hypercellular stroma (Fig. 12). Adenosarcoma can arise within an otherwise banal endometrial polyp (Fig. 13).

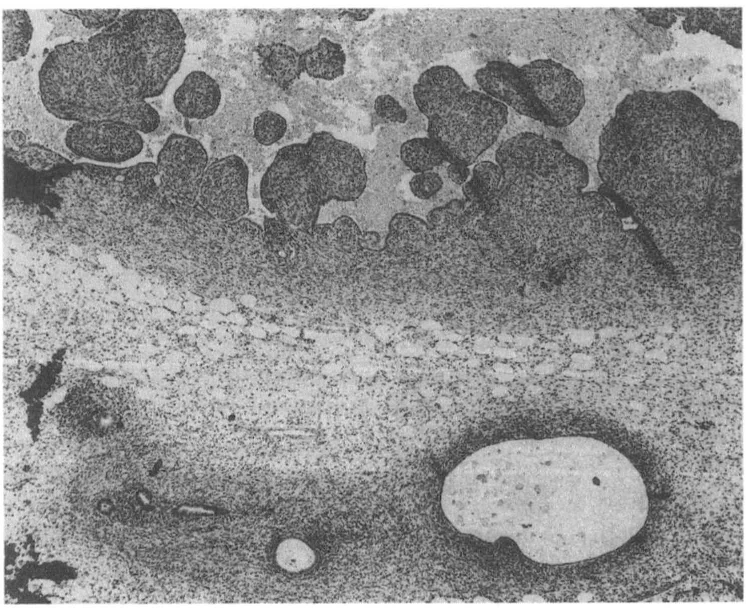

**Fig. 12.** Adenosarcoma. Low-power photomicrograph demonstrates papillae at surface and underlying benign glands, some cystically dilated, cuffed by hypercellular stroma. H&E, original magnification. × 40

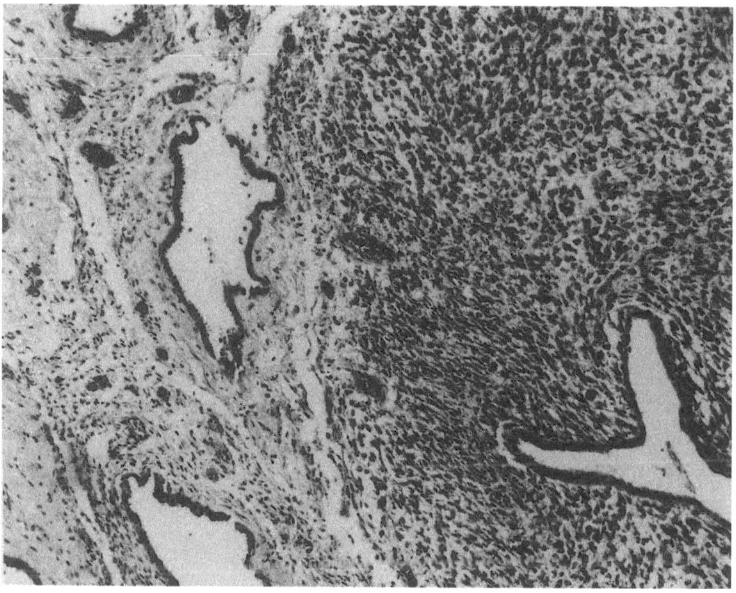

**Fig. 13.** Adenosarcoma (*right*) arising in banal endometrial polyp (*left*). H&E, original magnification. × 100

The epithelial component of adenosarcoma, by definition benign, is often characteristic because of the presence of papillary processes (Fig. 12), cystically dilated glands (Fig. 12), and compressed slitlike glands which may form complex anastomoses (Fig. 14). The glandular epithelium may cytologically resemble normal proliferative endometrium, but may also be flattened or show various types of metaplasic changes (Fig. 14). Although cytologic atypia may be present, by definition invasive carcinoma is absent.

The stromal component, which also by definition is cytologically malignant, is composed in homologous cases of spindle or round cells resembling fibroblasts, endometrial stromal cells, or both (Figs. 13, 14). Focally denser cuffs of hypercellular stroma surrounding glands are an almost invariable finding (Figs. 12, 13). Nuclear atypia is usually mild to moderate, and the mitotic count is greater than in adenofibroma (i.e., more than 2 or 3 per 10 high-power fields) but generally lower than in carcinosarcomas (which usually demonstrate 20 or more mitotic figures per 10 high-power fields). Frequent focal findings include stromal fibrosis and hyalinization, hemorrhage, foam cells, smooth muscle cells, and necrosis. A heterologous component—usually rhabdomyosarcoma or chondrosarcoma—may be present, and should be noted in the diagnosis. We have not encountered eosinophilic hyaline droplets in the cytoplasm of the stromal cells of adenosarcoma, although they are frequent in carcinosarcomas. Rarely, adenosarcomas contain sex cordlike elements within the stromal

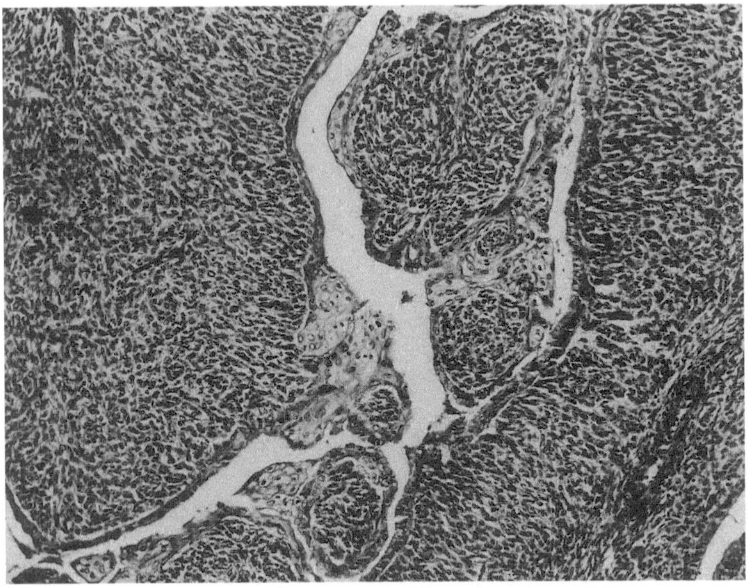

**Fig. 14.** Adenosarcoma. Slitlike anastomosing and branching glandular lumina are lined by proliferative endometrium with focal squamous metaplasia, and surrounded by a densely cellular low-grade sarcoma of endometrial stromal type. H&E, original magnification. × 100

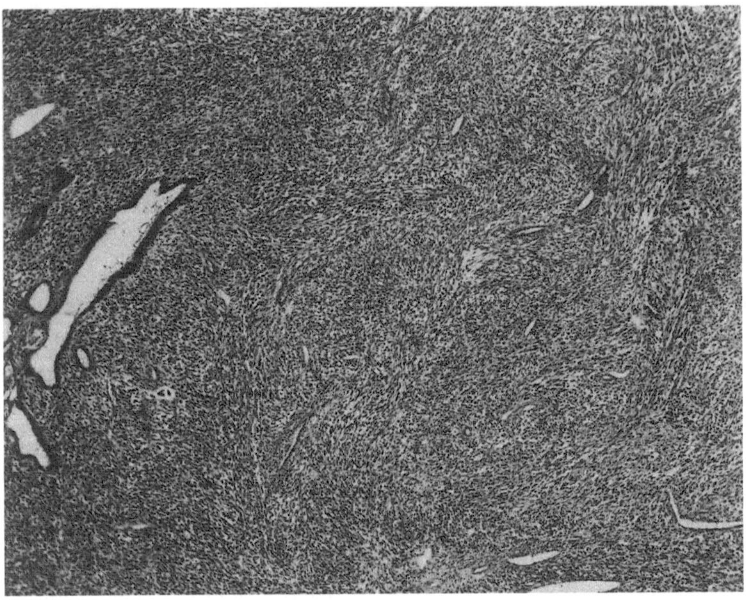

**Fig. 15.** Adenosarcoma with stromal overgrowth. Only a few benign glands remain in this field (*far left*), whereas most of the tumor illustrated consists of pure sarcoma. H&E, original magnification ×40

component, consisting of solid nests, trabeculae, and solid or hollow tubules composed of benign-appearing epithelial-type cells (CLEMENT and SCULLY 1989). The clinical and pathologic features of the tumors containing these elements are otherwise similar to those of typical adenosarcomas.

An important variant with profound clinical implications is *adenosarcoma with sarcomatous overgrowth* (CLEMENT 1990; KAKU et al. 1991). This is defined by the presence of a pure sarcoma—usually but not necessarily of higher grade and mitotic rate—that overgrows the typical adenosarcoma to account for at least 25% of total tumor volume (Fig. 15). The true frequency of this phenomenon is not yet known, since it has been reported only in two large series, and represented 10 of 125 cases in one (CLEMENT 1989) and 17 of 31 in the other (KAKU et al. 1991). Sarcomatous overgrowth may have been underrepresented in the former series, which consisted primarily of cases referred for pathologic consultation, and overrepresented in the second series, which consisted of cases entered into a Gynecologic Oncology Group protocol for staging laparotomy. We suspect, therefore, that the true frequency is probably intermediate between the two figures quoted.

More importantly, despite the difference in frequency quoted, sarcomatous overgrowth was an ominous prognostic sign in both series, with tumor recurrence developing in 44%–70% of cases, compared with 14%–25% of cases without sarcomatous overgrowth.

## 5.2 Differential Diagnosis

The main differential diagnosis of adenosarcoma is with adenofibroma on the one hand and carcinosarcoma on the other. As mentioned above, carcinosarcoma should be diagnosed when even a single small focus of adenocarcinoma is positively identified. CLEMENT and SCULLY (1990b) have recommended diagnosing adenosarcoma rather than adenofibroma when one or more of the following are present: (a) a stromal mitotic count of 2 or more mitotic figures per 10 high-power fields; (b) marked stromal cellularity; and (c) more than mild degrees of stromal nuclear atypia. We believe that the presence of periglandular stromal cuffing is also a useful differential diagnostic feature, which is almost always seen in adenosarcoma and never in adenofibroma.

In extrauterine sites, a differential diagnosis with endometriosis also exists, but this should not be important in an endometrial polypoid lesion. Endometrial polyps and adenomyomas should also not pose a significant problem.

## 5.3 Prognosis and Treatment

In most series, the majority of cases of adenosarcoma have not invaded the myometrium and have not recurred following surgical excision. In the large series of CLEMENT and SCULLY (1990b), recurrences developed in approximately

25% of cases, usually within the vagina, pelvis, or abdomen, and often appearing at an interval of 5 years or more after hysterectomy; distant metastases occurred in less than 5% of cases. In the series of ZALOUDEK and NORRIS (1981), recurrence occurred in 40% of cases, with a median interval of 5 years, and death from tumor progression occurred in 24%. In the study of KAKU et al. (1991), 30% of cases recurred and 20% of patients died of tumor progression.

The two histologic features of the primary tumor which have been associated with an increased risk of recurrence whenever they were analyzed are myometrial invasion and sarcomatous overgrowth. Other features which have been reported in some but not all series as unfavourable prognostic factors include the presence of extrauterine spread at the time of diagnosis, necrosis in the primary tumor, the presence of heterologous elements (particularly rhabdomyosarcoma), high sarcoma grade, and high mitotic index of the stromal component (CLEMENT and SCULLY 1990b; KAKU et al. 1991; HARIRI 1983; VELLIOS 1980). In the series of KAKU et al., the triad of stromal overgrowth, rhabdomyosarcomatous differentiation, and lymphatic/vascular space invasion predicted the 2 of 31 cases in which lymph node metastases were present at the time of exploratory laparotomy with pelvic and para-aortic lymph node dissection. Since these two cases were the only ones in the series with these three findings in the hysterectomy specimen itself, it was suggested that lymphadenectomy might be reserved in the future for cases displaying all three findings.

In general, the treatment of adenosarcoma has to date been almost exclusively surgical, with some patients receiving radiation or chemotherapy for recurrent disease. As mentioned above, patients whose tumors do not invade the myometrium and do not display sarcomatous overgrowth usually do well. Among those cases which have recurred, many of the recurrences have been vaginal, and these have been composed of either pure sarcoma or adenosarcoma; distant metastases are generally composed of pure sarcoma (CLEMENT and SCULLY 1990b). Carcinosarcomas diagnosed on the basis of a few foci of carcinoma in a tumor which otherwise resembles adenosarcoma may also develop sarcomatous metastases, in contradistinction to the usual carcinomatous appearance of early metastates in carcinosarcoma.

## References

Abell MR (1971) Papillary adenofibroma of the uterine cervix. Am J Obstet Gynecol 110:990–993

Amr SS, Tavassoli FA, Hassan AA, Issa AA, Madanat FF (1986) Mixed mesodermal tumor of the uterus in a 4-year-old girl. Int J Gynecol Pathol 5:371–378

Auerbach HE, LiVolsi VA, Merino MJ (1988) Malignant mixed müllerian tumors of the uterus: an immunohistochemical study. Int J Gynecol Pathol 7:123–130

Bitterman P, Chun BK, Kurman RJ (1988) Uterine carcinosarcomas: a clinicopathologic and immunohistochemical study providing evidence that these are biphasic carcinomas. Lab Invest 58:10A

Chung M-T, Mukai K, Teshima S, Kishi K, Shimosato K (1988) Expression of various antigens by different components of uterine mixed müllerian tumors. An immunohistochemical study. Acta Pathol Jpn 38:35–45

Clement PB (1989) Müllerian adenosarcoma of the uterus with sarcomatous overgrowth. A clinicopathological analysis of 10 cases. Am J Surg Pathol 13:28–38

Clement PB, Scully RE (1974) Müllerian adenosarcoma of the uterus. A clinicopathologic analysis of ten cases of a distinctive type of müllerian mixed tumor. Cancer 34:1138–1149

Clement PB, Scully RE (1978) Extrauterine mesodermal (müllerian) adenosarcoma. A clinicopathologic analysis of five cases. Am J Clin Pathol 69:276–283

Clement PB, Scully RE (1988) Uterine tumors with mixed epithelial and mesenchymal elements. Semin Diagn Pathol 5:199–222

Clement PB, Scully RE (1989) Müllerian adenosarcoma of the uterus with sex cord-like elements. A clinicopathologic analysis of eight cases. Am J Clin Pathol 91:664–672

Clement PB, Scully RE (1990a) Müllerian adenofibroma of the uterus with invasion of myometrium and pelvic veins. Int J Gynecol Pathol 9:363–371

Clement PB, Scully RE (1990b) Müllerian adenosarcoma of the uterus. A clinicopathological analysis of 100 cases with a review of the literature. Hum Pathol 21:363–381

de Brito PA, Orenstein JM, Silverberg SG (1991) Carcinosarcoma of the female genital tract: immunohistochemical and ultrastructural analysis of 28 cases. (submitted for publication)

Deligdisch L, Plaxe S, Cohen CJ (1988) Extrauterine pelvic malignant mixed mesodermal tumors. A study of 10 cases with immunohistochemistry. Int J Gynecol Pathol 7:361–372

Dictor M (1982) Ovarian malignant mixed mesodermal tumor. The occurrence of hyaline droplets containing α-1-antitrypsin. Hum Pathol 13:930–933

Dinh TV, Slavin RE, Bhagavan BS, Hannigan EV, Tiamson EM, Yandel RB (1989) Mixed müllerian tumors of the uterus: a clinicopathologic study. Obstet Gynecol 74:388–392

Geisinger KR, Dabbs DJ, Marshall RB (1987) Malignant mixed müllerian tumors. An ultrastructural and immunohistochemical analysis with histogenetic considerations. Cancer 59:1781–1790

Gersell DJ, Duncan DA, Fulling KH (1989) Malignant mixed müllerian tumor of the uterus with neuroectodermal differentiation. Int J Gynecol Pathol 8:169-178

Hariri J (1983) Müllerian adenosarcoma of the endometrium. Review of the literature and report of two cases. Int J Gynecol Pathol 2:182–191

Ishiwata I, Ishiwata C, Nagayama T, Ishikawa H (1981) Histogenesis and culture of human uterine carcinosarcoma: Cancer 41:1978–1983

Ishiwata I, Ono I, Ishiwata C et al. (1987) Heterotransplantation of mixed mesodermal tumor cells in nude mouse—histology of metastatic foci. Gynecol Oncol 27:189–196

Kaku T, Silverberg SG, Blessing J et al. (1991) Adenosarcoma of the uterus. A Gynecologic Oncology Group clinico-pathologic study of 31 cases. Int J Gynecol Pathol, in press

Kao GF, Norris HJ (1978) Benign and low grade variant of mixed mesodermal tumor (adenosarcoma) of the ovary and adnexal region. Cancer 42:1314–1324

Masuda A, Takeda A, Fukami H, Yamada C, Matsuyama M (1987) Characteristics of cell lines established from a mixed mesodermal tumor of the human ovary. Cancer 60:2696–2703

Mazur MT (1981) Atypical polypoid adenomyomas of the endometrium. Am J Surg Pathol 5:473–482

Nielsen SN, Podratz KC, Scheithauer BW, O'Brien PC (1989) Clinicopathologic analysis of uterine malignant mixed müllerian tumors. Gynecol Oncol 34:372–378

Noorduyn LA, Herman CJ (1987) The relation between mixed mesodermal tumors and adenocarcinomas of the ovary. An immunopathologic study. Eur J Cancer Clin Oncol 23:157–162

Norris HJ, Taylor HB (1966) Mesenchymal tumors of the uterus. III. A clinical and pathological study of 31 carcinosarcomas. Cancer 19:1459–1465

Norris HJ, Roth E, Taylor HB (1966) Mesenchymal tumors of the uterus. II. A clinical pathologic study of 31 mixed mesodermal tumors. Obstet Gynecol 28:57–63

Östör AG, Fortune DW (1980) Benign and low grade variant of mixed müllerian tumor of the uterus. Histopathology 4:369–382

Peters WA III, Rivkin SE, Smith MR, Tesh DE (1989) Cisplatin and adriamycin combination chemotherapy for uterine stromal sarcomas and mixed mesodermal tumors. Gynecol Oncol 34:323–327

Podozaski ES, Woomert CA, Stevens CH Jr et al. (1989) Management of malignant, mixed mesodermal tumors of the uterus. Gynecol Oncol 32:240-244

Press MF, Scully RE (1985) Endometrial "sarcomas" complicating ovarian thecoma, polycystic ovarian disease and estrogen therapy. Gynecol Oncol 21:135–154

Silverberg SG, Major FJ, Blessing JA et al. (1990) Carcinosarcoma (malignant mixed mesodermal tumor) of the uterus: a Gynecologic Oncology Group pathologic study of 203 cases. Int J Gynecol Pathol 9:1–19

Spanos WJ Jr, Peters LJ, Osward MJ (1986) Patterns of recurrence in malignant mixed müllerian tumor of the uterus. Cancer 57:155–159

Tenti P, Babilonti L, La Fianza A et al. (1989) Cytology of malignant mixed mesodermal tumour of the uterus: experience of 10 cases. Eur J Gynaecol Oncol 10:125–128

Vellios F (1980) Papillary adenofibroma-adenosarcoma. The uterine cystosarcoma phyllodes. Prog Surg Pathol 1:205–219

Vellios F, Ng ABP, Reagan JW (1973) Papillary adenofibroma of the uterus; a benign mesodermal mixed tumor of müllerian origin. Am J Clin Pathol 60:543–551

Young RH, Treger T, Scully RE (1986) Atypical polypoid adenomyoma of the uterus. A report of 27 cases. Am J Clin Pathol 86:139–145

Zaloudek CJ, Norris HJ (1981) Adenofibroma and adenosarcoma of the uterus: a clinicopathologic study of 35 cases. Cancer 48:354–366

# Cervical Intraepithelial Neoplasia and Microinvasive Carcinoma of the Cervix

K. NODA



## 1 Cervical Intraepithelial Neoplasia

### 1.1 Terminology and Definition

Various epithelial abnormalities may appear in the uterine cervix. Most are only benign changes, such as reserve cell hyperplasia, mature or immature squamous metaplasia, basal cell hyperplasia, ascending healing, and reactive proliferation for inflammation. However, a group of intraepithelial lesions with malignant potential known as dysplasia or carcinoma in situ (CIS) may also occur in the cervix.

The term "dysplasia" was introduced into the field of gynecologic pathology by REAGAN et al. (1953), who likened it to an atypical hyperplasia of the cervical squamous epithelium. Later, at the 1st International Congress of Exfoliative Cytology in Vienna (International Committee on Histological Terminology), the histologic classification and terminology for "dysplasia" were internationally discussed for the first time. Although dysplasia was defined then as "all other disturbances of differentiation of the squamous epithelium of lesser degree than carcinoma in situ," that definition was vague and without specific

Current Topics in Pathology
Volume 85, Ed. N. Sasano

description of the features of the lesion, and therefore could not gain support from pathologists who required precision in diagnosis.

In 1975, the World Health Organization (WHO) (POULSEN et al. 1975) defined dysplasia anew, as "a lesion in which part of the thickness of the epithelium is replaced by cells showing varying degrees of atypia." This definition is more concrete than the previous one and has been adopted for pathologic classification in recent work. Generally, dysplasia can be further subdivided into mild, moderate, and severe degrees (REAGAN and HAMONIC 1956). This subclassification is based upon the nature of cellular atypia and differentiation, and upon the number and location of mitoses. However, precise guidelines for these subdivisions have not been defined and this grading has always been subjective.

The definition of "carcinoma in situ" is relatively clear; the 1st International Congress of Exfoliative Cytology in Vienna in 1961 established it as replacement of the full thickness of the epithelium by undifferentiated cells. Because of many suggestions that the lesion with a certain degree of cell differentiation should also be included in the criteria, however, the WHO proposed, in 1975, a revised definition of CIS, i.e., "a lesion in which all or most of the epithelium shows the cellular features of carcinoma," which also allows for some differentiation on the surface. Although this definition is now used to define CIS in the cervix, objective diagnosis cannot be accomplished using it. Moreover, discrepancies in diagnosis between different pathologists observing the same slide, as well as between diagnostic results obtained at different times by the same pathologist examining identical material, have been pointed out (COCKER et al. 1968; BELLINA et al. 1982).

Classifying cervical intraepithelial abnormalities into dysplasia and CIS may give clinicians the impression that CIS and dysplasia have different disease processes, the former being malignant and the latter benign. This perception may lead to different treatments for each. Significant problems may occur, however, if therapeutic choices are based upon histologic diagnostic criteria which lack objectivity.

Many attempts have been made to classify these intraepithelial abnormalities using histologic findings as objective as possible and to clarify the biologic behavior of each lesion by long-term follow-up. Because dysplasia and CIS are not comparable in terms of subsequent occurrence of invasive carcinoma or spontaneous regression, some pathologists still prefer to use the dysplasia/CIS terminology. In fact, the revised draft of the WHO classification, which will be issued soon, seems to adopt this dysplasia/CIS terminology as it is.

In the last 20 years, studies using electron microscopy (SHINGLETON et al. 1968), autoradiography (RICHART 1963), microspectrophotometry (WILLBANKS et al. 1967), tissue culture (RICHART et al. 1967), or cytogenetics (KIRKLAND et al. 1967; SPRIGGS et al. 1971) have proven that there is no definite difference between dysplasia and CIS, suggesting that these two lesions are part of one continuous pathologic spectrum. It may, therefore, be impossible to clearly differentiate dysplasia from CIS. In 1967, RICHART suggested "cervical intraepithelial neoplasia" (CIN) as a name for both these lesions. This classification is now widely accepted. Cervical intraepithelial neoplasia is usually divided into three grades, CIN I, CIN II and CIN III; CIN I represents the well-differentiated lesions, previously categorized as mild dysplasia, and CIN III the poorly differentiated lesions corresponding in the old terminology to severe dysplasia or carcinoma in situ. CIN II is the intermediate category, loosely equivalent to moderate dysplasia (Fig. 1). Obviously, the borders between these grades are not always clear.

The nomenclature of CIN reflects the concept of tumor progression and progressive loss of differentiation with increasing malignancy, which fits in well with the current understanding of the biology of carcinogenesis. This CIN terminology uniquely regards dysplasia as a neoplastic process and is useful for understanding that both dysplasia and CIS are parts of a single disease process. An intraepithelial lesions from mild dysplasia to CIS may therefore clinically be dealt with in a similar way.

The Ninth Study Group of the Royal College of Obstetricians and Gynaecologists (Jordan et al. 1982) has recommended that all grades of CIN be regarded as a continuum and that CIN I lesions should be treated as seriously as CIN III lesions. Hence the diagnosis of CIN of any grade may have serious treatment implications for the patient.

As discussed in the section on natural history, however, CIN I has a relatively high probability of spontaneous regression, while CIN III has a relatively high probability of progression. There is also a great difference between CIN I and CIN III in the period preceding progression.

The dysplasia/CIS terminology has made it clear that severe treatment is required for CIS, and that different therapies are indicated for dysplasia

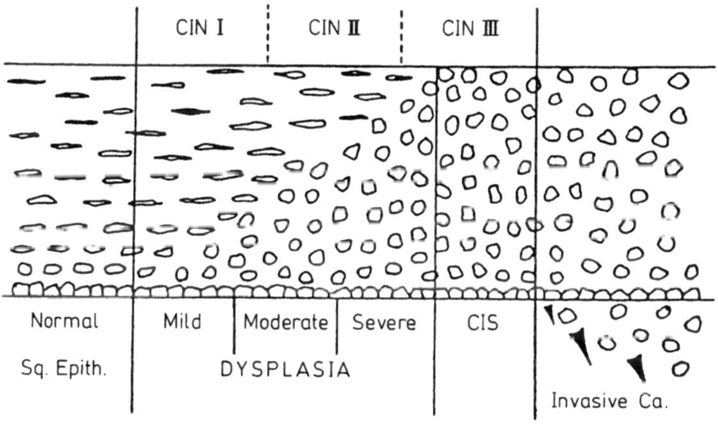


**Fig. 1.** Schematic diagram comparing CIN terminology with dysplasia/CIS terminology. No attempt is made to depict cytologic atypia, disorganization, and mitotic activity which characterize CIN. The histologic grade is based upon the degree to which the abnormal basal-type cells occupy the epithelium. (Richart 1976)

depending upon grade. Using the CIN terminology, however, the same type of treatment would be used for CIN I, CIN II, or CIN III on the basis of our understanding of their pathologic nature. This approach has become more widely used as therapy using local destruction with laser vaporization has become popular. This treatment is technically simple and requires little time. In addition, the long-term effects, particularly those related to pregnancy and delivery, appear to be less following local destruction than following conization (ANDERSON 1982). However, this type of treatment requires close observation with colposcopy to define the extension of the lesion and to rule out the possibility of invasive cancer. Even in cases where these requirements are met, close follow-up is needed to check for residual lesions.

The principal objection to CIN terminology has been that low-grade lesions, most of which are likely to be reversible, also take the name "neoplasia"; overtreatment may therefore result, or the patient may be caused unnecessary anxiety. This is because the CIN classification lacks histologic criteria to clearly rule out reactive, nonneoplastic changes from the category.

Recently, in 1989, ISMAIL et al. questioned the ability of histopathologists to differentiate CIN I and reactive proliferation and demonstrated poor interobserver agreement on CIN grading. Agreement occurred for most cases of invasive carcinoma, but not for many cases of CIN I, II and III. Of greater clinical significance, however, was the finding that CIN I and reactive proliferation could not be distinguished. According to the authors, this indicates that the current policy of adopting identical therapeutic approaches for CIN I and CIN III may result in overtreatment. The poor agreement among observers is largely caused by shortcomings in the morphologic criteria used to diagnose CIN and in the current grading system. ISMAIL et al. suggested further that an inaccurate, poorly reproducible grading system, which in any case is not essential to current clinical management, should be altogether abandoned, that the three subdivisions of CIN should be abolished, and that pathologists should be prepared to diagnose and gynecologists to accept a borderline category.

Consequently, additional methods are needed to improve the accuracy of the diagnosis of the preinvasive stage of cervical carcinoma and to determine the prognosis of morphologic abnormalities. A study on the prognostic importance of measurements of nuclear DNA showed that 91% of diploid or polyploid lesions regress and 9% persist (FU et al. 1981). In contrast, 81% of aneuploid lesions in this series persisted, 12% progressed to invasive carcinoma, and 7% showed normal results on follow-up. BIBBO et al. (1989) have suggested that the DNA profile yields significant information on prognosis. CIS with a polyploid DNA profile is more likely to regress than is that with an aneuploid pattern. However, some CIN lesions with polyploid DNA profiles progress and some CIN lesions with aneuploid patterns regress. The DNA profile therefore certainly provides important information on the prognosis, but is not determinative. The best morphologic indicator of aneuploidy was the presence of abnormal mitotic figures. REID et al. (1984) have suggested that abnormal mitotic figures are also useful for determining CIN prognosis. Abnormal mitotic figures have been noted in 19% of CIN cases with the aneuploid pattern. However, abnormal mitotic figures are of limited use for differentiating benign lesions from malignant ones, especially in cases of low-grade CIN. Abnormal mitotic figures are commonly observed in high-grade CIN but rarely in low-grade CIN. Thus, abnormal mitotic figures do not always represent a useful criterion in the differential diagnosis of low-grade lesions (WILLETT et al. 1989).

At present, pathologists cannot identify a fully transformed malignant cell prior to the occurrence of invasion. WILLETT et al. (1989) have proposed that the CIN terminology should be expanded to include all atypical proliferative lesions, and that CIN does not necessarily imply a malignant lesion, merely a proliferative process displaying varying degrees of cytologic atypia with uncertain malignant potential.

Recent data are consistent with the concept that human papillomavirus (HPV) is etiologically important in the causation of cervical squamous cell carcinoma and adenocarcinoma. There appear to be certain important events in the process of HPV infection and neoplasia.

Considering these arguments, RICHART (1990) made certain proposals regarding CIN terminology: It is suggested that the terminology of the HPV-related precursor lesions be modified and that two terms, rather than three, would best satisfy the requirements of both science and clinical care. The "early" lesions should be referred to as "low-grade cervical intraepithelial neoplasia (CIN) with HPV-related changes" and "high-grade CIN." Lesions diagnosed by the pathologist as "high-grade CIN" would be evaluated appropriately using colposcopy, biopsy, and endocervical curettage to rule out invasion, and then treated based on well-established protocols. Lesions diagnosed by the pathologist as "low-grade CIN with HPV-related changes" would be understood by the clinician to have uncertain potential, and the patient could be treated or followed, after ruling out invasive cancer and performing HPV typing, as the clinician thought appropriate.

RICHART'S suggestion seems to deny the concept of CIN as a single disease process, which is a conclusion drawn from data collection about histologic features of HPV infection.

## 1.2 Etiology

It has long been known that epidemiologic risk factors for cervical cancer include first intercourse at early ages, high parity, multiple sexual partners, prostitution, lower socioeconomic status, and smoking. These factors are considered to be related to the frequency and timing of exposure of the cervix to carcinogens (HERRERO et al. 1990).

Various factors are suspected to be potentially carcinogenic in the development of CIN and invasive carcinoma of the cervix, including transmissible agents such as smegma, spermatozoa, herpesvirus type 2 (HSV-2), and HPV, as well as smoking, contraceptive pills, and other factors.

Because the occurrence of cervical cancer is very much lower in women whose husbands have been circumcised, it has been suspected that accumulated smegma in uncircumcised men may act as a chemical carcinogen. There is certainly a correlation between phimosis and penile cancer. There have been reports that cervical cancer occurs at a higher rate in women whose husbands have penile cancer (GRAHAM et al. 1979; SMITH et al. 1980). However, considering the recent evidence that HPV plays a role in the etiology of both cervical and penile cancer (COCKS et al. 1980), the HPV in smegma seems likely to be responsible for cancerous changes. The chemical constituents of smegma cannot be exonerated; HSV-2 has been isolated from smegma (RAWLS et al. 1968).

COPPLESON and REID (1967) have presented evidence incriminating spermatozoa in the development of cervical cancer. It would seem important to consider the possibility of an interaction of sperm DNA with cervical epithelial cells. The number of their experiments was small, however, and their results have not yet been verified by other workers.

A relationship of HSV-2 infection to development of cancer was first suggested by NAIB et al. (1966), and later by many other workers reporting seroepidemiologic evidence for it. A considerable number of reports have shown that antibodies against HSV-2 are more frequently found in women with cervical neoplasia both intraepithelial and invasive in nature (MELNICK et al. 1974), although there have been wide variations in the proportion of cervical neoplasia patients and control women with HSV antibodies (RICHART and CRUM 1982).

In addition, there have been many investigations using tissue culture, animal experiments, or molecular biology. The data on the relation between HSV-2 infection and the development of CIN and cervical cancer can be summed up as follows:

1. Studies in the United States and Europe [NAIB et al. (1969) in Atlanta; RAWLS et al. (1969) in Texas; ROYSTON and AURELIAN (1970) in Maryland] reported that a high percentage (8%–100%) of patients with cervical cancer had HSV-2 antibodies in serum.
2. When women with positive HSV-2 were followed up, the incidences of dysplasia, CIS, and invasive carcinoma were significantly higher (NAIB et al. 1969).
3. Hela cells which are cultured cells of human cervical cancer origin have HSV antigenicity (MCKENNA and DAVIS 1966).
4. The interval to the development of methylcholanthrene-induced tumor in mice could be shortened by HSV infection (TANAKA and SOUTHAM 1965).
5. HSV infection into the genital organ induced cervical dysplasia in mice (NAHMIAS et al. 1967).
6. HSV-2 virus could be isolated from the smegma of the husbands of patients with cervical cancer (RAWLS et al. 1968).

7. The age of a peak incidence of HSV-infected cells which are detected in vaginal smears is 10 years lower than that of CIS and 20 years lower than that of invasive cancer (Naib et al. 1969).
8. Epidemiologically, cervical cancer more frequently occurs in women of the low socioeconomic bracket, which corresponds to the epidemiologic tendency of HSV-2 infection (Ory et al. 1975).
9. Epidemiology of cervical cancer indicates that a sexually transmitted agent may cause cervical cancer.

These findings suggest an undeniable role of HSV-2 infection in the development of cervical cancer, although we still do not have decisive data to justify this conclusion.

A hit-and-run mechanism for HSV has been hypothesized by Galloway and McDougall (1985), postulating that HSV may cause transformation without continued viral presence or expression by activating cellular oncogenes, mediating gene amplification, or acting as a mutagen.

Recently, Iwasaka et al. (1988) suggested in a study with culture cells that HSV-2 acts as an initiator and HPV 16 as a promoter to complete the transformation.

The association of HPV with cervical cancer is one of the current topics of interest in the field of gynecological pathology. As this subject is detailed in an other chapter, I shall discuss it only briefly here. A substantial amount of evidence has been gathered to establish a relationship between HPV and the development of cervical cancer. The data to date indicate that HPV types 6, 11, 16, 18, 31, 33, and 35, and several more recently described types (Yajima et al. 1988), are all involved in cervical neoplasia. It is also known that types 6 and 11 are usually associated with condyloma acuminatum and low-grade intraepithelial lesions, and that types 16, 18, and 31 are often associated with high-grade intraepithelial lesions and invasive carcinoma. These observations have promoted the concept that there may be "low-risk" and "high-risk" HPV types in cervical carcinogenesis.

Woodworth et al. (1988) established HPV-immortalized human exocervical epithelial cell lines after transfection with HPV 16 or 18. All the lines contained integrated HPV 16 or 18 sequences and expressed HPV mRNAs. However, HPV-immortalized cell lines were not tumorigenic in nude mice. Colgan et al. (1989) reported that HPV 16 infection of apparently normal cervical epithelium can occur in association with the onset of CIN and invasive carcinoma. Nuovo et al. (1989) found that about 10% of women over a wide range of ages are infected by HPV but have no clinical or histologic evidence of the infection.

These results suggest that HPV types 16 and 18 are not carcinogenic on their own, requiring other cofactors and breakdown of local immunity and other defense mechanisms as well. Winkelstein (1977) pointed out for the first time the relation between cigarette smoking and the development of cervical cancer, and subsequently there were many other epidemiologic studies on the subject

(Winkelstein 1986; WHO 1986). Wigle et al. (1980) and Harris et al. (1980) reported that the risk of cervical cancer or CIN is twice as high in woman smokers as in nonsmokers of the same sex. However, no reports have directly proved such an association. Zur Hausen (1982) has suggested that HSV-2 or perhaps cigarette smoking may act synergistically as an initiator or promoter in HPV-stimulated epithelium, providing for more efficient cellular transformation.

## 1.3 Histogenesis and Natural History

Cervical intraepithelial neoplasia and invasive cancer each occur in the transformation zone of the uterine cervix. This has been demonstrated in many investigations of the location of CIN and microinvasive carcinoma in the cervix. During adolescence, as the cervix everts, the columnar epithelium in the cervical canal is exposed to the vaginal cavity. The transformation zone is initially covered only by this columnar epithelium which, mainly in response to the acidity of the vaginal environment, undergoes reserve cell hyperplasia to squamous metaplasia. If a coitally transmitted carcinogen is present during this early metaplastic process, the epithelium may be transformed, resulting in a neoplastic process (CIN). At which stage in the metaplastic process the epithelial cells are most susceptible is still unknown. It is believed that mature metaplastic epithelium, original squamous epithelium, and original columnar epithelium are resistant to mutagenic changes, while active immature metaplastic epithelium is susceptible to them.

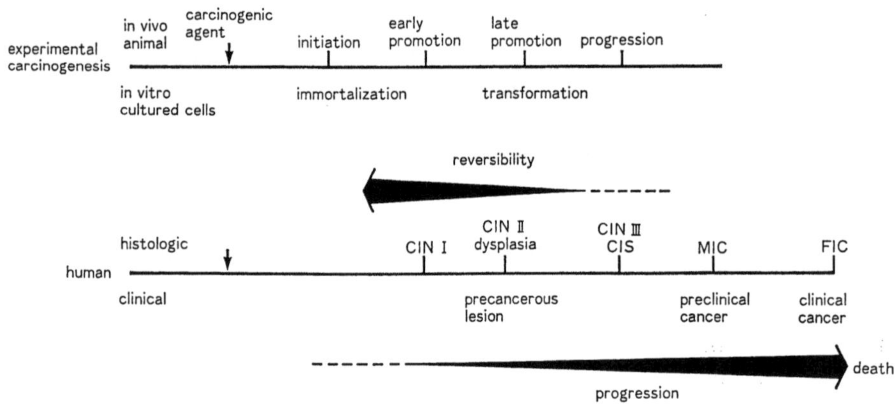


**Fig. 2.** Schematic comparison of experimental carcinogenesis in animals and cultured cells with histologic and clinical progressing patterns of human cervical cancer. *FIC*, frank invasive cancer; *MIC*, microinvasive cancer

Although the interaction between carcinogens and susceptible cells seems to be momentary, a time span of weeks or even years may be needed before carcinogen-stimulated cells undergo morphologic transformation through genetic or epigenetic changes within the cells. Since cell transformation is established in the two steps of initiation and promotion, even the mildest CIN should take quite a long time to form. Further progress in grade to CIN II or CIN III may require repeated steps of initiation and promotion in the course of development.

It is reasonably predicted that the number of women who have been exposed to carcinogens of CIN should greatly outstrip the number of those who in fact generate CIN. It seems that transformed cells occur in only a portion of women whose susceptible cells have contacts with carcinogens. This suggests that the defense mechanism, along with dying of some of the stimulated cells, may work to prevent the development of CIN so that even atypical cells are not established in the tissue.

Figure 2 compares the data obtained in experimental studies on carcinogenesis in animals and cultured cells with histologic and clinical progressing patterns of cancer observed in the human cervix. In vitro studies using cultured cells have made great progress thanks to the advancement of molecular biology. To give an example, HPV type 16 genome transfected into immortalized cells, NIH3T3, may produce transformed cells having tumorigenicity. The same virus transfected into the primary culture of human keratinocytes may induce immortalization but not transformation. These findings have helped somewhat in clarifying the mechanisms of immortalization and transformation in cultured cells.

Comparison of the data obtained in these cultured cell systems to the two steps of initiation and promotion observed in experimental animal models is illustrated in Fig. 2. As mentioned above, whether CIN is cumulatively promoted in such early and late promotion or whether initiation and promotion in the case of CIN are repeated stepwise is still unknown. In addition, it is also unclear whether the early and late promotions are continuously linked in a single series of carcinogenic stimulation or whether they are triggered by different agents. Anyway, it can be concluded that initiation in animal experiments is a change corresponding to immortalization in cultured cells.

In humans, histologically detectable CIN may further progress to microinvasive carcinoma (MIC), to frank invasive carcinoma (FIC), and finally to clinical carcinoma which causes the host's death. Each grade of CIN, MIC, and FIC is compared with experimental cancers in Fig 2. Above and below the comparison, the degrees of reversibility and progressibility of each lesion are added. The period from a hit of carcinogenic stimulation to the development of histologically detectable mild CIN varies in patients. As described later, the progress of CIN grades greatly depends on each individual patient.

It still has to be elucidated what can be initiators or promoters for the development of intraepithelial neoplasia and invasive carcinoma in the uterine cervix. As for histogenesis of CIN and invasive carcinoma, however, according to Anderson (1987) conceptual ideas at the present time can be summarized as follows: First, an initiating agent primes susceptible cells, such as immature metaplastic cells in the transformation zone of the uterine cervix. Next, a promoting agent transforms a single cell in the primed field (Park and Jones 1968; Smith et al. 1971; Spriggs et al. 1971). This transformed cell proliferates and escapes from the local control mechanism. If the defense mechanisms of the host are overcome, the transformed cells proliferate, replacing the surrounding normal epithelium and in addition displaying increased histologic atypia. In other words, severer forms of CIN occupy a larger area with deeper crypts compared with milder forms (Abdul-Karim et al. 1982). Severer forms of CIN established in this way further break through the basement membrane to infiltrate into the stroma and develop into MIC. Unless the proliferation is suppressed by the host defense mechanism the tumor nest continues to grow and progress to become FIC, which finally acquires metastatic potential, ultimately causing host death.

### *1.3.1 Follow-up Studies*

There are many reports describing the natural history of CIN; such follow-up studies entail several controversies, as discussed below:

The histopathologic criteria used for the diagnosis differ among the investigators. Although many of the studies have adopted the dysplasia/CIS terminology, these results cannot exactly be converted into the CIN terminology. The dissected lesion is subject to microscopic examination while the remaining part is followed up; within this context it is necessary to rule out precisely the presence of invasive carcinoma in the patient. If conization is performed for the purpose of entire observation of the transformation zone, a follow-up study will be impossible. Although cytologic and colposcopic examinations may help overcome these disadvantages, the former does not differentiate precise histologic backgrounds of CIN I, II, and III, MIC, and FIC, and the latter does not provide observations of endocervical lesions. Therefore, the results of short-term or small-scale studies have little credibility.

The most important points in follow-up studies are accuracy of the initial diagnosis and prevention of removal of the target lesion, although these two points contradict each other. Careful follow-up studies taking both points into account can be divided into two groups. One group comprises studies which use only cytologic techniques without biopsy, at the expense of some degree of accuracy in the initial diagnosis. The other group comprises studies in which a small biopsy is performed to obtain an initial diagnosis, and the region with the similar colposcopic appearance to the initial biopsy is followed up with cytologic examinations and colposcopy.

Richart and Barron (1969) observed a total of 557 patients with dysplasia over several years using only cytologic and colposcopic examinations. To exclude false-positive cytologic findings, patients were admitted to the study only if they showed abnormal cytology twice. The end point for follow-up was the development of CIS. The median transit time from mild lesions to moderate lesions, to severe lesions, and to CIS was 58 months, 38 months, and 12 months respectively. Only 6% of the total were regressed cases. The authors emphasized that these results depended largely on the follow-up methods and that even a small biopsy would have a great effect on the natural history of CIN.

Nasiell et al. (1983) compared progress rates in patients with dysplasia when the initial diagnosis was made with a small biopsy and when it was made only on the basis of cytologic examination. Although the progress rate was 27% in the former cases and 35% in the latter, the difference did not seem to be as large as Richart asserted it to be.

On the other hand, Johnson et al. (1968) reported that 50.4% of patients with dysplasia who had been followed up for 10 years using cytologic and biopsy examinations experienced regression of the lesion and that dysplasia progressed into CIS in only 1.4%. Galvin et al. (1955) reported that regression was noted in 53.9% of patients with mild dysplasia and that 17.1% of patients with severe dysplasia had regression and 65.7% progressed into CIS. Similar results have been described in many other reports, e.g., a biopsy study by Hall and Walton (1968) and a cytology study by Fox (1967). Burghardt (1973) reported that milder lesions were more likely to regress and that highly atypical lesions progressed at a high rate.

We previously conducted a follow-up study (Noda et al. 1976; Noda 1979) in patients with abnormal cytology who were selected through mass population screening. Under careful colposcopic observation, a small biopsy was taken in these patients to determine the initial diagnosis. To exclude invasive carcinoma from the study, patients were considered to be eligible if their cervical lesion was localized within the ectocervix. Except for the initial biopsy, only cytology and colposcopy were used for patient follow-up in order to keep the lesion out of any intervention. A large number of patients were included in the study to compensate as much as possible for diagnostic errors.

Epithelial lesions with any cellular atypia were histologically classified into mild dysplasia, severe dysplasia, and CIS according to the following criteria. Mild dysplasia indicated a mild degree of cellular and nuclear atypia, preserved stratification of the epithelium despite some delay in lining differentiation, mild disturbances in cell polarity, and mitoses localized within the lower third of the epithelium. Severe dysplasia indicated severe cellular and nuclear atypia, marked disturbances in cell polarity, and impaired lining differentiation. CIS was diagnosed if one or more of the following four findings were noted in a lesion which met the criteria of severe dysplasia: (a) replacement of an entire layer of epithelium with cells which had lost their polarity and displayed lack of differentiation; (b) lateral invasion or invasive growth into surrounding normal epithelium; (c) many abnormal mitoses (at least two per high power field); (d) mesenchymolysis, namely, unclear basement membrane accompanied by edematous and resolved stroma.

Between 1962 and 1973, 691 patients with mild dysplasia, 735 with severe dysplasia, and 46 with CIS were included in this follow-up study. All the data obtained were analyzed in 1979. Mild dysplasia developed into severe dysplasia in 17 patients (2.5%) and CIS in two (0.3%), while it disappeared in 652 patients (94.3%); in most of the latter cases the lesion disappeared within 18 months of the start of follow-up. Severe dysplasia developed into CIS in 112 patients and further into invasive carcinoma, mostly microinvasive carcinoma, in 80 patients. Progress was thus detected in 26.1% of the patients and required a period of 6–120 months, mean of 34.6 months. Spontaneous regression was confirmed in 490 patients (66.6%), taking a period of 6–84 months, with a mean of 30.0 months. Of 46 cases of CIS, 37 (80.4%) progressed into invasive carcinoma over 13–64 months. In seven patients (15.2%), the lesion extended into the endocervix during the follow-up period, which made the colposcopic observation impossible. Hysterectomy was performed. The other two patients (4.3%) experienced spontaneous regression.

We did not use CIN terminology in this study, and it is difficult to translate our results into CIN terminology. However, this study had the following characteristics:

1. Assuming that it is impossible to differentiate reactive proliferation of cervical epithelium and CIN I mild dysplasia was defined as including nonneoplastic lesions. As a result, 97% of the lesions were reversible. In other words, most mild dysplasia lesions which were diagnosed based on these criteria were nonneoplastic and reversible.

2. Severe dysplasia in this study may have included lesions which would have been classified as CIN II or CIN III. About a quarter of these lesions progressed further and the rest regressed. Therefore, several additional steps of progression were considered to be necessary for the lesions to show malignant behavior.

3. When CIS was diagnosed based on the four specific findings mentioned above, this group of lesions developed into invasive carcinoma with very little expectation of spontaneous regression, indicating that these intraepithelial lesions had already acquired malignant properties.

Because these results were strictly dependent on the histologic criteria we used in the study, direct comparisons with other studies are regrettably difficult.

Green and Donovan (1970) reported that only 0.17% of CIS lesions became invasive. However, they conducted cone biopsy in the subjects and it seems that the target lesions were dissected in the biopsy. Kinlen and Spriggs (1978) reported that when patients with positive cytology had been followed up with neither biopsy nor treatment, 19% of them developed invasive carcinoma while 36.6% became negative cytologically.

The reported rate of progression of CIS to invasive carcinoma varies from the aforementioned 0.17% to 80.4%, probably reflecting the differences in the accuracy of the initial diagnosis, the follow-up methods, and so on.

Because there is not yet any means of identifying CIN with the potential for progression, it is clinically mandatory that all patients with CIN be treated on the assumption that the lesions have the potential to invade, even though some of them may regress. This consistent approach should be taken in respect of all CIN cases, whether the risk of progression is 5% or 40%.

Another factor of importance for a screening program and patient management is the duration of the preinvasive phase. A cytologic follow-up study by RICHART and BARRON (1969) and an epidemiologic study by FIDLER et al. (1968) showed that it may take at least 10 years for CIN III to develop into invasive carcinoma. Using statistical analysis, BARRON et al. suggested in 1978 that the CIS phase may last 3–10 years. We observed that approximately 9 years had passed before a severe dysplasia lesion progressed into invasive carcinoma. These findings are further supported by many reports that patients with CIN III are on average about 10 years younger than those with invasive carcinoma.

Exceptionally it has been reported that a young woman with negative cytology suddenly developed an invasive cancer (BERKELEY et al. 1980; PRENDIVILLE et al. 1980). With a small number of exceptions, however, it is reasonable to consider that CIN may need at least 10 years to develop into invasive carcinoma. Great differences in the natural history between patients are probably related to how the CIN lesion behaves and exists in the host individual.

On the basis of the results of studies of the natural history of cervical cancer, it should again be emphasized that milder CIN lesions have a high potential to regress, partly because some of them inevitably include reactive proliferation, while severe CIN lesions, when untreated, develop into invasive carcinoma at a significantly high rate. In addition, invasive carcinoma goes through a phase of CIN before demonstrating its invasion. These results form the basis for a cancer control program aimed at drastically reducing the mortality and morbidity of cervical cancer by discovering CIN lesions at the preinvasive stage by means of cytology and treating them.

## 1.4 Histology

Histologic features of CIN were mentioned in the preceding section. In CIN lesions, various degrees of atypical cells occupy the space within the epithelium. Atypical cells are identified on the basis of microscopic findings, including differentiation such as impaired maturation and stratification, nuclear abnormalities such as hyperchromasia and a coarse chromatin pattern, an increase in the nuclear cytoplasmic ratio, nuclear pleomorphism, and anisonucleosis (BUCKLEY et al. 1982). In CIN I, mild cellular and nuclear atypia and abnormalities of cytoplasmic differentiation are observed, although stratification is generally maintained. Hyperchromasia and a coarse chromatin pattern in larger nuclei are also noted but are limited to the lower third of the epithelium. Superficial cells have a normal degree of cytoplasm. Differential diagnosis from benign lesions such as immature metaplasia, reactive changes to inflammation, and tissue repair is important but actually quite difficult in many cases.

Basically, CIN II is similar to CIN I except that cells having pleomorphic nuclei occupy about two-thirds of the epithelium, are variously differentiated, and retain stratification. Mitoses are often observed.

In one type of CIN III, depolarized immature basal type cells with a high nuclear-cytoplasmic ratio replace the entire layer of the epithelium. Cell nuclei show most conspicuous pleomorphism and hyperchromasia. This type is called small cell type undifferentiated CIS, and is often found in the endocervix. Another type of CIN III is large cell keratinizing type CIS, which has large cells with a clear cell border and intensive parakeratosis in the superficial layer; cell polarity and stratification are lacking. Mitoses or abnormal mitoses may be found through the full thickness. The third type of CIN III is called severe dysplasia; the nuclear–cytoplasmic ratio is relatively low and stratification is lacking in spite of polarity being slightly maintained. This type is often located in the mid transformation zone. As indications of the cancerous nature of the epithelium, lateral invasion and mesenchymolysis should receive special attention. The existence of many abnormal mitoses is significant because it demonstrates an aneuploid DNA pattern.

## 1.5 Cytology

In dysplasia, cytology reveals the appearance of dyskaryotic cells (DCs), which have normally differentiated cytoplasm containing enlarged hyperchromatic nuclei. The nucleus of a dyskaryotic cell is large and hyperchromatic. The chromatin pattern is irregular in the sense that it shows a granular condensation of chromatin but the arrangement of condensed chromatin is usually uniform. The nucleus is round or oval and the nuclear outline can be smooth or finely wrinkled. Based on the morphology and characteristics of the cytoplasm, these cells are divided into superficial, intermediate, and parabasal types. Each type is additionally classified into mild and severe according to the degree of nuclear atypia. Mild and severe DCs are observed in mild and severe dysplasia, respectively. The former often consists of superficial DCs, while severe DCs in accordance with the maturation of the tissue pattern appear in the latter. Although it is impossible to read the biologic behavior of the epithelium by analyzing the cell patterns, close cytologic observation reveals that the proportion of parabasal type DCs in relation to the total number of DCs in preparations is certainly increased as the CIN grade increases.

Cytologic features of small cell type undifferentiated CIS—in which there is a high density of hyperchromatic nuclei occupying the full thickness of the epithelium, cell differentiation is poor, and stratification and polarity are absent—are as follows: Cells have round enlarged hyperchromatic nuclei with an extremely high nuclear-cytoplasmic ratio. Cytoplasm is cyanophilic and cell borders are unclear. These cells are uniform and lack pleomorphism and diversity of intranuclear structures.

In the tissue of invasive carcinoma, malignant cells appear in the superficial, middle, and deep layers of the epithelium. These cells are characterized by their diversity, i.e., the appearance of bizarre cells such as tadpole and fiber types. Tumor diathesis is noted in the background.

When a cytologic technique is used for the diagnosis of cervical neoplasia, fairly accurate differential diagnosis of dysplasia, CIS, and invasive carcinoma is possible through close observation of dyskaryotic or malignant cells in the whole preparations and degrees of cellular differentiation and atypia. However, the diagnostic accuracy of cytology depends on not only microscopic criteria but also technique and methods of cell sampling, fixation, and staining. Skills of cytoscreeners are also relevant.

Recently, a working group in the National Cancer Institute (NCI) has proposed a new cytologic classification named the "Bethesda System" (1988)

**Table 1.** The Bethesda system for reporting cervical/vaginal cytologic diagnosis (1988)

I STATEMENT ON SPECIMEN ADEQUACY
II GENERAL CATEGORIZATION
III DESCRIPTIVE DIAGNOSES
- (1) INFECTION
- (2) REACTIVE AND REPARATIVE CHANGES
- (3) EPITHELIAL CELL ABNORMALITIES

*Squamous Cells*
- Atypical squamous cells of undetermined significance (recommended follow-up and/or type of further investigation):
- Squamous intraepithelial lesion (SIL)
  [comment on presence of cellular changes associated with HPV if applicable]
- Low-grade squamous intraepithelial lesion, encompassing:
  - (1) Cellular changes associated with HPV
  - (2) Mid (slight) dysplasia/cervical intraepithelial neoplasia grade 1 (CIN 1)
- High-grade squamous intraepithelial lesion, encompassing:
  - (1) Moderate dysplasia/CIN 2
  - (2) Severe dysplasia/CIN 3
  - (3) Carcinoma in situ/CIN 3
- Squamous cell carcinoma

*Glandular cells*
- Presence of endometrial cells in one of the following circumstances:
  - Out-of-phase in a menstruating woman
  - In a postmenopausal woman
  - No menstrual history available
- A typical glandular cells of undetermined significance (recommended follow-up and/or type of further investigation)
  - Endometrial
  - Endocervical
  - Not otherwise specified
- Adenocarcinoma
  - Specify probable site of origin: endocervical, endometrial, extrauterine
  - Not otherwise specified
- Other epithelial malignant neoplasm

(4) NONEPITHELIAL MALIGNANT NEOPLASM
(5) OTHERS

and a corresponding report form at based on comprehensive discussions on a cytopathologic approach. The report format consists of the following three elements: (a) a statement on the adequacy of the specimen for diagnostic evaluation, (b) a general categorization of the diagnosis, and (c) the descriptive diagnosis. The third element is further divided into (a) infection, (b) reactive and reparative changes, (c) epithelial cell abnormalities, (d) nonepithelial malignant neoplasm, and (e) others. Of these, epithelial cell abnormalities are listed in Table 1.

The Bethesda System limits use of the term "atypical cells" to those cases in which the cytologic findings are undetermined significance. "Atypia" should not be used as a diagnosis for otherwise defined inflammatory, preneoplastic, or neoplastic cellular changes. To assist the referring physician, a report in which cells are described as "atypical" should include a recommendation for further evaluation that may help to determine the significance of the atypical cells.

The only new diagnostic terms in the Bethesda System are low-grade squamous intraepithelial lesion (SIL) and high-grade SIL. They encompass the spectrum of terms currently used for squamous cell precursors to invasive squamous cell carnicoma, including the grades of CIN, the degrees of dysplasia, and CIS.

While low-grade SIL and high-grade SIL are preferred, use of these new terms does not preclude the addition of the degree of "dysplasia" or grade of "CIN" by cytopathologists who wish to retain these designations. Examples are "low-grade squamous intraepithelial lesion: cellular changes associated with human papillomavirus," "low-grade squamous intraepithelial lesion: mild dysplasia and cellular changes associated with human papillomavirus," and "high-grade squamous intraepithelial lesion: cervical intraepithelial neoplasia, grade 3 (CIN 3)."

The statement "cellular changes associated with human papillomavirus" is added to the report of either low-grade SIL or high-grade SIL when appropriate. "Cellular changes associated with human papillomavirus" (without features of "dysplasia" or "CIN") may be used as a separate diagnostic phrase, although it is recommended that it be included under the designation low-grade SIL. Terms such as koilocytic atypia, keratinizing atypia, and dyskaryosis are not included in the Bethesda system.

## 2 Microinvasive Carcinoma of the Cervix

### 2.1 Terminology and Definition

A neoplastic process starting in the epithelium of the uterine cervix invades through the basement membrane into the stroma with destructive growth to end up as a frank invasive cancer. In this process of invasion, a small lesion which has just started invasion is called microinvasive carcinoma. The definition of microinvasive carcinoma has been ambiguous and controversial for a long time and there is still no clear international agreement on its terminology. Usually, a small invasive lesion grows very slowly over a relatively long period with no visible clinical signs until it finally develops into invasive carcinoma. It has a relatively good prognosis, being a peculiar type of cervical cancer for gynecologists.

Invasive carcinoma located within the uterine cervix is clinically classified as stage I [International Federation of Gynecology and Obstetrics, (FIGO)]. Since a stage I lesion at a quite early stage has an extremely good prognosis and is subjected to various treatments depending on the institution, the early stage of stage I should be separately discussed and compared in terms of clinical results. Thus, stage I carcinoma is subclassified into Ia and Ib.

Subclassification of stage I invasive carcinoma was adopted by FIGO in 1961 for the first time, when Ia was defined as early stromal invasion. In 1970, FIGO revised the definition, classifying stage Ia as cancer which cannot be diagnosed by clinical examination, encompassing (a) early stromal invasion and (b) occult cancer. With another change in 1973,Ia was redefined as microinvasive carcinoma (early stromal invasion).

Within these frequent changes in the definition of stage Ia by FIGO, one can recognize two different concepts; one is "preclinical carcinoma" that cannot be detected by routine clinical examinations and the other, "early stromal invasion" that is histopathologically determined. In spite of the fact that these terms are sometimes used in confusion, they belong to different orders when used as diagnostic criteria.

A very important role of clinical stage classification is to make possible the accurate comparison of clinical results between different institutions. For this purpose, the classification needs to be simple and well defined, as well as universal. In addition, the classified materials have to have a certain uniformity. The definition of "preclinical carcinoma" does not meet these requirements.

In particular, precise diagnostic criteria are essential in order to confine stage Ia to the cancer stage in which a high rate of cure can be achieved even with relatively conservative treatments, rather than radical ones. This seems to be the reason why the FIGO classification has always referred to histopathologic criteria (early stromal invasion) in its revisions. However, "early stromal invasion" also has several problems as the criterion of stage Ia. First, the histology of early stromal invasion is undefined. For the sake of universality, it has to be clarified what degree of cancerous invasion should be included in this category, i.e., how to confirm the invasion, what differentiates the lesion from CIS, and how to define the border between stage Ia and Ib. Some investigators recommend using the depth of invasion in order to achieve a universal criterion. However, what depth should be adopted is another controversial point; some argue 5 mm (Mestwerdt 1958) and others 3 mm (Moore 1961).

In measuring the depth of invasion, results may be greatly affected by the fixation methods, the preparation technique, the baseline of measurement, the way of determining a leading point of invasion, and so forth. In addition, the thickness of the cervical wall varies for each individual. In the elderly, a depth of 5 mm may be more than half the total thickness of the cervical wall. Some argue that such interpersonal differences should be considered in determining the depth of invasion (KURIHARA 1975). Even with the same depth of invasion, cancerous lesions can take many different invading forms. Some may show quite similar invading patterns to advanced cancer though they are shallow in depth. Therefore, strong opposition is also presented against defining stage Ia lesions by measuring the depth of invasion (NODA 1975; YAMABE 1974).

In 1978, the Cancer Committee of the Japan Society of Obstetrics and Gynecology (JSOG) defined stage Ia as epidermoid carcinoma (squamous cell carcinoma) with histologically confirmed stromal invasion to a depth of 3 mm or less, measured from the basement membrane of the overlying surface layer. Even in cases with the deepest focus of invasion at 3 mm or less, those with confluent invasion or vessel permeation are excluded from stage Ia and considered as stage Ib (NODA et al. 1979). This definition has been in use in Japan since 1 January 1979.

In 1985, FIGO again changed the definition of stage Ia, including measurements for the first time (FIGO Cancer Committee 1986). The new definition states that stage Ia comprises preclinical carcinomas of cervix, that is, those diagnosed only by microscopy. Stage Ia is divided into two groups: stage Ia1, minimal microscopically evident stromal invasion, and stage Ia2, lesions detected microscopically that can be measured. The upper limit of the measurement should not show a depth of invasion greater than 5 mm taken from the base of the epithelium, either surface or glandular, from which it originates, and a second dimension, the horizontal spread, must not exceed 7 mm. Larger lesions should be staged as Ib. Vascular space involvement, either venous or lymphathic, should not alter the staging.

## 2.2 Histology

### *2.2.1 Growth Pattern*

A carcinomatous lesion which has just started growing from within the epithelium into the stroma is detected as small bud- or finger-like invasion, which corresponds to early stromal invasion (HAMPERL 1959) or "*tropfige Infiltration*" (FETTIG 1964). Usually, it starts as a bud or pinpoint invasion from an intraepithelial lesion with simple replacement or gland involvement. In some cases, migration may be the first form of discontinuous invasion.

In the invading part, differentiation of epithelium is usually observed. Compared with the area of CIN, cytoplasm is more eosinophilic and enlarged, containing a clear nucleus (LOHE 1978; BURGHARDT 1982). Edema and lymphocyte infiltration are often noted in the invaded stromal tissue. These findings support the diagnosis of early stromal invasion. Accelerated by breakdown of host defense mechanisms, this early stromal invasion may further expand and fuse in a pattern of confluent invasion ("*netzige Infiltration*"), developing into advanced cancer.

BOYES et al. (1970) first promoted the idea that confluent masses of cancer cells were more likely to be associated with metastatic spread. A confluent pattern is related to the tumor size, being more conspicuous with larger tumors. According to ROCHE and NORRIS (1975), a confluent growth pattern is independent of vessel permeation and has little significance in cases of cancer with a depth of 5 mm or less.

The value of recognizing microinvasive carcinoma (stage Ia) lies in defining a category of invasive cancer with a negligible risk of metastasis. BENSON and NORRIS (1977) reported that metastasis was detected in dissected lymph nodes at a frequency of less than 1%.

### *2.2.2 Vessel Permeation*

Lymph vessel permeation by tumor cells is considered to be associated with a higher frequency of lymph node metastasis and a poor prognosis. However, the relation between vessel permeation and lymph node metastasis is more complex. ROCHE and NORRIS (1975) examined 30 cases of microinvasive cancer 2–5 mm in depth from the surface epithelium in step-sections and found cancerous involvement in capillary-like spaces in 57% of them. However, radical hysterectomy and lymph node dissection in these patients failed to reveal lymph node metastasis in any of them. They concluded that vessel permeation by cancer cells does not increase the risk of lymph node metastasis. Contrary to this, BURGHARDT (1982), HOLZER (1982), and KOLSTAD et al. (1982) have argued that lymphatic channel involvement significantly increases the risk of metastasis. The difference in clinical results seems to be caused by a discrepancy in the diagnostic criterion of lymphatic channel involvement. Only endothelium-lined spaces around cancer nests should be considered. Care should be taken not to confuse lymphatic channels with spaces produced by surrounding tissue shrinkage in the preparation process.

### *2.2.3 Tumor Dimensions*

Generally, if the tumor invades deep into the tissue, radical treatment is selected because of the poor prognosis. As for microinvasive cancer which allows conservative treatment, there has been no agreement for a long time on how to define the maximum depth of invasion. As mentioned above, the JSOG (1978) determined it to be 3 mm while FIGO (1985) defined microinvasion in two dimensions, namely a depth no greater than 5 mm and horizontal spread no greater than 7 mm.

It has already been pointed out that the definition of stage Ia (microinvasive carcinoma) proposed by the JSOG in 1978 stipulates a depth of invasion of 3 mm or less from the surface basement membrane and excludes lesions with vessel permeation, evident confluent type invasions, and adenocarcinoma. The definition proposed by FIGO in 1985, on the other hand, classifies microinvasion further into Ia1 and Ia2 by measuring the invasion depth (5 mm or less) and horizontal spread (7 mm or less), paying no regard to the presence of vessel permeation, adenocarcinoma, and other histologic features. This definition seems to be based on the volume concept proposed by Austrian and German investigators (BURGHARDT and HOLZER 1977; LOHE 1978). However, FIGO did not give any reason or provide data to explain why the above-mentioned measurements were chosen. The upper limits of stage Ia2 are clear; however, the border between Ia1 and Ia2 is not at all clear. In its notes to the staging, FIGO stated that "stage Ia should be divided into those lesions with minute foci of invasion visible only microscopically as stage Ia1, and the macroscopically measurable microcarcinomas as stage Ia2." Stage Ia1 is defined as "minimal microscopically evident stromal invasion." This is a vague as "early stromal invasion!" In 1974, the Society of Gynecologic Oncologists (SGO) proposed that microinvasive carcinoma be defined as a lesion that invades the cervical stroma to a depth of 3.0 mm or less below the base of the epithelium and in which there is no evidence of lymphovascular space invasion. This is probably the most widely accepted definition of stage Ia. Several papers have claimed that patients who satisfy the SGO definition may be safely treated by simple hysterectomy (CREASMAN et al. 1985; VAN NAGELL et al. 1983; SIMON et al. 1986).

In Japan, the JSOG definition has been used since 1979. This definition is similar to that of the SGO except that the former excludes cases with a confluent pattern, as stated above. The main aim of the JSOG definition was to exclude from stage Ia those cases of invasive cervical cancer with a possibility of lymph node metastasis. When this definition was proposed in 1978, 164 hospitals in Japan, which were registered with the Uterine Cancer Registry Committee of the JSOG, were asked to report any cases of cervical cancer with stromal invasion of 5 mm or less that had lymph node metastasis and/or recurred after treatment (TAKI 1979). One hundred and three institutions replied; 22 replied that they had experienced such a case, while 81 replied that they had not. Sixteen of the aforementioned 22 institutions sent appropriate slides to the Committee for review. A total of 40 cases were accessioned. Of the 40 cases, 23 had pelvic lymph node metastases at initial surgery and 17 cases recurred after treatment.

The proposed JSOG Ia definition was applied to these 40 cases. Three were excluded because they were adenocarcinoma. Fourteen cases had stromal invasion greater than 3 mm and 12 cases with stromal invasion of 3 mm or less had lymphatic permeation and/or confluent invasion. These 26 cases were excluded. The remaining 11 cases satisfied the JSOG definition of stage Ia and none of them had lymph node metastasis. They were all cases of vaginal stump recurrence, mainly of carcinoma in situ.

TSUKAMOTO et al. (1989) reported that the depth of stromal invasion is clearly correlated with the horizontal spread of the lesion, suggesting that the depth measurement is sufficient to indicate the tumor volume.

The results in our hospital are as follows. A total of 766 patients with stage I cervical cancer breaks down into 418 with Ia and 348 with Ib using the JSOG definition, and 468 with Ia1, 30 with Ia2, and 268 with Ib using the 1985 FIGO definition. The 468 patients with FIGO: Ia1 include 49 with cancer invasion of confluent pattern and one with vessel permeation. The 30 patients with FIGO Ia2 include 13 with confluent invasion and five with vessel permeation (IKEDA et al. 1988).

Cervical cancer of stage Ia according to the new FIGO classification is not, as such, an indication for conservative therapy. Although Ia1 may be an indication, the ill-defined borderline between Ia1 and Ia2 gives rise to problems. In order to use the diagnosis of microinvasive cancer as a yardstick for the safe application of conservative therapy, the depth of invasion, vessel permeation, and confluent growth pattern should be included in the definition. If stage Ia1 is defined according to the FIGO classification as cancer invasion of 3 mm or less in depth, excluding lesions with vessel permeation and/or a confluent growth pattern, there is no problem with conservative therapy for Ia1 lesions.

## References


Abdul-Karim FW, Fu YS, Reagan JW, Wentz WB (1982) Morphometric study of intraepithelial neoplasia of uterine cervix. Obstet Gynecol 60:210–214

Adelusi B, Osunkoya BO, Fabiyi A (1975) Antibodies to herpesvirus type 2 in carcinoma of the cervix uteri in Ibadan, Nigeria. Am J Obstet Gynecol 123:758–761

Anderson MC (1982) Difficulties in colposcopic and histological interpretation. In: Anderson MC (ed) Proceedings of the fourth world congress for cervical pathology and colposcopy. Churchhill Livingstone, London

Anderson MC (1987) Obstetrical and gynecological pathology. Churchill Livingstone, London

Barron BA, Cahill MC, Richart RM (1978) A statistical model of the natural history of cervical neoplastic disease. The duration of carcinoma in situ. Gynecol Oncol 6:196–205

Bellina JH, Dunlop WP, Riopelle MA (1982) Reliability of histopathologic diagnosis of cervical intraepithelial neoplasia. South Med J 75:6–8

Benson WL, Norris HJ (1977) A critical review of the frequency of lymph node metastases and death from microinvasive carcinoma of the cervix. Obstet Gynecol 49:632–638

Berkeley AS, LiVolsi VA, Schwartz PE (1980) Advanced squamous cell carcinoma of the cervix with recent normal Papanicolaou tests. Lancet II:375–376

Bibbo M, Dytch HE, Alenhhat E, Bartels PH, Wied G (1989) DNA ploidy profiles as prognostic indicators in CIN lesions. Am J Clin Pathol 92:261–265

Boyes DA, Worth JA, Fidler HK (1970) The results of treatment of 4389 cases of preclinical cervical squamous carcinoma. J Obstet Gynaecol Br Commonw 77:769–780

Buckley CH, Butler EB, Fox H (1982) Cervical intraepithelial neoplasia. J Clin Pathol 35:1–13

Burghardt E (1973) Early histological diagnosis of cervical cancer. Friedman EA (ed) Major problems in obstetrics and gynecology, vol 6. Saunders, Philadelphia

Burghardt E (1982) Diagnostic and prognostic criteria in cervical microcarcinoma. Clin Oncol 1:323–333

Burghardt E, Holzer E (1977) Diagnosis and treatment of microinvasive carcinoma of the cervix uteri. Obstet Gynecol 49:641–653
Cocker J, Fox H, Langley FA (1968) Consistency in the histological diagnosis of epithelial abnormalities of the cervix uteri. J Clin Pathol 21:67–70
Cocks PS, Peel KR, Cartwright RA, Adib R (1980) Carcinoma of the penis and cervix (letter). Lancet II:855–856
Colgan TJ, Percy ME, Suri M, Shier RM, Andrews DR, Lickrish GM (1989) Human papillomavirus infection of morphologically normal cervical epithelium adjacent to squamous dysplasia and invasive carcinoma. Hum Pathol 20:316–319
Coppleson M, Reid B (1967) Preclinical carcinoma of the cervix uteri. Pergamon, Oxford
Creasman WT, Fetter BF, Clarke-Pearson DL et al. (1985) Management of stage IA carcinoma of the cervix. Am J Obstet Gynecol 153:164–172
Fettig O (1964) Zur morphologischen und klinischen Problematik des Makrocarzinoms (Kollum Carzinom Stadium Ia). Arch Gynäkologie 199:571–608
Fidler HK, Boyes DA, Worth AJ (1968) Cervical cancer detection in British Columbia. J Obstet Gynaecol Br Commonw 75:392–404
FIGO Cancer Committee (1986) Staging announcement. Gynecol Oncol 25:383–385
Fox CH (1967) Biologic behaviour of dysplasia and carcinoma in situ. Am J Obstet Gynecol 99:960–974
Fu YS, Regan JW, Richart RM (1981) Definition of procursors. Gynecol Oncol 12:S220–S223
Galloway DA, McDougall JK (1985) The oncogenic potential of herpes simplex viruses: evidence for a 'hit-and-run' mechanism. Nature 302:21–24
Galvin GA, Jones HW, TeLinde RW (1955) The significance of basal cell hyperactivity in cervical biopsies. Am J Obstet Gynecol 70:808–821
Graham S, Priore R, Graham M, Browne R, Burnett W, West D (1979) Genital cancer in wives of penile cancer patients. Cancer 44:1870–1874
Green GH, Donovan JW (1970) The natural history of cervical carcinoma in situ. J Obstet Gynaecol Br Commonw 77:1–9
Hall JE, Walton L (1968) Dysplasia of the cervix: a prospective study of 206 cases. Am J Obstet Gynecol 100:662–671
Hamperl H (1959) Definition and classification of the so-called carcinoma in situ. Symposion Ciba Foundation study group No.3, "cancer of the cervix", S.2. Churchill, London.
Harris RWC, Brinton LA, Cowdell RH et al. (1980) Characteristics of women with dysplasia or carcinoma in situ of the cervix uteri. Br J Cancer 42:359–369
Herrero R, Brinton LA, Reeves WC et al. (1990) Sexual behavior, venereal diseases, hygiene practice, and invasive cervical cancer in a high-risk population. Cancer 65:380–386
Holzer E (1982) Microinvasive carcinoma of the cervix: clinical aspects, treatment and follow-up. Clin Oncol 1:315–322
Ikeda M, Inoue T, Noda K (1988) On the new FIGO classification of the stage Ia of uterine cervix (in Japanese). Obstet Gynecol 55:1647–1651
International Committee on Histological Definition (1961) Acta Cytol 6:235–236
Ismail SM, Colclough AB, Dinnen JKS et al. (1989) Observer variation in histopathological diagnosis and grading of cervical intraepithelial neoplasia. Br Med J 298:707–710
Iwasaka T, Yokoyama M, Hayashi Y et al. (1988) Combined herpes simplex virus type 2 and human pap. virus 16 or 18 leads to oncogenic transformation. Am J Obstet Gynecol 159:1251–1255
Johnson LD, Nickerson RJ, Easterday CL, Stuart RS, Hertig AT (1968) Epidemiological evidence for the spectrum of change from dysplasia through carcinoma in situ to invasive cancer. Cancer 22:901–914
Jordan JA, Sharp F, Singer A (eds) (1982) Proceedings of the Ninth Study Group of the Royal College of Obstetricians and Gynaecologists. Royal College of Obstetricians and Gynaecologists, London, pp 299–300
Josey WE, Nahmias AJ, Naib ZM (1972) The epidemiology of type 2 (genital) herpes simplex virus infection. Obstet Gynecol Surv 27:295–302
Kinlen LJ, Spriggs AI (1978) Women with positive cervical smears but without surgical intervention. Lancet II:463–465
Kirkland JA, Stanley MA, Cellier KM (1967) Comparative study of histologic and chromosomal abnormalities in cervical neoplasia. Cancer 20:1934–1952
Kolstad P, Abeler V, Iversen T, Kjorstad K (1982) Microinvasive carcinoma of the cervix: definition and treatment problems. Clin Oncol 1:335–347

Kurihara S (1975) On the stage Ia cancer of the uterine cervix (in Japanese). World Obstet Gynecol 27:707–712
Lohe KJ (1978) Early squamous cell carcinoma of the uterine cervix. 1. Definition and histology. Gynecol Oncol 6:10–30
McKenna JM, Davis FE (1966) Induction of neoantigen (G) in human amnion ("WISH") cells by herpes virus A. Nature 212:1602–1603
Melnick JL, Adam E, Rawls WE (1974) The causative role of herpes virus type II in cervical cancer. Cancer 34:1375–1385
Mestwerdt G (1947) Die Frühdiagnose des Kollumkarzinoms, Zbl. Gynäkologie 69:198–203
Moore JG (1961) Management of early carcinoma. Am J Obstet Gynecol 85:1175–1182
Nahmias AJ, Naib AM, Highsmith AK, Josey WE (1967) Experimental genital herpes simplex infection in the mouse. Pediatr Res 1:209
Naib ZM, Nahmias AJ, Josey WE (1966) Cytology and histopathology of cervical herpes simplex infection. Cancer 19:1026–1031
Naib ZM, Nahmias AJ, Josey WE, Kramer JH (1969) Genital herpetic infection association with cervical dysplasia and carcinoma. Cancer 23:940–945
Nasiell K, Nasiell M, Vaclavinkova V (1983) Behavior of moderate cervical dysplasia during long-term follow-up. Obstet Gynecol 61:609–614
National Cancer Institute Workshop (1989) The Bethesda system for reporting cervical/vaginal cytologic diagnosis. Acta Cytol 33:567–574
Noda K (1975) Diagnosis and treatment of Ia cancer of the cervix (in Japanese). Obstet Gynecol Ther 30:268–272
Noda K (1979) Dysplasia of the cervix. Gynecology and obstetrics. Proceedings of the IX World Congress of Gynecology and Obstetrics. Excerpta Medica, Tokyo
Noda K, Yajima A, Higashiiwai H, Sato A, Teshima K (1976) Histopathologic criterion of dysplasia of the cervix and its biological nature. Acta Cytol 20:224–228
Noda K, Taki I, Takeuchi S et al. (1979) A new proposal regarding criteria for stage Ia cancer in the uterine cervix, Gynecol Oncol 8:353–369
Nuovo GJ, Cottral S, Richart RM (1989) Occult human papillomavirus infection of the uterine cervix in postmenopausal women. Am J Obstet Gynecol 160:340–344
Ory HW, Jenkins RJ, Byrd JY, Nahmias AJ, Tyler CW Jr, Allen DT, Conger SB (1975) The epidemiology and interrelationship of cervical dysplasia and type 2 herpesvirus in a low-income housing project. Am J Obstet Gynecol 123:269–274
Park IJ, Jones HW (1968) Glucose-6-phosphate dehydrogenase and the histogenesis of epidermoid carcinoma of the cervix. Am J Obstet Gynecol 102:106–109
Poulsen HE, Taylor CW, Sobin LH (1975) Histological typing of female genital tract tumors. International histological classification of tumors, No. 13. World Health Organization, Geneva
Prendiville W, Guillebaud J, Bamford P, Beilby J, Steel SJ (1980) Carcinoma of the cervix with recent normal Papanicolaou tests. Lancet II:835–854
Rawls WE, Laurel D, Melnick JL, Glicksman JM, Kaufman RH (1968) A search for viruses in smegma, premalignant and early malignant cervical tissues. The isolation of herpesviruses with distinct antigenic properties. Am J Epidemiol 87:647–655
Rawls WE, Tompkins WAF, Melnick JL (1969) The association of herpesvirus type 2 and carcinoma of the uterine cervix. Am J Epidemiol 89:547–554
Reagan JW, Hamonic MJ (1956) Dysplasia of the uterine cervix. Ann NY Acad Sci 63:1236–1244
Reagan JW, Seidemand IL, Saracusa Y (1953) The cellular morphology of carcinoma in situ and dysplasia or atypical hyperplasia of the uterine cervix. Cancer 6:224–235
Reid R, Fu YS, Herschman BR et al. (1984) Genital warts and cervical cancer. Am J Obstet Gynecol 150:189–199
Richart RM (1963) A radioautographic analysis of cellular proliferation in dysplasia and carcinoma in situ of the uterine cervix. Am J Obstet Gynecol 86:925–930
Richart RM (1967) Natural history of cervical intraepithelial neoplasia. Clin Obstet Gynecol 10:748–784
Richart RM (1976) Cervical intraepithelial neoplasia and the cervicologist. Can J Med Technol 38:177
Richart RM (1990) A modified terminology for cervical intraepithelial neoplasia. Obstet Gynecol 75:131–132

Richart RM, Barron BA (1969) A follow-up study of patients with cervical dysplasia. Am J Obstet Gynecol 105:386–393
Richart RM, Crum CP (1982) The role of infective agents in the genesis of cervical intraepithelial neoplasia. In: Anderson MC (ed) Proceedings of the fourth world congress for cervical pathology and colposcopy. Churchill Livingstone, London
Richart RM, Lerch V, Barron BA (1967) A time-lapse cinematographic study in vitro of mitoses in normal human cervical epithelium, dysplasia and carcinoma in situ. JNCI 39:571–577
Roche WD, Norris HJ (1975) Microinvasive carcinoma of the cervix. The significance of lymphatic invasion and confluent patterns of stromal growth. Cancer 36:180–186
Royston I, Aurelian L (1970) The association of genital herpesvirus with cervical atypia and carcinoma in situ. Am J Epidemiol 91:531–538
Shingleton HM, Richard RM, Wiener J, Spiro D (1968) Human cervical intraepithelial neoplasia: fine structure of dysplasia and carcinoma in situ. Cancer Res 28:695–706
Simon NL, Gore H, Shingleton HM, Soong SJ, Orr JW, Hatch KD (1986) Study of superficially invasive carcinoma of the cervix. Obstet Gynecol 68:19–24
Smith JW, Townsend DE, Sparkes RS (1971) Genetic variants of glucose-6-phosphate dehydrogenese in the study of carcinoma of the cervix. Cancer 28:529–532
Spriggs AI, Bowey CE, Cowdell H (1971) Chromosomes of precancerous lesions of the cervix uteri. Cancer 27:1239–1254
Taki I (1979) The report of the Cancer Committee of the Japan Society of Obstetrics and Gynecology (in Japanese). Acta Obstet Gynaecol Jpn 30:1755–1756
Tanaka S, Southam CM (1965) Joint action of herpes simplex virus and 3-methylcholanthrene in production of papillomas in mice. JNCI 34:441–451
Tsukamoto N, Kaku T, Matsukuma K, Matsuyama T, Kamura T, Saito T, Suenaga T (1989) The problem of stage Ia (FIGO 1985) carcinoma of the uterine cervix. Gynecol Oncol 34:1–6
van Nagell JR, Greenwell N, Powell DF, Donaldson ES, Hanson MB, Gay EC (1983) Microinvasive carcinoma of the cervix. Am J Obstet Gynecol 145:981–991
Wigle DT, Mao Y, Grace M (1980) Re: 'Smoking and cancer of the uterine cervix: hypothesis' (letter). Am J Epidemiol 111:125–127
Willbanks GD, Richart RM, Terner JY (1967) DNA content of cervical intraepithelial neoplasia studied by two-wave length Feulgen cytophotometry. Am J Obstet Gynecol 98:792–799
Willett GD, Kurman RJ, Reid R, Greenberg M, Jenson AB, Lorincz AT (1989) Correlation of the histologic appearance of intraepithelial neopolasia of the cervix with human papillomavirus types. Emphasis on low-grade lesions including so-called flat condyloma. Int J Gynecol Pathol 8:18–25
Winkelstein W (1986) Cigarette smoking and cancer of the uterine cervix. Banbury Report 23:329–341
Winkelstein W Jr (1977) Smoking and cancer of the uterine cervix: hypothesis. Am J Epidemiol 106:257–259
Woodworth CD, Bowden PE, Doniger J, Pirisi L, Barnes W, Lancaster WD, DiPaolo JA (1988) Characterization of normal human exocervical epithelial cells immortalized in vitro by papillomavirus types 16 and 18 DNA. Cancer Res 48:4620–4628
World Health Organization/International Agency for Research on Cancer (1986) Epidemiological studies of cancer in humans. In: IARC monograph on the evaluation of the carcinogenic risk of chemicals to humans: tobacco smoking. International Agency for Research on Cancer, Lyon, pp 199–308
Yajima H, Noda T, de Villiers EM, Yajima A, Yamamoto K, Noda K, Ito Y (1988) Isolation of a new type of human papillomavirus (HPV52b) with a transforming activity from cervical cancer tissue. Cancer Res 48:7164–7172
Yamabe T (1974) Histological criteria of Ia cancer of the cervix (in Japanese). Acta Obstet Gynaecol Jpn 26:641–644
Zur Hausen H (1982) Human genital cancer: synergism between two virus infections or synergism between a virus infection and an initiating agent. Lancet II:1370–1372

# Cervical Adenocarcinoma

R. KUDO



## 1 Introduction

Adenocarcinoma of the uterine cervix appears to be increasing in prevalence, and it currently accounts for about 10%–20% of invasive cervical cancers owing to the relative decrease in invasive squamous carcinoma resulting from detection and treatment of intraepithelial squamous neoplasia.

The detection and diagnosis of cervical adenocarcinoma, whose preinvasive lesions arise within the endocervical canal, are often more difficult than those of squamous carcinoma, because the location of the lesions impedes direct visualization and cytologic sampling, thus allowing relatively high false-negative rates. In addition, diagnostic problems arise in cases with very well differentiated morphologic features.

On the other hand, the epidemiology, histogenesis, natural history, histologic criteria of precancerous legions for cervical adenocarcinoma, and early stages of cervical adenocarcinoma have not been clearly elucidated compared with those of squamous carcinoma. The above aspects and the diagnostic pathology of cervical adenocarcinoma and other glandular carcinomas are discussed in this chapter.

Current Topics in Pathology
Volume 85, Ed. N. Sasano

## 2 Epidemiology

In recent reports, the relative incidence of cervical adenocarcinoma has been cited as 18.5% (SHINGLETON et al. 1981), 18.2% (BEREK et al. 1985), 17.5% (DUK et al. 1989), 18.3% (VESTERINEN et al. 1989), and 20% (GOODMAN et al. 1989). The incidences reported from the institutions of these authors are higher than the frequency of cervical adenocarcinoma observed at the author's institution, which was 88 of 1015 cases (8.7%) between 1966 and 1977, and 72 of 548 cases (13.1%) between 1978 and 1989. In the large population of Los Angeles County, adenocarcinomas made up 10.6% of all invasive carcinomas (PETERS et al. 1986).

The author has also estimated the worldwide incidence from the large number of cases which were reported in the series *Annual Report on the Results of Treatment in Gynecological Cancer* (KOTTMEIER et al. 1979, 1982; PETTERSSON et al. 1985, 1988). The reported incidence of cervical adenocarcinoma from institutions worldwide was 5.79% (1969–1972), 7.0% (1973–1975), 8.28% (1976–1978), and 8.83% (1979–1981) (Table 1).

These incidence ratios and the absolute numbers of cases suggest relative increase in the occurrence of cervical adenocarcinoma. Proportionally, the incidence in women under the age of 35 years increased more than twofold between 1973 and 1982, with an estimated annual increase of about 10% (SCHWARTZ and WEISS 1986).

As to the factors accounting for the increase, PETERS et al. (1986) hypothesized that oral contraceptives might have a carcinogenic effect on glandular cells of the cervix if given during periods of active metaplasia. A relationship between the long-term use of oral contraceptives and development of cervical adenocarcinoma has been reported by several authors (CZERNOBILSKY et al. 1974; BOUSFIELD et al. 1980; DALLENBACH-HELLWEG 1984), and BRINTON et al. (1987) found extended use of oral contraceptives to be a risk factor for all types of cervical carcinoma, especially adenocarcinoma. However, there is not yet evidence of a direct link between oral contraceptive use and cervical adenocarcinoma (VALENTE and HANJANI 1986). JONES and SILVERBERG (1989) have found

**Table 1.** Incidence of adenocarcinoma of the uterine cervix (based on *Annual Report on the Results of Treatment in Gynecological Cancer*, vols. 17–20)

| Year treated | Total No. of Cervical ca. | No. of adenocarcinomas | % | No. of institutions |
|---|---|---|---|---|
| 1969–72 | 24 712 | 1431 | 5.79 | 71 |
| 1973–75 | 19 623 | 1374 | 7.00 | 82 |
| 1976–78 | 20 944 | 1735 | 8.28 | 93 |
| 1979–81 | 23 804 | 2103 | 8.83 | 114 |
| Total | 89 083 | 6643 | 7.46 | |

no evidence of an etiologic relationship between either contraceptive usage or microglandular hyperplasia and cervical adenocarcinoma.

Recent epidemiologic studies also suggest a risk for long-term oral contraceptive users, but it is usually of borderline statistical significance and severely confounded by sexual factors. Despite the suggested association of some cases of adenocarcinoma in situ and invasive adenocarcinoma with oral contraceptive use in young women, one should be cautious in drawing conclusions from a limited population already preselected for closer surveillance of cervical smears than the general population. Further epidemiologic and experimental studies on the effect of long-term oral contraceptive use on endocervical epithelium are certainly warranted to determine whether oral contraceptives promote cervical adenocarcinoma either independently or synergistically with other carcinogenic factors.

In addition, TAKAHASHI et al. (1984) made a comparison of the prevalence of different types of cervical neoplasm in Japanese and New Zealand women. The frequency of adenocarcinoma in the two groups was not significantly different despite the much higher oral contraceptive usage in New Zealand. The incidence of adenosquamous carcinoma, however, was significantly higher in oral contraceptive users than in nonusers, and in New Zealand women as compared with Japanese women.

In other epidemiologic studies, HOROWITZ et al. (1988) found that patients with epidermoid carcinoma were frequently unemployed or earned a lower income than those with adenocarcinoma of the cervix. From these results, they suggested that patients with adenocarcinoma might be of a more affluent socioeconomic background.

Cigarette smoking increases the risk of developing cervical squamous cell carcinoma, but not adenocarcinoma. Women with adenosquamous carcinoma of the cervix appear to have some of the risk factors for squamous carcinoma, including a high number of sexual partners and low level of education (BRINTON et al. 1987).

There have been many reports in the recent literature about the role of human papillomavirus (HPV) infection in the development of cervical squamous carcinoma. Because the issue of HPV infection is discussed in detail in the chapter by T. OKAGAKI, I will not elaborate on this subject except for a few comments concerning cervical adenocarcinoma.

High positive rates of HPV infection in endocervical adenocarcinoma, as well as in squamous cell carcinoma, have been reported by TASE et al. (1988a, b, 1989) and LORINCZ et al. (1987). The detection rate of HPV 16 and HPV 18 in adenocarcinoma was 33% in each instance, and these percentages were similar to those in respect of squamous carcinoma for Washington, D.C. (LORINCZ et al. 1987). On the other hand, the positive rates of HPV 16 and HPV 18 were 2.5% and 40%, respectively, in Minnesota (TASE et al. 1988a). In addition, in Japan, HPV 18 DNA was detected in 5 of 11 cases (45%) of adenocarcinoma, one case of adenocarcinoma in situ, and two of three cases of adenosquamous carcinoma. In contrast, HPV 16 DNA was detected in 2 of 11 cases (18%) of adenocarcinoma and three of seven cases (43%) of squamous carcinoma (TASE et al. 1988b).

These results suggest that HPV 16 and HPV 18 have a high oncogenic association in endocervical adenocarcinoma. The differences in the frequency of the type of DNA sequences may be due to geographic factors. However, whether there is a special type of HPV with an affinity for the oncogenesis of endocervical adenocarcinoma needs to be studied further. It is considered that the oncogenic association of HPV type and lifestyle may also be an important factor in the development of cervical adenocarcinoma.

## 3 Histogenesis

TESHIMA et al. (1985), on the basis of histopathologic analyses and the localization of early stage adenocarcinoma, suggested that most adenocarcinomas of the uterine cervix originate from endocervical glands adjoining the transformation zone, and that they might develop directly from normal-appearing epithelium without passing through adenomatous or dysplastic changes. On the other hand, NODA et al. (1983) suggested that endocervical adenocarcinoma originates from the primary cleft, and that adenocarcinoma of the endometrioid type might arise in ectopic endometrial glands, based on their observations on the location of early-stage adenocarcinoma. However, the cellular origin of endocervical adenocarcinoma has not yet been clarified.

Endocervical adenocarcinoma has many unusual features. It has long been recognized as occurring in association with squamous neoplasia (CHRISTOPHERSON et al. 1979; MAIER and NORRIS 1980; SHINGLETON et al. 1981). These observations have been explained by the postulation of a common carcinogenic stimulus to the subcolumnar reserve cell, which is capable of differentiation to both squamous and glandular epithelium. Furthermore, the atypical reserve cell was suggested as having the role of a primitive stem cell with a capacity for squamous or columnar differentiation (BOON et al. 1981b).

The author has observed ultrastructural features of normal endocervical columnar epithelium, adenocarcinoma in situ, and microinvasive adenocarcinoma with a view to elucidating the cellular origin of cervical adenocarcinoma. In adenocarcinoma in situ and microinvasive adenocarcinoma, tonofibers and secretory granules are contained in the same cell. Reserve cells in the endocervical columnar epithelium contained both tonofilaments present as aggregates or small bundles and secretory granules. From these findings, it seems likely that most adenocarcinomas of the endocervical type originate from the reserve cell passing through glandular atypia.

As to the histogenesis of mixed cervical carcinoma, ALVA and LAUCHLAN (1975) reported the theory of reserve cell origin. This theory suggests that the derivatives of the reserve cell develop to form squamous dysplasia and carcinoma in situ, and, on the glandular side, progress to adenocarcinoma in situ. These epidermoid carcinomas in situ and adenocarcinomas in situ could develop to mixed forms.

A reserve cell origin is also postulated for adenoid cystic carcinoma and adenoid basal carcinoma of the uterine cervix. Because of their content basaloid, squamous, and glandular cells may share their origin with the pluripotent reserve cells (FERRY and SCULLY 1988). In addition, a myoepithelial origin has been suggested for adenoid cystic carcinoma at various sites. However, myoepithelium has not been identified in cervical adenoid cystic carcinoma (LAWRENCE and MAZUR 1982) and is consequently considered improbable as its histogenetic precursor.

## 4 Natural History

Because follow-up studies of patients with glandular dysplasia or adenocarcinoma in situ have not yet been performed, only a few retrospective observations concerning the natural history have been reported.

BOUSFIELD et al. (1980) presented their cases of microinvasive adenocarcinoma that had cytologic findings of adenocarcinoma in situ on smears taken

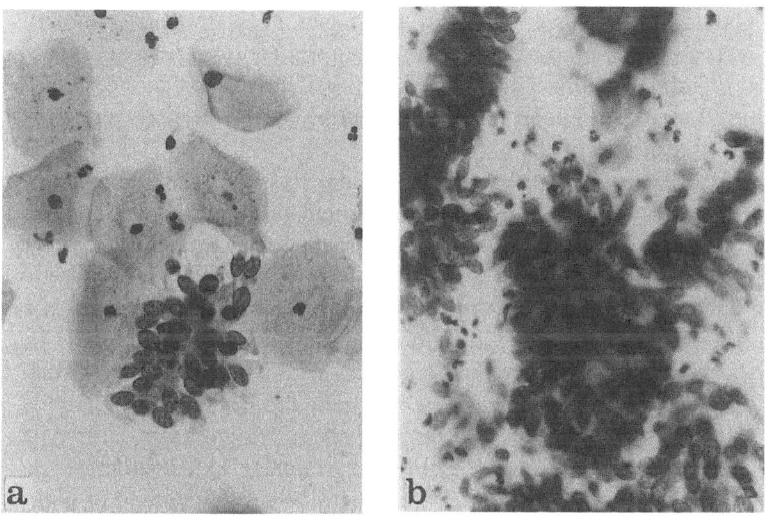


**Fig. 1. a** Cytologic features in a smear which was taken 4 years before the diagnosis of microinvasive adenocarcinoma. × 340. **b** Same patient as in **1a**: Cytologic features from which microinvasive adenocarcinoma was suspected. × 340

5–10 years previously. Boddington et al. (1976) also reported reviewed cases. In their six patients, a subsequent review showed that cells, with hindsight, could be called either clearly malignant or at least suspicious of adenocarcinoma. The interval during which the lesions were evidently present was 7–8 years.

In a review of 18 cervical biopsies which were performed 3–7 years prior to the detection of invasive cervical adenocarcinoma and which were originally reported as negative for malignancy, five were found to contain adenocarcinoma in situ (Boon et al. 1981a).

The author had a patient with adenocarcinoma in situ that showed cytologic findings suggestive of adenocarcinoma in situ for at least 4 years, and a case of microinvasive adenocarcinoma in which cytologic features continued to be suggestive of adenocarcinoma in situ for 4 years and then became suspicious for microinvasive adenocarcinoma (Fig. 1).

These studies may indicate that there is a latent period of several years before progression to invasive adenocarcinoma from adenocarcinoma in situ.

## 5 Glandular Dysplasia

Endocervical dysplasia was the name given to an atypical glandular lesion with less atypia than adenocarcinoma in situ (Bousfield et al. 1980). The existence of precancerous lesions for cervical adenocarcinoma is controversial, because there are no follow-up studies concerning glandular dysplasia. The histologic criteria for glandular dysplasia have not been generally defined, although Brown and Wells (1986) proposed histologic criteria of low-grade and high-grade cervical glandular atypia. This histologic classification was based mainly on the location of stratified nuclei in the epithelium, nuclear atypia, frequency of mitoses, and irregularity of the glands.

Gloor and Hurlimann (1986) brought glandular dysplasia and adenocarcinoma in situ together under the heading of cervical intraepithelial glandular neoplasia (CIGN) and, analogous to cervical intraepithelial squamous neoplasia, classified these lesions into grades I–III (CIGN I–III). In their histologic criteria for CIGN I, the nuclei are slightly hyperchromatic and arranged in a single row at the base of the cells, with a few mitoses being seen. In CIGN II, the nuclei are oval, hyperchromatic, and crowded, with some pseudostratification (two rows of nuclei). Mitoses are more frequent and intracellular mucin is diminished. CIGN III corresponds to classical adenocarcinoma in situ. It is often thicker than normal columnar epithelium, nuclear hyperchromasia is distinct, and the densely crowded nuclei are generally very elongated or cigar shaped. Nuclear pseudostratification is marked, as three or more rows of nuclei are counted. Mitoses are numerous, while intracellular mucin is scant or completely missing.

TASE et al. (1989) indicated that glandular dysplasia could not be classified as a precursor of adenocarcinoma of the uterine cervix because most cases of glandular dysplasia did not contain either HPV 16 or HPV 18 DNA, although these HPV DNAs were detected in other coexisting adenocarcinomas in situ, microinvasive adenocarcinomas, and squamous intraepithelial neoplasms of grade III at a high frequency.

Further investigation of the biologic behavior and histologic criteria of glandular dysplasia is needed in order to validate this terminology and grading system.

## 6 Early Cervical Adenocarcinoma

### 6.1 Adenocarcinoma In Situ

Adenocarcinoma in situ (AIS) of the cervix is an uncommon lesion that is most often discovered histologically concomitant with squamous abnormality or at the edge of an invasive adenocarcinoma. In a minority of cases, AIS is found alone. Ratios of AIS to squamous carcinoma in situ have been given as 1:26 (BOON et al. 1981a) and 1:104 (BROWN and WELLS 1986).

The diagnosis of AIS should be based on strict criteria supported by at least cervical conization rather than direct biopsy.

Some authors have found AIS to be a mostly multifocal lesion (GLOOR and RUZICKA 1982; BROWN and WELLS 1986), often located high in the endocervical canal (BROWN and WELLS 1986). But others (TESHIMA et al. 1985; ANDERSEN and ARFFMANN 1989) have found that AIS occurs in the transformation zone and that most cases are unifocal. In addition, there is controversy concerning curative conization in AIS. However, ANDERSEN and ARFFMANN (1989) have indicated that conization with uninvolved margins is a sufficient therapy in cases of AIS without associated early invasive lesions.

In terms of its microscopic features, AIS is confined to the surface, the underlying glands, or both. The abnormal epithelium grows within the preexisting glands, which retain the normal branching pattern. The glandular morphology is abnormal with complex folding, outpouching, and intraluminal papillary projections. Most commonly, the neoplastic epithelium consists of pseudostratified tall columnar cells. The lining epithelium shows an increased nuclear–cytoplasmic ratio, increased nuclear length, nuclear stratification, and frequent mitoses.

The cytoplasm usually shows reduced mucin production. A single gland shows as abrupt change to normal epithelium or features an intermediate zone of transitional cervical glandular atypia (Fig. 2a). AIS is usually divided into endocervical and endometrioid types. Negative cytoplasmic mucin staining is

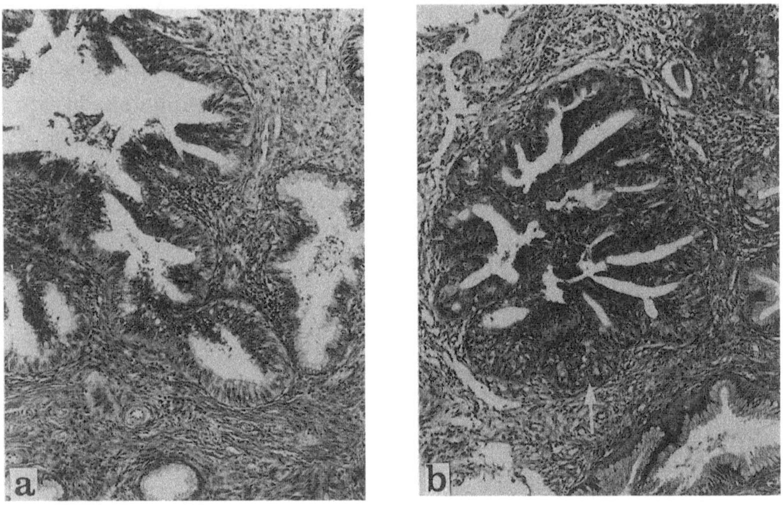


**Fig. 2 a, b.** Microscopic features of adenocarcinoma in situ and microinvasive adenocarcinoma. **a** adenocarcinoma in situ. × 85. **b** Microinvasive adenocarcinoma. The *white arrow* shows the budding region. × 85

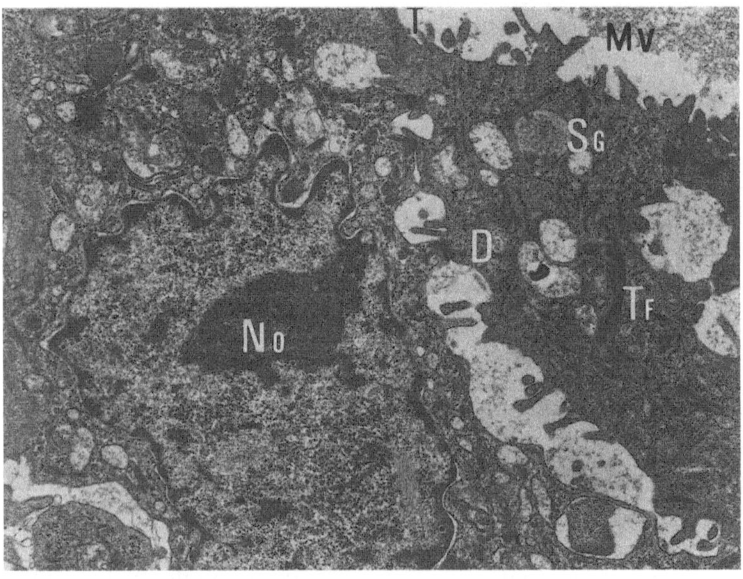


**Fig. 3.** Electron micrograph of adenocarcinoma in situ. *TF*, tonofibers; *SG*, secretory granules; *No*, nucleolus; *D*, desmosome; *T*, tight junction; *Mv*, microvilli. × 9200

required for definitive classification of endometrioid AIS. The ratios of these types differ from series to series.

GLOOR and RUZICKA (1982) have introduced two variant morphologies described as type I (columnar epithelial type), which is the one documented extensively in the literature, and the less common type II, with ballooned cells. The second type displays a conspicuous structural disorder with unequal and large, often clear, nuclei containing enlarged nucleoli.

In addition, JAWORSKI et al. (1988) have classified AIS into endocervical, endometrioid, intestinal, and miscellaneous types. They prefer to regard the endometrioid type of AIS as a manifestation of differentiation and mucus depletion.

Immunohistochemically, positive staining for carcinoembryonic antigen (CEA) in AIS has been mixed: 67% in a study by HURLIMANN and GLOOR (1984), but only 1 of 11 cases in a study by TOBON and DAVE (1988).

As regards ultrastructural features, the nuclei are elongated and occupy the basal half or two-thirds of the cell area. The cell membrane displays irregularly shaped microvilli. Cilia are not seen at any luminal side of these cells. A few

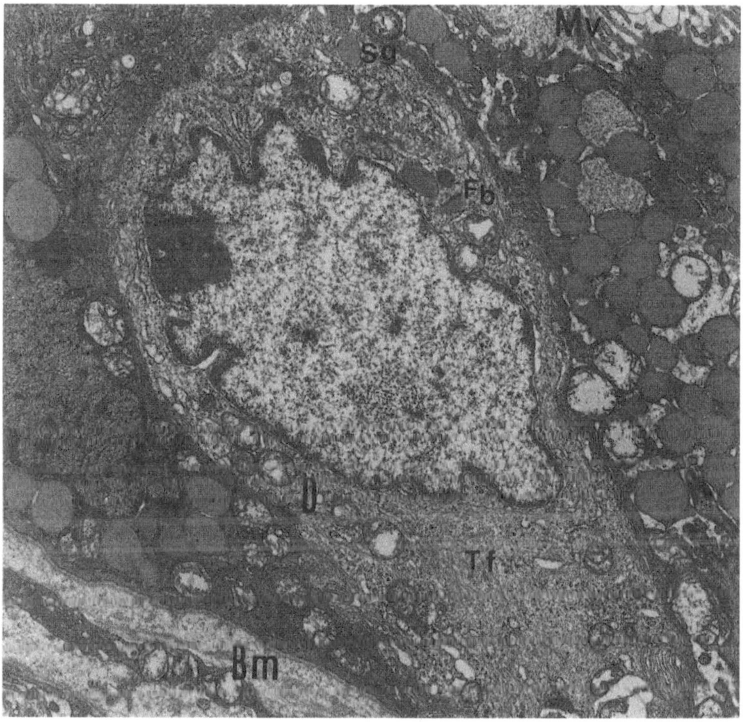


**Fig. 4.** Electron micrograph of reserve cell. *Sg*, secretory granules; *Fb*, fibrillar bodies; *Tf*, tonofilaments; *Mv*, Microvilli; *Bm*, basement membrane; *D*, desmosome. × 8500

secretory granules are distributed in the cytoplasm and the basement membrane is intact. A few cells of AIS contain tonofibers and a few secretory granules in the same cytoplasm. These cells are joined with neighboring cells by junctional complexes comprising tight junctions, zonulae adherens, and desmosomes (Fig. 3). The ultrastructural findings indicate that squamous and adenomatous features exist within the same cells. These findings are also observed in the reserve cells (Fig. 4); therefore, from these findings, it is considered that an origin of cervical adenocarcinoma is the reserve cells.

## 6.2 Microinvasive Adenocarcinoma

The definition and morphologic criteria of microinvasive adenocarcinoma (MIA) have not yet been clarified. TESHIMA et al. (1985) defined early adenocarcinoma as involving stromal invasion of 5 mm or less as measured from the mucosal surface. After hysterectomy, however, 1 of 30 patients with this early adenocarcinoma developed tumor recurrence. BUSCEMA and WOODRUFF (1984) reported a superficially invasive adenosquamous carcinoma that had widely metastasized.

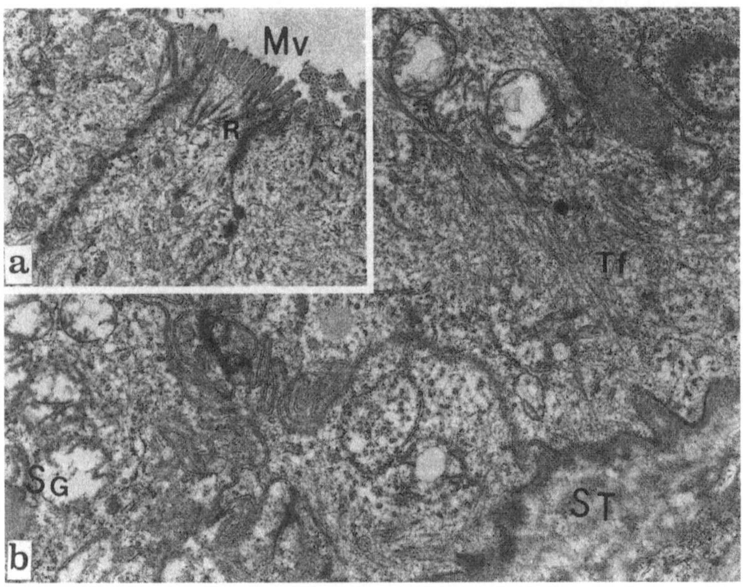


**Fig. 5 a, b.** Electron micrograph of microinvasive adenocarcinoma. **a** Luminal side. *Mv*, microvilli with core filaments; *R*, rootlets (cytoplasmic tonofilaments are continuous with internal filaments of luminal microvilli). × 8500. **b** Basal side. *ST*, stroma; *Tf*, tonofilaments; *SG*, secretory granules. × 10 300

In adopting morphologic criteria for MIA, the criteria should be useful for determining the method of treatment or be related to prognosis. From this point of view, it is considered that histologic criteria based only on depth of invasion are not sufficient as the morphologic criteria of MIA.

Fu and Reagan (1989) proposed the term of MIA for an early adenocarcinoma arising directly from AIS at the site of invasion, and in which the smooth configuration of the gland is distorted by one or a few tongue-like processes that are surrounded by desmoplastic stroma. The depth of invasion as measured from the point of invasion is less than 1 mm. None of the cases based on their definition have pelvic nodal metastases or recurrence after surgery.

Japan Society of Obstetrics and Gynecology, the Japanese Pathological Society, and Japan Radiological Society (1987) have defined the following criteria for MIA: "Adenocarcinoma is located within the normal endocervical gland area. At the site of invasion, budding is observed from a part of the adenocarcinoma in situ. The budding is observed as a smooth configuration." The micrograph of MIA in Fig. 2b is based on these histologic criteria.

The ultrastructural features of MIA include rounded nuclei with a convoluted outline. The cell membrane displays irregularly shaped microvilli from the free surface of the cells. Cells having microvilli with core filaments, rootlets, and secretory granules in the cytoplasm are observed. These ultrastructural features are characteristic findings in intestinal metaplastic cells. Such features have been observed by Shingleton et al. (1981) in invasive cervical adenocarcinoma.

Fine tonofilaments and secretory granules are distributed in some cells. The basement membrane is partially disrupted at the budding lesions, whereas the basement membrane is intact at an AIS lesion (Fig. 5). These findings indicate that MIA has the characteristic features of invasive adenocarcinoma.

## 7 Invasive Adenocarcinoma

The following criteria for the identification of primary adenocarcinoma were suggested by Maier and Norris (1980): (a) transition from normal endocervical glands identified in a specimen, (b) normal endometrium present in a curettage or hysterectomy specimen, (c) adenocarcinoma present in a cervical stump 5 or more years after removal of the corpus, and (d) gross tumor located on the cervix of a normal-sized uterus and absence of gross tumor in the endometrial cavity. The first criterion is appropriate for early endocervical adenocarcinoma but is not fulfilled by advanced cervical adenocarcinoma.

Many histologic classifications of cervical adenocarcinoma have been based on the cell type and the degree of differentiation of the growth pattern. In this chapter, histologic classification is mainly based on the cell type and the histologic grade.

## 7.1 Adenocarcinoma, Endocervical Type

In terms of microscopic features, endocervical adenocarcinoma is composed of cells that resemble endocervical columnar cells or, less frequently, intestinal cells.

The tumors are subdivided into three differentiated types. Tumors with a mostly glandular pattern and mild nuclear atypia are classified as well-differentiated adenocarcinoma. Those with a solid pattern and marked nuclear atypia are classified as poorly differentiated adenocarcinoma. Those with a combination of glandular and solid pattern and moderate nuclear atypia are classified as moderately differentiated adenocarcinoma.

Among the tumors with a predominantly glandular pattern, the glands are divided into small and closely packed groups in a back-to-back pattern with large, cystic spaces. In the mucinous tumors, the malignant tumor cells form abundant intra- and extracellular mucin. In the poorly differentiated tumors, the malignant cells form nests or solid sheets with few glandular spaces. In these cases, mucus staining is helpful in confirming their endocervical differentiation.

Because of the importance of detecting cells of cervical adenocarcinoma in the cervical smears, a brief cytologic description of these cells is appropriate. The characteristic cytologic features according to the degree of histologic differentiation can be summarized as follows (KUDO et al. 1987). The cells of well-differentiated adenocarcinoma are usually columnar in shape and there are exfoliated palisades, glandular rosettes, acinar, sheet-like arrangements showing a grape-like formation and forming irregularly shaped, overlapping clusters. In moderately differentiated adenocarcinoma, solitary cells with markedly atypical nuclei are combined with multilayered cell clusters. The cells from poorly differentiated adenocarcinoma are roundish, occurring as solitary cells or irregularly overlapping cell clusters, and show markedly atypical nuclei.

The authors of several recent studies have commented on the utility of immunohistochemical staining for the differential diagnosis of cervical adenocarcinoma. WAHLSTRÖM et al. (1979) first commented on the use of anti-CEA staining to distinguish between adenocarcinomas of endocervical and endometrial origin; over 80% of the former were positively stained, in contrast to only 8% of the latter. The high positive rates of immunohistochemical localization of CEA have been reported by several authors (COHEN et al. 1982; HURLIMANN and GLOOR 1984). However, numerous other studies have not noted any difference in CEA reactivity in endocervical and endometrial adenocarcinomas; these studies have been summarized most recently by MAES et al. (1988), who also found no difference between the two carcinomas regardless of whether polyclonal or monoclonal antibodies to CEA were used.

Using immunohistochemical staining, HURLIMANN and GLOOR (1984) performed a comparative study on the distribution of CEA, secretory component, fat globule membrane antigens (FGMAs), and keratin in cervical adenocarcinoma tissue. They found that 77% of invasive adenocarcinomas were positive for CEA, 47% for secretory component, 77% for FGMAs, and 89% for keratin. They noted no specific relationship between the reactivity with any of these markers and the differentiation of the tumors studied.

GRIFFIN et al. (1989) have presented immunohistochemical reactivity using a polyclonal antisalivary α-amylase antibody in normal cervical epithelium, cervical glandular atypia, adenocarcinoma in situ, and invasive adenocarcinoma. Immunoreactive amylase was detected in 39 of 40 cases of invasive cervical adenocarcinoma, six of seven cases of adenocarcinoma in situ, all six cases of high-grade cervical glandular atypia, 12 of 14 cases of low-grade cervical glandular atypia, and only 2 of 18 cases of normal secretory columnar epithelium. However, all 13 tubal metaplasias and all eight reserve cell hyperplasias in the cervix were positively stained. From their results, it is considered that this staining is not useful for differential diagnosis of cervical adenocarcinoma. In addition, GRIFFIN et al. suggested that high-grade cervical glandular atypia and adenocarcinoma in situ show the same pattern of reactivity as adenocarcinoma, in keeping with their proposed role as precursor lesions. They also pointed out that the finding that immunoreactive amylase is present in reserve cells is interesting in view of the hypothesis that adenocarcinoma may arise from reserve cells.

1C5 is a murine monoclonal antibody that has been produced with fused spleen cells obtained from mice immunized with a 10% formalin-fixed cell line derived from human uterine cervical adenocarcinoma (KOIZUMI et al. 1988). The antigen defined by 1C5 was found to have a molecular weight of 26,000, and an epitope of this antigen has a carbohydrate moiety. In this study, approximately 87% of adenocarcinomas of the uterine cervix were strongly stained by 1C5 (Fig. 6) and 40% of endometrial adenocarcinomas were weakly stained only at the luminal side of the gland. It thus appears that this monoclonal antibody is useful for differential diagnosis of cervical adenocarcinoma.

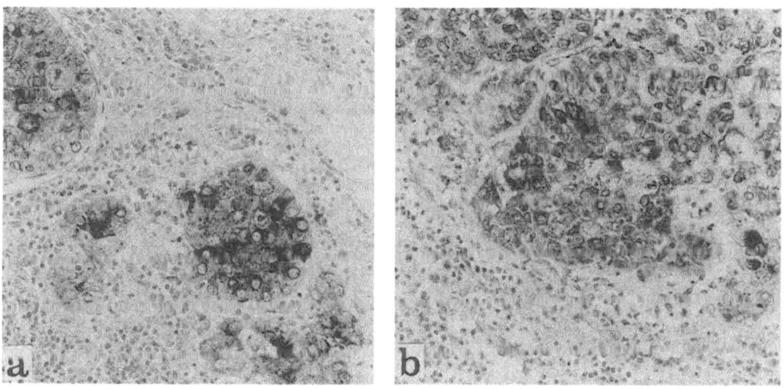


**Fig. 6 a, b.** Poorly differentiated adenocarcinoma showing strong cytoplasmic staining by monoclonal antibody 1C5. × 170

Ultrastructurally, the tumor cells have long and relatively irregular microvilli at the luminal side. Some specimens have cells with microvilli having core microfilaments, rootlets in the cytoplasm, and filaments connected to the terminal webs. These microvilli have not been observed in any benign glandular proliferations or in normal columnar epithelium. There is ordinarily a decrease in the number of secretory granules as the tumors become more poorly differentiated. The cellular organelles are more prominent in the differentiated type than in the poorly differentiated type.

Ultrastructural studies are useful for differential diagnosis of poorly differentiated neoplasm in which the cell type is not identified. Adenocarcinoma is considered in those cases in which microvilli, intercellular or intracytoplasmic lumina, cellular connections with tight junctions and junctional complexes, and secretory granules are observed.

### *7.1.1 Minimal Deviation Adenocarcinoma (Adenoma Malignum)*

Minimal deviation adenocarcinoma is a variant of the endocervical type of adenocarcinoma. The term "adenoma malignum" of the cervix was formerly used to refer to a group of extremely well-differentiated mucinous adenocarcinomas. However, it has become a confusing term. "Adenoma" characterizes the histologically benign appearance, and "malignum" refers to the highly virulent and almost invariably fatal progression of this tumor. Silverberg and Hurt (1975) proposed the term "minimal deviation adenocarcinoma" for this neoplasm.

Some cases of this tumor have been found to combine with Peutz–Jeghers syndrome (Gilks et al. 1989).

Cytologic examination is very important for detection of minimal deviation adenocarcinoma because the lesion does not express the usual abnormal colposcopic findings. Slightly atypical tall columnar or cuboidal epithelial cells of an endocervical type are arranged in grape-like clusters, branching, honeycomb, palisading, sheet-like or syncytium-like arrangements, and glandular rosettes. The monolayered or slightly multilayered cellular clusters are composed of columnar cells that have round or oval nuclei, sometimes with prominent nucleoli. The chromatin is distributed in a fine granular or moderately coarse granular pattern and the size of the nuclei is rather uniform (Kudo et al. 1990a).

Microscopically, each gland is lined by a single layer of cells or a few stratified cells, and the appearance approximates that of normal cervical glands. The characteristic features are represented by randomly disposed or variably apposed glandular structures in the fibromuscular stroma. The glands tend to be more irregular in size and shape than normal glands. They occasionally exhibit intraluminal papillary projections with cores of fine fibrous connective tissue producing characteristic bridging and branching shapes. The most characteristic pattern is the sharp points projecting from the glands as though

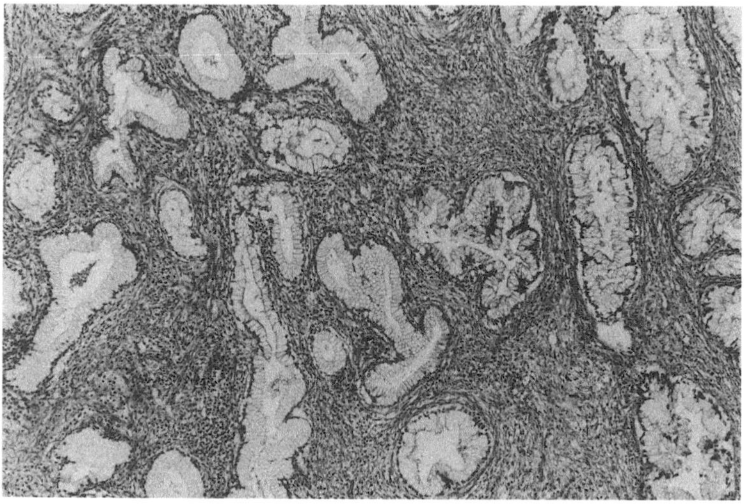

**Fig. 7.** Minimal deviation adenocarcinoma. Each gland is lined by a single layer of cells or a few stratified cells and approximates the appearance of a benign endocervical gland. × 85

pushing into the connective tissues. There is a discrete rim of periglandular stromal edema. Chronic inflammatory infiltration and necrosis are usually absent (Fig. 7).

Many authors, however, have indicated the difficulty of histologic differential diagnosis for minimal deviation adenocarcinoma. In the series of GILKS et al. (1989), 10 of 26 cases were diagnosed only after hysterectomy. In another case, the diagnosis was not made until 13 months after hysterectomy, when the presence of adenocarcinoma at the apex prompted review of the slides of the uterus. These facts indicate that cervical biopsy specimens and endocervical curettings have frequently been misinterpreted as benign.

Immunohistochemical staining for CEA has been suggested as useful for the differential diagnosis of minimal deviation adenocarcinoma from benign endocervical glandular proliferations or confusing benign lesions (STEEPER and WICK 1986). This neoplasm has also been positively stained with monoclonal antibody 1C5 (KOIZUMI et al. 1988).

Electron microscopic observations were first reported by KUDO et al. (1990). The characteristic features include the presence of intestinal metaplastic cells that have microvilli with core filaments and cytoplasmic tonofilaments that connect to the terminal web at the base of the microvilli. This structure is observed in well-differentiated adenocarcinoma of the endocervical type. Furthermore, there is a complete absence of ciliated cells in this tumor. It appears that the presence of the aforementioned structure in minimal deviation adenocarcinoma is a malignant rather than a benign feature (Fig. 8).

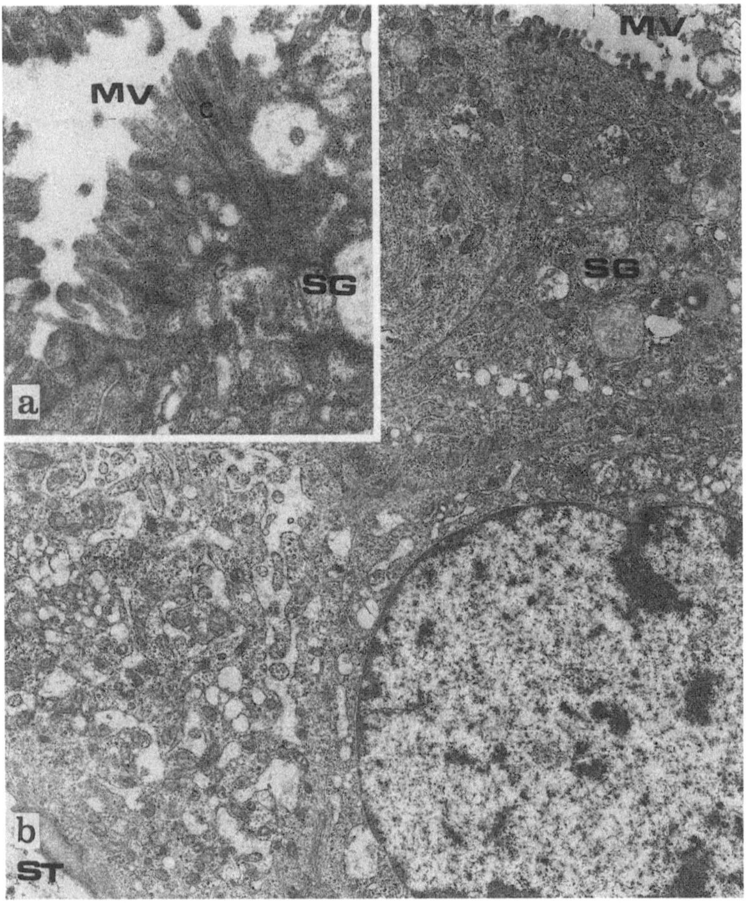


**Fig. 8 a, b.** Electron micrograph of minimal deviation adenocarcinoma. **a** Luminal side. *Mv*, microvilli; *c*, core filaments; *SG*, secretory granules. × 15,600. **b** Whole cell. *ST*, stroma. × 7100

## 7.2 Adenocarcinoma, Endometrioid Type

The diagnosis of primary endometrioid adenocarcinoma of the cervix should be made only if the endometrium is entirely normal.

The frequency of this endometrioid type in cervical adenocarcinoma has been reported as 0% (Shingleton et al. 1981), 4.3% (Fu et al. 1982), 16.9% (Hurt et al. 1977), 24% (Saigo et al. 1986), and 40% (Teshima et al. 1985). The different frequencies may be due to slightly different histologic criteria for its diagnosis.

Microscopically, the glandular cells are tall and columnar. The lining cells have densely basophilic rather than pale-stained, vacuolated cytoplasm.

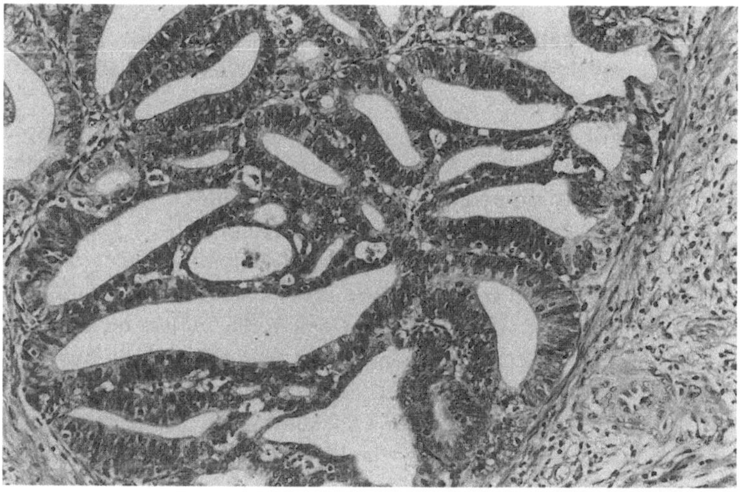

**Fig. 9.** Microscopic features of adenocarcinoma, endometrioid type. × 170

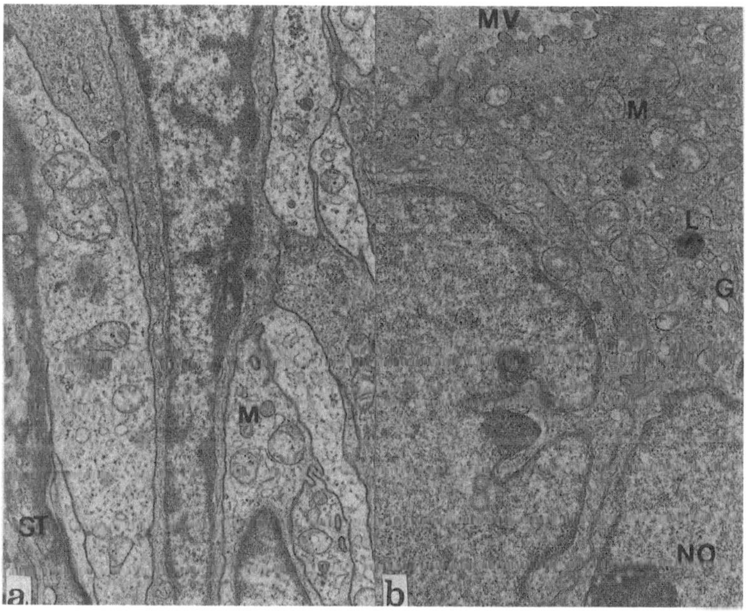


**Fig. 10 a, b.** Electron micrograph of adenocarcinoma, endometrioid type. **a.** Basal side. *ST*, stroma; *M*, mitochondria. × 7400. **b** Luminal side. *MV*, microvilli; *L*, lysosome; *G*, Golgi apparatus; *NO*, nucleolus. ×10 300

Mucicarminophilic material is present in the glands, but not in the cytoplasm. The predominant growth pattern is glandular or, less commonly, papillary. Occasionally, mature squamous metaplasia occurs as well-defined solid nests within the lumen (Fig. 9).

KOIZUMI et al. (1988) found that two out of four cases of endometrioid adenocarcinoma were not stained with the monoclonal antibody 1C5, while the other two cases were weakly stained only at the luminal side.

Ultrastructurally, at the luminal side there are short microvilli. In a few cells, microvilli with core filaments and cytoplasmic tonofilaments connected to the terminal web at the base of the microvilli are also observed. The nuclei are elongated and show more or less deep invaginations of the nuclear membranes. The nucleolus is prominent. Secretory granules are not observed in any neoplastic cells. The Golgi apparatus is not well developed compared with that of adenocarcinoma of the endocervical type. Lysosomes and dense bodies are found in greater number than in the endocervical type. There is marked variation in the development of rough endoplasmic reticulum. The cell membranes are sinuous and sporadically reveal desmosomes. The basement membrane is intact in some places; however, tumor cells are in direct contact with stroma at other places (Fig. 10).

The ultrastructural features of adenocarcinoma of the endometrioid type are similar to those of well-differentiated endometrial adenocarcinoma.

### 7.3 Clear Cell Adenocarcinoma

Diethylstilbestrol (DES)-related carcinomas have mainly been found in a younger age group, but there is a bimodal age distribution of clear cell adenocarcinoma (CCA) of the cervix unrelated to DES in women younger than 24 years and those older than 45 years (KAMINSKI and MAIER 1983). In addition, the cumulative proportion of women with cervical or vaginal clear cell cancer is in the range of 0.5–2.0 per 1000 DES-exposed women (EDELMAN 1989).

Clear cell adenocarcinoma accounts for 2%–3% of cervical adenocarcinomas and was originally thought to arise in mesonephric remnants. The histologic features of CCA of the cervix, however, are similar to those of clear cell carcinoma of the endometrium and ovary, which is derived from müllerian epithelium, and electron microscopic study of these neoplasms has documented them as having müllerian characteristics (DICKERSIN et al. 1980). Therefore, the lesion presumably arises from tuboendometrial-type gland cells within the endocervical mucosa.

Microscopically, carcinoma cells are arranged in a solid, tubular, microcystic, or papillary pattern. The major growth patterns include a tubular cystic or solid pattern. Some neoplasms contain a single pattern, although a mixture of several patterns is not uncommon. The predominant cells have abundant clear cytoplasm and enlarged, hyperchromatic nuclei, some of which project into the apical cytoplasm, giving a hobnail appearance. Mitotic figures are usually not

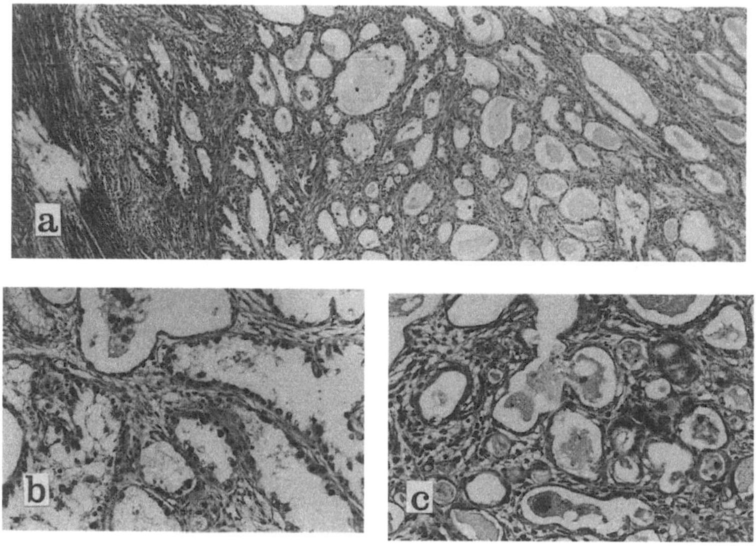

**Fig. 11 a–c.** Microscopic features in a cervical adenocarcinoma believed to have arisen from the mesonephric duct. This case was diagnosed after 8 years from pathologic definition of mesonephric hyperplasia. **a** Microscopic appearance found deep in the lateral wall of the cervix. ×70. **b** The neoplastic cells consist of hobnail cells. × 170. **c** Fine tubules and follicles. ×170. (Courtesy of Dr. Ikuyo Takamura, Department of Obstetrics and Gynecology, Aomori Prefectural Central Hospital, Japan)

abundant. Special stains, such as PAS stain and diastase digestion, are helpful in confirming glycogen particles in the cytoplasm. Mucicarminophilic material cannot be found in the cytoplasm.

As a rare variant of clear and hobnail cell type adenocarcinoma, mesonephroma of the uterine cervix has been reported (Woyke et al. 1972). The histogenesis of this tumor has not been clarified. However, it may be suspected that this tumor, like clear cell carcinoma, is of müllerian origin.

In addition, true mesonephric adenocarcinomas are found deep in the lateral wall of the cervix in a site corresponding to the location of mesonephric duct remnants (Fig. 11). The histologic transition from mesonephric duct remains to carcinomas has been demonstrated (Rosen and Dolan 1975).

The typical microscopic appearance of mesonephroma consists of tubules and fine follicles, lined by one layer of relatively low cells of hobnail shape, together with structures resembling primitive glomeruli. In the histochemical staining of mesonephroma of the cervix, a PAS-positive substance is found at the matrix of the invaginating and surrounding stroma of tubules and epithelial nests. Mucicarmine staining is faintly positive. Intracytoplasmic glycogen and mucin are absent (Woyke et al. 1972).

The characteristic ultrastructural feature of CCA is the presence of glycogen particles in the cytoplasm. The glycogen particles are most conspicuous in the

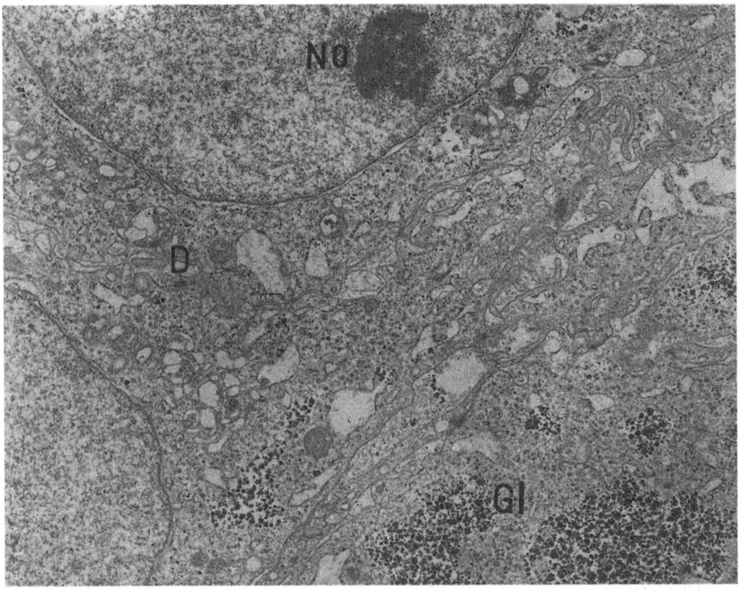


**Fig. 12.** Electron micrograph of clear cell adenocarcinoma. *Gl,* glycogen particles; *NO*, nucleolus; *D*, desmosome. × 6800

clear cells within solid areas, but are also evident in lining tubules and cysts. The glycogen particles are distributed in the supranuclear or apical areas of the hobnail and cuboidal cells. The free surface of the lining cells and intracellular canaliculi has numerous blunt microvilli. Cilia are not observed on any neoplastic cells. The composition of the cytoplasmic organelles in the cells depends on the amount of glycogen present. In those cells having abundant glycogen, other organelles and inclusions appear to be decreased and displaced. The nuclei are oval and large, with the nucleoli also being large, and there are multiple nucleoli in some cells. The glands and the solid groups of cells are surrounded by a double-layered basement membrane that is often discrete. The ultrastructural features are similar to those of clear cell carcinoma of the endometrium and ovary (Fig. 12).

On the other hand, mesonephroma of the uterine cervix has a peculiar type of basement membrane composed of numerous stratified basal laminae (Woyke et al. 1972). This appearance may be useful for differential diagnosis of clear cell carcinoma and mesonephroma of the cervix.

## 7.4 Adenosquamous Carcinoma

The reported relative frequency of adenosquamous carcinoma among cervical cancers is highly variable, from 1.7% (Korhonen 1978) to 10.5% (Yajima et al. 1984). The major reason for the discrepancies may be the definition of glandular differentiation by special staining in poorly differentiated carcinoma, which is usually diagnosed as squamous cell carcinoma with regular H&E staining. Benda et al. (1985) reported that 18 of 55 (33%) cases of squamous cell carcinoma, which were originally diagnosed from H&E-stained sections, contained mucinous material in the cytoplasm. If all these tumors were classified as adenosquamous carcinoma, the frequency of adenosquamous carcinoma would increase to 26%.

Microscopically, the well-differentiated mixed carcinoma is characterized in the mature type of adenosquamous carcinoma by glandular and squamous elements that are readily recognized on regular H&E-stained sections. The poorly differentiated mixed carcinoma is characterized in the mucoepidermoid type or signet-ring type by the tumor cells growing in solid nests and sheets closely resembling nonkeratinizing squamous cell carcinoma. These cells have basophilic, vacuolated, or clear cytoplasm. With mucicarmine and PAS stains, the mucous droplets can be confirmed. In immunohistochemical staining with monoclonal antibody 1C5, six of six specimens of adenosquamous carcinoma were positively stained, with the immature type also being clearly stained (Kudo et al. 1990b). It is suggested that this antibody may be helpful for recognition of the cervical adenomatous pattern, even in a solid sheet-like structure (Fig. 13).

Glassy cell carcinoma has been considered to be the most poorly differentiated variant of adenosquamous carcinoma. This type of lesion accounts for about 1%–2% of cervical adenocarcinomas and has an extremely aggressive clinical course. Because of its poor prognosis, it should be distinguished from large cell nonkeratinizing squamous carcinoma. However, Maier and Norris (1982), in their review of the material, questioned whether glassy cell carcinoma, as described, exists as a "meaningful entity," and further suggested that "the most likely categories to contain examples of glassy cell carcinoma are nonkeratinizing large-cell carcinoma and undifferentiated carcinoma."

The tumor is made up of small separated sheets and nests of neoplastic cells with extensive invasion of the stroma. The fibrous stroma is heavily infiltrated by lymphocytes, plasma cells, and eosinophils. These neoplastic cells have abundant eosinophilic, granular, and ground-glass cytoplasm and distinct cell borders. Nuclei are usually oval or round with prominent nucleoli. Numerous mitotic figures are noted (Fig. 14).

Scant intracellular glycogen is demonstrated in a few neoplastic cells by PAS following diastase digestion. Mucin is not revealed by any of the stains.

Ultrastructural studies of glassy cell carcinoma have denostrated the presence of glandular cells with intracytoplasmic lumina and additional cells which

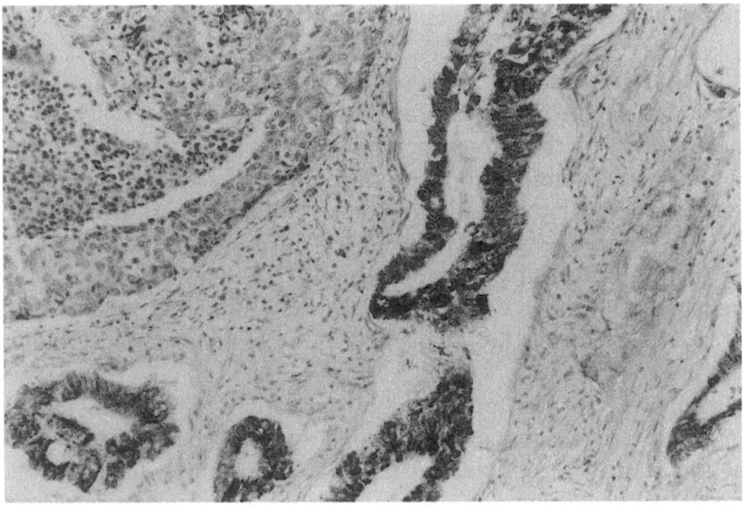

**Fig. 13.** Immunohistochemical staining of adenosquamous carcinoma by monoclonal antibody 1C5. Part of the squamous carcinoma is not stained (*upper left*). Adenocarcinoma showing strongly positive staining. × 170

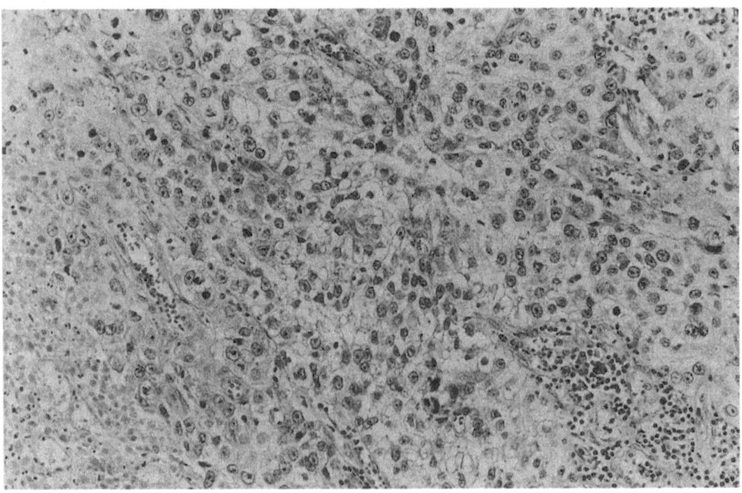

**Fig. 14.** Glassy cell carcinoma. The tumor cells have abundant, eosinophilic, granular, and ground glass cytoplasm and distinct cell borders. Nuclei are oval or round with prominent nucleoli. In the stroma, lymphocytes are abundant. × 170

are rich in tonofilaments, suggesting squamous differentiation (RICHARD et al. 1981; ULBRIGHT and GERSELL 1983).

As characteristic features of glassy cell carcinoma, RICHARD et al. (1981) presented evidence of cytofilaments of about 80 Å in diameter and glycogen granules, both of which were interspersed or in clusters, although they were rarely seen. They also indicated that glassy cell carcinoma closely resembles poorly differentiated adenosquamous carcinoma of the endometrium, including glandular lumen-forming and malignant squamous cells.

## 7.5 Adenoid Cystic Carcinoma

Adenoid cystic carcinoma (ACC) is indistinguishable from that occurring in the salivary gland and rarely involves the uterine cervix. This neoplasm occurs in postmenopausal women, most commonly in their seventh decade of life, and thus occurs later than adenoid basal carcinoma.

Microscopically, most ACCs exhibit a cribriform appearance characterized by small cells with sparse cytoplasm arranged around cystic glands like lumina. These microcystic spaces are empty or contain a basophilic substance or eosinophilic hyaline material. The nuclei are usually small, uniform, and hyperchromic. Mitotic figures are frequently observed. Squamous differentiation is observed in many cases. The cells lining the cysts do not differ significantly from those forming the solid sheets and cords (Fig. 15).

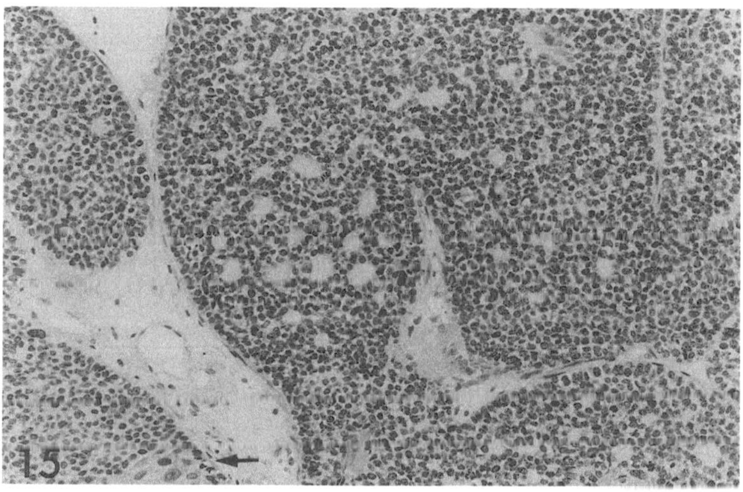


**Fig. 15.** Microscopic features of adenoid cystic carcinoma composed of large nests with a cribriform pattern. Hyaline or mucinous material occupies the lumina of the cribriform areas within nests of tumor. The *arrow* indicates minute foci of squamous differentiation. × 170

Adenoid cystic carcinoma is associated with squamous carcinoma in situ, other types of adenocarcinoma, and undifferentiated carcinoma (Lawrence and Mazur 1982; Ferry and Scully 1988).

In an immunohistochemical study, the presence of S-100 protein was not confirmed, so there is no immunohistochemical evidence of myoepithelial differentiation in this neoplasm (Ferry and Scully 1988).

Ultrastructurally, the cells that compose microcysts have aboundant microvilli at the luminal side and contain secretory granules. The common feature of ACC in various organs is the pattern of intercellular spaces with pseudocysts (Lawrence and Mazur 1982).

The cluster of cells is surrounded by multiple layers of redundant basal lamina and joined by desmosomes. Some of the cells in the solid area of this cytoplasm contain tonofilaments. On the other hand, only some cervical ACCs contain cells that have the appearance of myoepithelial cells with myofilaments and dense bodies (Ferry and Scully 1988).

### 7.6 Adenoid Basal Carcinoma

Adenoid basal carcinoma (ABC), which was initially described by Baggish and Woodruff (1966), has occasionally been confused with ACC. Most women with the tumor are in their fourth to seventh decades and are confined to clinical stage I (Ferry and Scully 1988).

The microscopic features of ABC show infiltrating growth with surface ulceration. Basaloid cells mostly form round or oval invasive solid nests with a distinct peripheral palisading. The nuclei are uniform and hyperchromatic; mitotic activity is low. There is a resemblance to basal cell carcinoma of the skin. These cells occasionally contain eosinophilic cytoplasm, suggesting individual cell keratinization.

Adenoid basal carcinoma rarely demonstrates a cribiform pattern. ABC has been referred to by one group as "basaloid carcinoma" (Daroca and Dhurandhar 1980). The tumors do not invade vascular or lymphatic channels, and the depth of invasion tends to be superficial. These histologic features may be correlated with the better prognosis of this neoplasm compared with that of ACC.

## 8 Prognosis

The 5-year survival rates reported for stage I endocervical adenocarcinoma vary from about 60% to 92% (Rutledge et al. 1975; Berek et al. 1981; Prempree et al. 1985; Saigo et al. 1986; Ireland et al. 1985; Moberg et al. 1986; Hopkins et al. 1988; Goodman et al. 1989). Most authors report 5-year survival rates of

**Table 2.** Five-year survival in patients with lymph node metastases and parametrial invasion (Sapporo Medical College, 1975–1983)

| | Squamous ca. | Adenosquamous | Adenosquamous ca. | Adenocarcinoma + adenosquamous ca. |
|---|---|---|---|---|
| Parametrial invasion | 20/28(71.4) | 1/3(33.3) | 0/2(0.0) | 1/5 (20.0) |
| Parametrial invasion and lymph node metastases | 8/15(53.3) | 0/3(0.0) | 0/2(0.0) | 0/5 (0.0) |
| Lymph node metastases | 11/17(64.7) | 2/3(66.6) | 1/1(100.0) | 3/4 (75.0) |
| Total | 39/60(65.0) | 3/9(33.3) | 1/5(20.0) | 4/14(28.6) |
| Invasion and metastases negative | 84/87(96.6) | 13/15(86.7) | | |

about 80%. It seems that the 5-year survival rate of stage I with adenocarcinoma is similar to that of squamous carcinoma. However, in stage II and more advanced disease, the 5-year survival rate after radiotherapy is lower for patients with adenocarcinoma than for those with squamous cell carcinoma. The poor prognosis of adenocarcinoma was also confirmed by a randomized comparative study between pure adenocarcinoma and squamous cell carcinoma (Moberg et al. 1986) and by matched-pair analysis (Kleine et al. 1989).

Concerning the frequency of lymph node metastases and grade of adenocarcinoma, Berek et al. (1985) found that lymph mode metastases occurred in 5.3% of patients with grade 1 tumors, 11.1% with grade 2 tumors, and 50.0% with grade 3 tumors. The 5-year survival rate of patients with lymph node involvement was 10%, compared with 91.7% in patients without lymph node involvement.

The relation between the degree of differentiation and survival has also been confirmed by several authors (Fu et al. 1982; Hopkins et al. 1987, 1988; Ireland et al. 1985; Saigo et al. 1986; Goodman et al. 1989). In the study by Goodman et al. (1989), the 5-year survival rate in stage I disease was 92% in patients with grades 1 and 2 lesions, in contrast with 68% in patients with grade 3 lesions.

The author examined the 5-year survival rates associated with lymph node metastases and parametrial invasion. The 5-year survival rate was 28.6% in adenocarcinoma cases having lymph node metastases and/or parametrial invasion. On the other hand, the survival rate in squamous carcinoma cases having lymph node metastases and/or parametrial invasion was 65%. These data indicate that adenocarcinoma cases that have extrauterine lesions are little improved by radiotherapy after surgery (Table 2).

As to the prognosis of adenocarcinoma of the endometrioid type, in general it is considered that it is better than that of the endocervical type (Saigo et al. 1986). This may be due to the grade of the tumor since there is a preponderance of well-differentiated tumors within the endometrioid type.

As regards the prognosis of cervical papillary adenocarcinomas of the villoglandular type, Young and Scully (1989) noted that this lesion has an

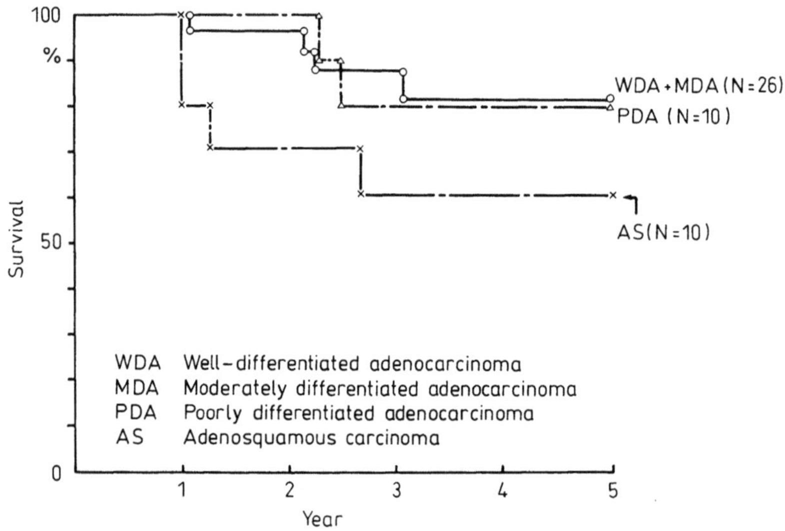


**Fig. 16.** Life table survival of patients (Sapporo Medical College, 1965–1983) with cervical adenocarcinoma and adenosquamous carcinoma (surgery group: stages I and II)

unusually favorable prognosis: none of 13 cases described in their series showed evidence of metastases.

For patients with minimal deviation adenocarcinoma, some authors have reported a dismal outcome (Kaku and Enjoji 1983; Szyfelbein et al. 1984). In a recent report, Gilks et al. (1989) have also indicated a poor prognosis of minimal deviation adenocarcinoma. Of their 22 patients, 13 died of recurrent tumor, four were alive with recurrent tumor at the time of the last follow-up examination, and only three were disease-free for 2 years or more. However, other authors have indicated that this tumor has a favorable survival rate (Silverberg and Hurt 1975; Kaminski and Norris 1983). An examination of the extent of the disease has revealed that survival in patients with stage I or II neoplasms without pelvic lymph node metastases is favorable after radical hysterectomy; however, most patients with clinical stage III or IV die. As mentioned above, there is no agreement on the biologic behavior of this tumor. However, it is evident that misdiagnosis of this tumor as a benign lesion due to the high degree of differentiation might lead to delayed treatment. With diagnostic delay, the prognosis of this tumor becomes poor (Kudo et al. 1990a).

For clear cell carcinoma, the prognosis in the less common cases, such as clear cell adenocarcinoma, is difficult to evaluate because of the small size of the treatment groups. The 5-year survival rates for stages I, IIA, IIB, III, and IV based on data accumulated by the Registry for Research on Hormonal Transplacental Carcinogenesis were 90%, 80%, 60%, 37% and 0%, respectively (Herbst and Anderson 1981).

The overall survival rate of 80% in DES-related carcinoma is higher than the 57% (KAMINSKI and MAIER 1983) or 64% (SAIGO et al. 1986) among non-DES-exposed women. From these 5-year survival rates, it appears that clear cell adenocarcinoma is associated with a more favorable prognosis than endocervical type or adenosquamous carcinoma.

As regards the mixed type of adenocarcinoma and squamous cell carcinoma, many authors have found the results of patients with adenosquamous carcinoma to be significantly worse than those of patients with pure adenocarcinoma (FU et al. 1982; GALLUP et al. 1985; SAIGO et al. 1986; BURKE et al. 1987).

The author performed a comparative study of life table survival of patients with cervical adenocarcinoma and adenosquamous carcinoma treated with surgery (Fig. 16). The prognosis of adenosquamous carcinoma was again found to be worse than that of cervical adenocarcinoma. However, GOODMAN et al. (1989) indicated that the histologic subtype reached significance as a prognostic factor, with the survival advantage in favor of adenosquamous lesions.

The frequency of lymph node metastases also contributes to a poor prognosis in the signet-ring variant. A higher incidence of lymph node metastases was reported in mucoepidermoid carcinoma (BENDA et al. 1985). The poor prognosis of mucoepidermoid carcinoma was also noted by IRELAND et al. (1987). These studies indicate that the identification of mucin production in squamous cell carcinoma is necessary for the definite diagnosis of poorly differentiated adenosquamous carcinoma.

Glassy cell carcinoma has been shown to have a poor response to surgery and/or radiotherapy, with 5-year survival rates in the range of 31%–33% (LITTMAN et al. 1976; PAK et al. 1983). This poor prognosis was thought to be related in part to radioresistance and its early dissemination (PAK et al. 1983; ULBRIGHT and GERSELL 1983).

TAMIMI et al. (1988) presented 29 undifferentiated large cell nonkeratinizing cervical carcinomas of stage Ib which had the histologic characteristics of glassy cell carcinoma; 28 of these cases were treated by radical hysterectomy. Fourteen of the patients developed recurrent carcinoma, and in all but one the interval to recurrence was less than 8 months. Only two survived after second-line salvage therapy. From these results, TAMIMI et al. suggested that the poor prognosis ascribed to the classically defined glassy cell carcinoma holds true for this extended group of large cell, undifferentiated cervical cancers that display similar histologic features and pursue a similarly aggressive clinical course.

As regards adenoid cystic carcinoma, in the series of PREMPREE et al. (1980) 5-year survival rates were 56% for patients with stage I disease, 27% for stage II, and 0% for stages III and IV. In the series of FERRY and SCULLY (1988), none of the women with stage II, III, or IV tumors lived. Metastases occurred most frequently in the lung and less commonly in the bone, liver, and brain. These data indicate that the prognosis of adenoid cystic carcinoma is worse than that of adenocarcinoma of the endocervical or endometrial type.

Only one of fourteen women with adenoid basal carcinoma died of their disease in the report of FERRY and SCULLY (1988). Their study indicates that the prognosis of adenoid basal carcinoma is favorable.

## References


Alva JA, Lauchlan SC (1975) The histogenesis of mixed cervical carcinomas. The concept of endocervical columnar cell dysplasia. Am J Clin Pathol 64:20–25

Andersen ES, Arffmann E (1989) Adenocarcinoma in situ of the uterine cervix: a clinico-pathologic study of 36 cases. Gynecol Oncol 35:1–7

Baggish MS, Woodruff JD (1966) Adenoid-basal carcinoma of the cervix. Obstet Gynecol 28:213–218

Benda JA, Platz CE, Buchsbaum H, Lifshitz S (1985) Mucin Production in defining mixed carcinoma of the uterine cervix: a clinicopathologic study. Int J Gynecol Pathol 4:314–327

Berek JS, Castaldo TW, Hacker NF, Petrilli ES, Lagasse LD, Moore JG (1981) Adenocarcinoma of the uterine cervix. Cancer 48:2734–2741

Berek JS, Hacker NF, Fu YS, Sokale JR, Leuchter RC, Laggase LD (1985) Adenocarcinoma of the uterine cervix: histologic variables associated with lymph node metastasis and survival. Obstet Gynecol 65:46–52

Boddington MM, Springgs AI, Cowdell RH (1976) Adenocarcinoma of the uterine cervix: cytological evidence of a long preclinical evolution. Br J Obstet Gynecol 83:900–903

Boon ME, Baak JPA, Kurver PJH, Overdiep SH, Verdonk GW (1981a) Adenocarcinoma in situ of the cervix: an underdiagnosed lesion. Cancer 48:768–773

Boon ME, Kirk RS, Rietveld-Scheffers PEM (1981b) The morphogenesis of adenocarcinoma of the uterine cervix— a complex pathological entity. Histopathology 5:565–577

Bousfield L, Pacey F, Young Q, Krumins I, Osborn R (1980) Expanded cytologic criteria for the diagnosis of adenocarcinoma in situ of the cervix and related lesions. Acta Cytol 24:283–296

Brinton LA, Tashima KT, Lehman HF, Levine RS, Mallin K, Savitz DA (1987) Epidemiology of cervical cancer by cell type. Cancer Res 47:1706–1711

Brown LJR, Wells M (1986) Cervical glandular atypia associated with squamous intraepithelial neoplasia: a premalignant lesion? J Clin Pathol 39:22–28

Buntine DW (1979) Adenocarcinoma of the uterine cervix of probable wolffian origin. Pathology 11:713–718

Burke TW, Hoskins WJ, Heller PB, Shen MC, Weiser EB, Park RC (1987) Clinical patterns of tumor recurrence after radical hysterectomy in stage I B cervical carcinoma. Obstet Gynecol 69:382–385

Buscema J, Woodruff JD (1984) Significance of neoplastic atypicalities in endocervical epithelium. Gynecol Oncol 17:356–362

Christopherson WM, Nealon N, Gray LA (1979) Noninvasive precursor lesions of adenocarcinoma and mixed adenosquamous carcinoma of the cervix uteri. Cancer 44:975–983

Cohen C, Shulman G, Budgeon LR (1982) Endocervical and endometrial adenocarcinoma. An immunoperoxidase and histochemical study. Am J Surg Pathol 6:151–157

Czernobilsky B, Kessler I, Lancet M (1974) Cervical adenocarcinoma in a woman on long-term contraceptives. Obstet Gynecol 43:517–521

Dallenbach-Hellweg G (1984) On the origin and histological structure of adenocarcinoma of the endocervix in women under 50 years of age. Pathol Res Pract 179:38–50

Daroca PJ, Dhurandhar HN (1980) Basaloid carcinoma of the cervix. Am J Surg Pathol 4:235–239

Davis JR, Moon LB (1975) Increased incidence of adenocarcinoma of uterine cervix. Obstet Gynecol 45:79–83

Dickersin GR, Welch WR, Erlandson R, Robboy SJ (1980) Ultrastructure of 16 cases of clear cell adenocarcinoma of the vagina and cervix in young women. Cancer 45:1615–1624

Duk JM, Aalders JG, Fleuren GJ, Krans M, DeBruijin HWA (1989) Tumor markers CA 125, squamous cell carcinoma antigen, and carcinoembryonic antigen in patients with adenocarcinoma of the uterine cervix. Obstet Gynecol 73:661–668

Edelman DA (1989) Diethylstilbestrol exposure and risk of clear cell cervical and vaginal adenocarcinoma. Int J Fertil 34:251–255

Ferry JA, Scully RE (1988) "Adenoid cystic" carcinoma and adenoid basal carcinoma of the uterine cervix. A study of 28 cases. Am J Surg Pathol 12:134–144

Fu YS, Reagan JW, Hsiu JG, Storaasli JP, Wents WB (1982) Adenocarcinoma and mixed carcinoma of the uterine cervix. I. A clinicopathologic study. Cancer 49:2560–2570

Fu YS, Reagan JW (1989) Benign and malignant epithelial lesions of the uterine cervix, vagina and vulva. Major problems in pathology, vol 21, Saunders, Philadelphia, pp 295–296

Gallup DG, Harper RH, Stock RJ (1985) Poor prognosis in patients with adenosquamous cell carcinoma of the cervix. Obstet Gynecol 65:416–422

Gilks CB, Young RH, Aguirre P, DeLellis RA, Scully RE (1989) Adenoma malignum (minimal deviation adenocarcinoma) of the uterine cervix. Am J Surg Pathol 13:717–729

Gloor E, Hurlimann J (1986) Cervical intraepithelial glandular neoplasia (adenocarcinoma in situ and glandular dysplasia). Cancer 58:1272–1280

Gloor E, Ruzicka J (1982) Morphology of adenocarcinoma in situ of the uterine cervix: a study of 14 cases. Cancer 49:294–302

Goodman HM, Buttlar CA, Niloff JM et al. (1989) Adenocarcinoma of the cervix: prognostic factors and patterns of recurrence. Gynecol Oncol 33:241–247

Griffin NR, Wells M, Fox H (1989) Modulation of the antigenicity of amylase in cervical glandular atypia, adenocarcinoma in situ and invasive adenocarcinoma. Histopathology 15:267–279

Herbst AL, Anderson D (1981) Clinical correlations and management of vaginal and cervical clear cell adenocarcinoma. In: Herbst AL, Bern HA (eds) Developmental effects of diethylstilbestrol (DES) in pregnancy. Thieme-Stratton, New York, pp 71–80

Hopkins MP, Sutton P, Roberts JA (1987) Prognostic features and treatment of endocervical adenocarcinoma of the cervix. Gynecol Oncol 27:69–75

Hopkins MP, Schmidt RW, Roberts JA, Morley GW (1988) Gland cell carcinoma (adenocarcinoma) of the cervix. Obstet Gynecol 72:789–795

Horowitz IR, Jacobson LP, Zucker PK, Currie JL, Rosenshein NB (1988) Epidemiology of adenocarcinoma of the cervix. Gynecol Oncol 31:25–31

Hurlimann J, Gloor E (1984) Adenocarcinoma in situ and invasive adenocarcinoma of the uterine cervix. An immunohistologic study with antibodies specific for several epithelial markers. Cancer 54:103–109

Hurt WG, Silverberg SG, Frable WJ, Belgrad R, Crooks LD (1977) Adenocarcinoma of the cervix: histopathologic and clinical features. Am J Obstet Gynecol 129:304–315

Ireland D, Hardiman P, Monaghan JM (1985) Adenocarcinoma of the uterine cervix: a study of 73 cases. Obstet Gynecol 65:82–85

Ireland D, Cole S, Kelly P, Monaghan JM (1987) Mucin production in cervical intraepithelial neoplasia and in stage Ib carcinoma of cervix with pelvic lymph node metastases. Br J Obstet Gynecol 94:467–472

Japan Society of Obstetrics and Gynecology, The Japanese Pathological Society, Japan Radiological Society (1987) The general rules for clinical and pathological management of uterine cervical cancer (in Japanese). Kanehara Shutupan, Tokyo, pp 56–57

Jaworski RC, Pacey NF, Greenberg ML, Osborn RA (1988) The histologic diagnosis of adenoca cinoma in situ and related lesions of the cervix. Adenocarcinoma in situ. Cancer 61:1171–1181

Jones MW, Silverberg SG (1989) Cervical adenocarcinoma in young women: possible relation to microglandular hyperplasia and use of oral contraceptives. Obstet Gynecol 73:984–989

Kaku T, Enjoji M (1983) Extremely well-differentiated adenocarcinoma ("adenoma malignum") of the cervix. Int J Gynecol Pathol 2:28–41

Kaminski PF, Maier RC (1983) Clear cell adenocarcinoma of the cervix unrelated to diethylstilbestrol exposure. Obstet Gynecol 62:720–727

Kaminski PF, Norris HJ (1983) Minimal deviation carcinoma (adenoma malignum). Int J Gynecol Pathol 2:141–152

Kjorstad KE, Bond B (1984) Stage I B adenocarcinoma of the cervix: metastatic potential and patterns of dissemination. Am J Obstet Gynecol 150:297–299

Kleine W, Rau K, Schwoeorer D, Pfleiderer A (1989) Prognosis of the adenocarcinoma of the cervix uteri: a comparative study. Gynecol Oncol 35:145–149

Koizumi M, Uede T, Shijubo N, Kudo R, Hashimoto M, Kikuchi K (1988) New monoclonal antibody, 1C5, reactive with human cervical adenocarcinoma of the uterus, with immunodiagnostic potential. Cancer Res 48:6565–6573

Korhonen MO (1978) Adenocarcinoma of the uterine cervix. Acta Pathol Microbiol Scand [Suppl] 264:1–59

Kottmeier HL, Kolstad P, McGarrity KA, Pettersson F, Ulfelder H (1979) Annual report on the results of treatment in gynecological cancer, vol 17. Pago, Stockholm, pp 37–44

Kottmeier HL, Kolstad P, McGarrity KA, Pettersson F, Ulfelder H (1982) Annual report on the results of treatment in gynecological cancer, vol 18. Pago, Stockholm, pp 44–59

Kudo R, Sagae S, Hayakawa O, Kusanagi T, Hashimoto M (1987) The cytological features and DNA content of cervical adenocarcinoma. Diagn Cytopathol 3:191–197

Kudo R, Sagae S, Kusanagi T, Mizuuchi H, Hayakawa O, Hashimoto M (1990a) Minimal deviation adenocarcinoma (adenoma malignum) of the uterine; four case reports. Eur J Obstet Gynecol Reprod Biol 34:179–188

Kudo R, Sasano H, Koizumi M, Orenstein JM, Silverberg SG (1990b) Immunohistochemical comparison of new monoclonal antibody IC5 and carcinoembryonic antigen in differential diagnosis of the uterine cervix. Int J Gynecol Pathol 9:325–336

Lawrence JB, Mazur MT (1982) Adenoid cystic carcinoma: a comparative pathologic study of tumors in salivary gland, breast, lung and cervix. Hum Pathol 13:916–924

Littman P, Clement PB, Henriksen B et al. (1976) Glassy cell carcinoma of the cervix. Cancer 37:2238–2246

Lorincz AT, Temple GF, Kurman RJ, Jenson AB, Lancaster WD (1987) Oncogenic association of specific human papillomavirus types with cervical neoplasia. JNCI 79:671–677

Maes G, Fleuren GJ, Bara J, Nap M (1988) The distribution of mucins, carcinoembryonic antigen, and mucus-associated antigens in endocervical and endometrial adenocarcinomas. Int Gynecol Pathol 7:112–122

Maier RC, Norris HJ (1980) Coexistence of cervical intraepithelial neoplasia with primary adenocarcinoma of the endocervix. Obstet Gynecol 56:361–364

Maier RC, Norris HJ (1982) Glassy cell carcinoma of the cervix. Obstet Gynecol 60:219–224

Michael H, Grawe L, Kraus FT (1984) Minimal deviation adenocarcinoma: clinical and histologic features, immunohistochemical staining for carcinoembryonic antigen, and differentiation from confusing benign lesions. Int J Gynecol Pathol 3:261–276

Moberg PJ, Einhorn N, Silfversward C, Soderberg G (1986) Adenocarcinoma of the uterine cervix. Cancer 57:407–410

Mullins JD, Hilliard GD (1981) Cervical carcinoid ("argyrophil cell" carcinoma) associated with an endocervical adenocarcinoma: a light and ultrastructural study. Cancer 47:785–790

Noda K, Kimura K, Ikeda M, Teshima K (1983) Studies on the histogenesis of cervical adenocarcinoma. Int J Gynecol Pathol 1:336–346

Pak HY, Yokota SB, Paladugu RR, Agliozzo CM (1983) Glassy cell carcinoma of the cervix. Cytologic and clinicopathologic analysis. Cancer 52:307–312

Peters RK, Chao A, Mack TM, Thomas D, Bernstein L, Henderson BE (1986) Increased frequency of adenocarcinoma of the cervix in young women in Los Angeles County. JNCI 76:423–428

Pettersson F, Coppleson M, Creasman W, Ludwig H (1985) Annual report on the results of treatment in gynecological cancer, vol 19, Panorama, Stockholm, pp 32–49

Pettersson F, Coppleson M, Creaman W, Ludwig H (1988) Annual report on the results of treatment in gynecological cancer, vol 20. Panorama, Stockholm, pp 34–53

Prempree T, Villasanta U, Tang C-K (1980) Management of adenoid cystic carcinoma of the uterine cervix (clindroma): report of 6 cases and reappraisal of all cases reported in the medical literature. Cancer 46:1631–1635

Prempree T, Amornmarn R, Wizenberg MJ (1985) A therapeutic approach to primary adenocarcinoma of the cervix. Cancer 56:1264–1268

Richard L, Guralnick M, Ferency A (1981) Ultrastructure of glassy cell carcinoma of cervix. Diagn Gynecol Obstet 3:31–38

Rosen Y, Dolan TE (1975) Carcinoma of the cervix with clindromatous features believed to arise in mesonephric duct. Cancer 36:1739–1747

Rutledge FN, Galakatos AE, Wharton JT, Smith JP (1975) Adenocarcinoma of the cervix. Am J Obstet Gynecol 122:236–245

Saigo PE, Cain JM, Kim WS, Gaynor JJ, Johnson K, Lewis JL (1986) Prognostic factors in adenocarcinoma of the uterine cervix. Cancer 57:1584–1593

Schwartz SM, Weiss NS (1986) Increased incidence of adenocarcinoma of the cervix in young women in the United States. Am J Epidemiol 124:1045–1047

Shingleton HM, Lawrence WD, Gore H (1977) Cervical carcinoma with adenoid cystic pattern. Cancer 40:1112–1121

Shingleton HM, Gore H, Bradley DH, Soong SJ (1981) Adenocarcinoma of the cervix. I. Clinical evaluation and pathologic feature. Am J Obstet Gynecol 139:799–814

Silverberg SG, Hurt WG (1975) Minimal deviation adenocarcinoma ("adenoma malignum") of the cervix: a reappraisal. Am J Obstet Gynecol 121:971–975

Steeper TA, Wick MR (1986) Minimal deviation adenocarcinoma of the cervix ("adenoma malignum"). Cancer 58:1131–1138

Szyfelbein WM, Young RH, Scully RE (1984) Adenoma malignum of the cervix. Cytologic findings. Acta Cytol 28:691–698

Takahashi M, Aoki K, Banham DG, McLean MR (1984) Some effects of long-term use of oral contraceptives on cervical neoplasia. Int Cong Ser 644:21–27

Tamimi SK, Ek M, Hesla J, Cain AM, Figge DC, Greer BE (1988) Glassy cell carcinoma of the cervix redefined. Obstet Gynecol 71:837–841

Tase T, Okagaki T, Clark BA, Manias DA, Ostrow RS, Twiggs LB, Faras AJ (1988a) Human papillomavirus types and localization in adenocarcinoma and adenosquamous carcinoma of the cervix: a study by in situ DNA hybridization. Cancer Res 48:993–998

Tase T, Sato S, Wada Y, Yajima A, Okagaki T (1988b) Prevalence of human papillomavirus type 18 DNA in adenocarcinoma and adenosquamous carcinoma of the uterine cervix occurring in Japan. Tohoku J Exp Med 156:47–53

Tase T, Okagaki T, Clark BA, Twiggs LB, Ostrow RS, Faros A (1989) Human papillomavirus DNA in glandular dysplasia and microglandular hyperplasia: presumed precursors of adenocarcinoma of the uterine cervix. Obstet Gynecol 73:1005–1008

Teshima S, Shimosato Y, Kishi K, Kasamatsu T, Ohmi K, Uei Y (1985) Early stage adenocarcinoma of the uterine cervix. Histopathologic analysis with consideration of histogenesis. Cancer 56:167–172

Tobon H, Dave H (1988) Adenocarcinoma in situ of the cervix. Clinicopathologic observations of 11 cases. Int J Gynecol Obstet 7:139–151

Trowell JE (1985) Intestinal metaplasia with argentaffin cells in the uterine cervix. Histopathology 9:551–559

Ulbright TM, Gersell DJ (1983) Glassy cell carcinoma of the uterine cervix. A light and electron microscopic study of five cases. Cancer 51:2255–2263

Valente PT, Hanjani P (1986) Endocervical neoplasia in long-term users of oral contraceptives: clinical and pathologic observations. Obstet Gynecol 67:695–704

Vesterinen E, Forss M, Nieminen U (1989) Increase of cervical adenocarcinoma: a report of 520 cases of cervical carcinoma including 112 tumors with glandular elements. Gynecol Oncol 33:49–53

Wahlström T, Lindgren J, Korhonen M, Seppala M (1979) Distinction between endocervical and endometrial adenocarcinoma with immunoperoxidase staining of carcinoembryonic antigen in routine histological tissue specimens. Lancet Dec 1 (No. 8153):1159–1160

Woyke S, Damagala W, Olszewski W (1972) Mesonephroma of the uterine cervix. Submicroscopical study and comparison with fine structure of endocervical adenocarcinoma. Virchows Arch [A] 355:29–40

Yajima A, Fukuda M, Noda K (1984) Histopathological findings concerning the morphogenesis of mixed carcinoma of the uterine cervix. Gynecol Oncol 18:157–164

Young RH, Scully RE (1989) Villoglandular papillary adenocarcinoma of the uterine cervix. A clinicopathologic analysis of 13 cases. Cancer 63:1773–1779

# Endocrine Tumors of the Ovary

R.H. YOUNG and R.E. SCULLY



Current Topics in Pathology
Volume 85, Ed. N. Sasano

# 1 Introduction

This chapter will emphasize aspects of the pathology of functioning ovarian tumors that have appeared in the literature of the last 10–15 years, with particular attention to problems in differential diagnosis. Since there is important recent information concerning a variety of ovarian neoplasms with paraendocrine manifestations, tumors in this category will also be discussed.

# 2 Sex Cord–Stromal Tumors

The category of ovarian neoplasms designated as sex cord–stromal tumors includes those that contain granulosa cells, theca cells and their luteinized derivatives, Sertoli cells, Leydig cells, and fibroblasts of gonadal stromal origin, singly or in various combinations and in varying degrees of differentiation. The classification of these tumors used here is similar to that currently being formulated by the International Society of Gynecological Pathologists under the auspices of the World Health Organization (WHO) (Table 1). These tumors account for approximately 8% of all ovarian tumors (YOUNG and SCULLY 1984c). Fibromas account for approximately half the cases and will not be discussed because they do not produce hormones. The remaining tumors in this category are usually associated with endocrine manifestations, which may be estrogenic, androgenic, or rarely progestagenic, or any combination of the above.

## 2.1 Granulosa Cell Tumors

Granulosa cell tumors that occur most often in women in the reproductive age group and in older women differ both clinically and pathologically from the much rarer form that occurs most often in the first two decades, and these two subtypes, the adult and juvenile granulosa cell tumors, respectively, will be discussed separately. The names of these tumors reflect only a strong tendency for them to occur at certain ages; adult granulosa cell tumors, however, occur very rarely in children and juvenile granulosa cell tumors are encountered very rarely in women over 30 years of age (YOUNG et al. 1984a).

### *2.1.1 Adult Granulosa Cell Tumor*

Adult granulosa cell tumor is the most common clinically estrogenic ovarian tumor. It accounts for 1%–2% of all ovarian tumors, and 95% of all granulosa cell tumors, occurring more often in postmenopausal than premenopausal

**Table 1.** Classification of sex cord–stromal tumors

Granulosa–stromal cell tumors
A. Granulosa cell tumor
    i) Adult type
    ii) Juvenile type

B. Tumors in the thecoma–fibroma group
    i) Thecoma
        a) Typical
        b) Luteinized
    ii) Fibroma–fibrosarcoma
        a) Fibroma
        b) Cellular fibroma
        c) Fibrosarcoma
    iii) Stromal tumor with minor sex cord elements
    iv) Sclerosing stromal tumor
    v) Unclassified

*Sertoli–stromal cell tumors*
A. Sertoli cell tumor
B. Leydig cell tumor
C. Sertoli–Leydig cell tumor
    i) Well differentiated
    ii) Of intermediate differentiation
    iii) Poorly differentiated
    iv) With heterologous elements
    v) Retiform
    vi) Mixed

*Gynandroblastoma*
*Sex cord tumor with annular tubules*
*Unclassified*

women and having a peak age incidence between 50 and 55 years. Women in the reproductive age group typically present with irregular, excessive uterine bleeding, but amenorrhea may precede the abnormal bleeding or may be the only hormonal manifestation. Postmenopausal bleeding is the most common endocrine symptom in older women. Rarely, the adult granulosa cell tumor is androgenic (Nakashima et al. 1984).

Adult granulosa cell tumors vary in size from those that are too small to be felt on pelvic examination (10%–15%) (Fathalla 1967) to large abdominal masses; the average diameter is approximately 12 cm. At operation the tumor may appear predominantly solid or predominantly cystic and is unilateral in over 95% of the cases; spread beyond the ovary at the time of presentation is uncommon. Most characteristically, the tumor is either predominantly cystic, with numerous locules that are typically filled with fluid or clotted blood and separated by solid tissue, or solid with large areas of hemorrhage. The solid tissue may be gray-white or yellow, depending on its lipid content, and soft or firm depending on its relative content of neoplastic cells and fibrothecomatous stroma. An interesting clinical corollary of the frequent hemorrhage seen in granulosa cell tumors is the presentation of approximately 10% of them as an acute abdominal disorder due to rupture and hemoperitoneum. A rare cystic tumor is thin-walled and unilocular or oligolocular, appearing indistinguishable grossly from a serous cystadenoma. Almost half the androgenic tumors have been in the thin-walled cystic category (NAKASHIMA et al. 1984).

Microscopic examination of an adult granulosa cell tumor reveals only granulosa cells or more often, an additional component of theca cells, fibroblasts, or both; in some cases, the latter cell types predominate. The granulosa cells grow in a wide variety of patterns. The better differentiated tumors have one or more of the following patterns: microfollicular, macrofollicular, insular, trabecular, solid-tubular, and rarely hollow-tubular. The microfollicular pattern is characterized by numerous small cavities simulating the Call–Exner bodies of the developing graafian follicle. These cavities may contain eosinophilic fluid and often one or a few degenerating nuclei, hyalinized basement membrane material, or rarely basophilic fluid. The microfollicles are separated typically by well-differentiated granulosa cells that contain scanty cytoplasm and pale, angular or oval, often grooved nuclei arranged haphazardly in relation to one another and to the follicles. The macrofollicular pattern, which is relatively uncommon, is characterized by cysts lined by well-differentiated granulosa cells, beneath which theca cells are usually present. The trabecular and insular forms of granulosa cell tumor are characterized by bands and islands of granulosa cells separated by a fibromatous or thecomatous stroma. In the solid tubular pattern the tubules may be uniformly cellular or contain peripheral nuclei and a central syncytial-like mass of pale cytoplasm; occasionally a few hollow tubules or glandlike structures are encountered.

The less well-differentiated forms of the adult granulosa cell tumor typically have a watered silk (moiré silk), gyriform, or diffuse (sarcomatoid) pattern, alone or in combination. The first two patterns are manifested by parallel undulating or zigzag rows of granulosa cells, generally in single file, whereas the diffuse pattern is characterized by a monotonous cellular growth; the cells usually have round to oval, pale, and often grooved nuclei but rarely the cells are spindle shaped, resembling a cellular fibroma or low-grade fibrosarcoma; mitotic figures may be numerous, but are rarely atypical.

Although the cells in most adult granulosa cell tumors usually have scanty cytoplasm, in some tumors they have moderate to abundant quantities of dense or vacuolated cytoplasm; the term luteinized granulosa cell tumor is appropriate when such cells predominate.

Approximately 2% of adult granulosa cell tumors contain mononucleate and multinucleate cells with large, bizarre, hyperchromatic nuclei (Fig. 1), the presence of which does not appear to worsen the prognosis on the basis of study of a small series of cases (YOUNG and SCULLY 1983b). Usually only small numbers of such cells are present but rarely they are a prominent feature of the tumor. In one granulosa cell tumor the stromal component of the neoplasm had the appearance of a high-grade sarcoma (SUSIL and SUMITHRAN 1987).

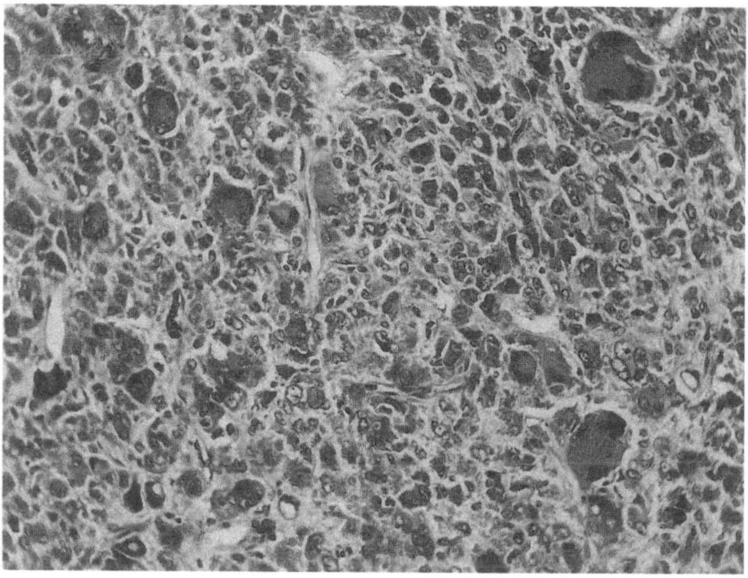

**Fig. 1.** Adult granulosa cell tumor with bizarre nuclei. Mononucleate and multinucleate cells exhibit conspicuous nuclear atypia. H&E, × 200

*2.1.1.1 Differential Diagnosis.* In some adult granulosa cell tumors, particularly those with a diffuse pattern, differentiation of granulosa cells and the cells of a thecoma or a cellular fibroma may be difficult or impossible on routine staining (Scully 1979). In such cases a reticulum stain may be helpful as the fibrils typically surround groups of granulosa cells but invest individually cells of stromal origin. The use of immunohistochemistry in the differential diagnosis of adult granulosa cell tumors has not been fully explored. All of them are vimentin positive (Chadha and van der Kwast 1989). Unlike thecomas and fibromas, however, occasional adult granulosa cell tumors are positive for various cytokeratins, but such tumors have epithelial patterns and are not of the diffuse type that is most apt to cause a problem in differential diagnosis. The misinterpretation of an undifferentiated carcinoma as a diffuse granulosa cell tumor is common. The single best criterion for distinguishing these two tumors is the appearance of the nuclei, which are hyperchromatic, usually of unequal size and shape, and rarely grooved in undifferentiated carcinomas; the latter with occasional exceptions have higher mitotic rates than diffuse granulosa cell tumors and atypical mitotic figures are often found as well. The presence of a desmoplastic stroma or identification of mucin or epithelial membrane antigen in the tumor cells makes the diagnosis of a diffuse granulosa cell tumor highly unlikely. The small cell carcinoma (Dickersin et al. 1982), which is usually associated with hypercalcemia, may also be misdiagnosed as a granulosa cell tumor, particularly since it almost always contains follicle-like structures.

However, other patterns of the granulosa cell tumor are not encountered, the nuclei are darker than granulosa cell nuclei and lack grooves, and mitotic figures are generally much more numerous than in the adult granulosa cell tumor, which has never been reported to have an association with hypercalcemia. Unlike the typically indolent clinical course of the adult granulosa cell tumor, the small cell carcinoma usually has an aggressive behavior and is associated with a high mortality. Rarely, an endometrioid carcinoma of the ovary has a microfollicular pattern with multiple, regularly distributed, uniform, small spaces containing eosinophilic material (Young et al. 1982a). In such cases, however, the nuclei are round and hyperchromatic, other patterns of endometrioid carcinoma are usually also present, and other features of granulosa cell tumor are absent. A diffuse granulosa cell tumor is occasionally confused with a primary endometrioid stromal sarcoma (Young et al. 1983b) or metastatic endometrial stromal sarcoma in the ovary, particularly when either of the latter tumors contains sex cord-like aggregates (Young and Scully 1990). A variety of clinical and pathologic findings, however, facilitate the differential diagnosis. The tumors of endometrial stromal type are frequently high stage and bilateral, typically contain numerous small arteries resembling the spiral arteries of the late secretory endometrium, and contain abundant intercellular reticulum. They do not produce steroid hormones. The sex cord-like formations of the stromal tumors typically have nuclei that are darker than those of the granulosa cell tumor and lack grooves; true Call–Exner bodies are not present.

The high degree of differentiation in the walls of the cysts of macrofollicular adult granulosa cell tumors may cause a problem in distinguishing them from nonneoplastic follicle cysts. In practice, however, this problem rarely exists if the cysts lined by granulosa and theca cells are viewed in the context of the clinical, gross, and microscopic findings. Except during pregnancy and the puerperium, nonneoplastic follicle cysts rarely exceed 8 cm in diameter. Microscopic examination reveals that the cystic granulosa cell tumors almost always exhibit at least small foci of solid neoplasia in their walls, often with the formation of solid tubules filled with vacuolated cells. The large luteinized follicle cyst of pregnancy and the puerperium is distinctive not only in its clinical setting but also in its apparently invariable context of large lutein cells with large, bizarre, hyperchromatic nuclei (Clement and Scully 1980).

A number of studies in the last 15 years have contributed information concerning the relation of various clinical and pathologic features of adult granulosa cell tumors to the prognosis (Fox et al. 1975; Bjorkholm and Pettersson 1980; Bjorkholm and Silfversward 1981; Stenwig et al. 1979). The stage of the tumor is the single most important prognostic feature, with the 10-year survival rate in one series falling from 86% in stage I cases to 49% when the tumor was present outside the ovary at the time of exploration (Stenwig et al. 1979). When only stage I tumors are considered, rupture is the major prognostic parameter, causing the 10-year survival rate to drop from 86% to 60% (Bjorkholm and Silfversward 1981). Microscopic features have not been very helpful prognostically in the experience of most investigators but two groups have found tumors with low-grade nuclear atypia to have a better prognosis than those with high-grade atypia (STENWIG et al. 1979; BJORKHOLM and SILFVERSWARD 1981).

### 2.1.2 Juvenile Granulosa Cell Tumor

Juvenile granulosa cell tumors occur within the first two decades in almost 80% of the cases and within the first three decades in 97% of the cases (YOUNG et al. 1984a). In prepubertal girls they typically result in isosexual pseudoprecocity (LACK et al. 1981; ZALOUDEK and NORRIS 1982; YOUNG et al. 1984a), accounting for 5%–10% of cases of sexual precocity in the female. In these cases breast development is followed by the appearance of pubic and axillary hair, stimulation and enlargement of the external and internal secondary sex organs, irregular uterine bleeding, and a whitish vaginal discharge. Somatic and skeletal development are typically also accelerated. In addition to growth of public and axillary hair, androgenic manifestations such as clitoromegaly may occur.

When the juvenile granulosa cell tumor occurs after normal puberty it usually presents with abdominal pain or swelling, and sometimes is associated with menometrorrhagia or amenorrhea. Approximately 6% of the patients present with acute abdominal symptoms due to rupture of the tumor and hemoperitoneum. An interesting clinical association of the juvenile granulosa cell tumor has been its occurrence in occasional patients with Ollier's disease (enchondromatosis) or Maffucci's syndrome (enchondromatosis and hemangiomatosis) (YOUNG et al. 1984a).

The juvenile granulosa cell tumor is bilateral in only about 2% of the cases. It appears ruptured at operation in approximately 10% of the cases, and ascites is present in a similar percentage. Spread beyond the ovary is unusual; in our series of 125 cases only three tumors were stage II (YOUNG et al. 1984a) and we have subsequently seen a single stage III tumor with omental spread. The diameter of the tumor has ranged from 3.0 cm to 32.0 cm with an average of 12.5 cm. Because of the usual moderate to large size of the tumor, an adnexal mass is almost always detectable clinically. Rarely, however, a mass has not been palpable preoperatively on bimanual rectal examination.

The range of gross appearances of the juvenile granulosa cell tumor is similar to that of the adult form. The single most common presentation is as a solid and cystic neoplasm (Fig. 2), in which the cysts may contain hemorrhagic fluid. Uniformly solid and uniformly cystic neoplasms are also encountered; the latter may be multilocular or rarely, unilocular. The solid component is typically yellow-tan or gray, and occasionally exhibits extensive necrosis, hemorrhage, or both.

Microscopic examination typically reveals a predominantly solid cellular tumor with focal follicle formation (Fig. 3), but occasionally a uniformly solid or uniformly follicular pattern is seen. In the solid areas the neoplastic cells may be arranged diffusely or as multiple nodules of various sizes; occasionally small clusters of tumor cells are present in a fibrous stroma. In the solid foci granulosa

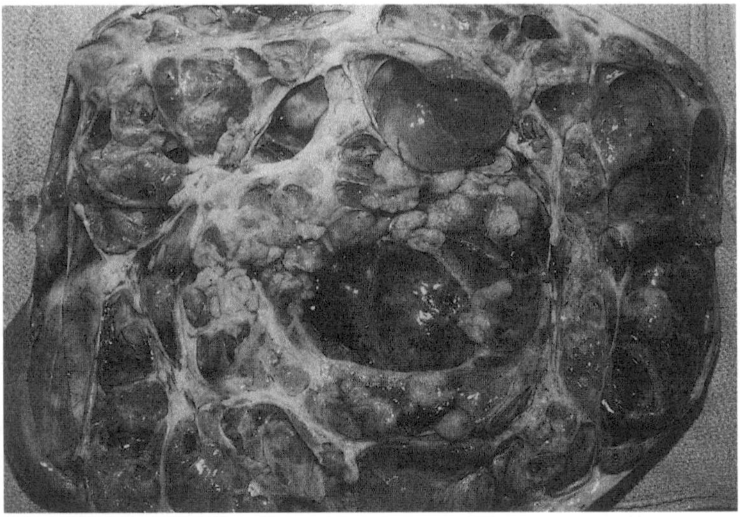

**Fig. 2.** Juvenile granulosa cell tumor. The sectioned surface has a variegated solid and cystic appearance

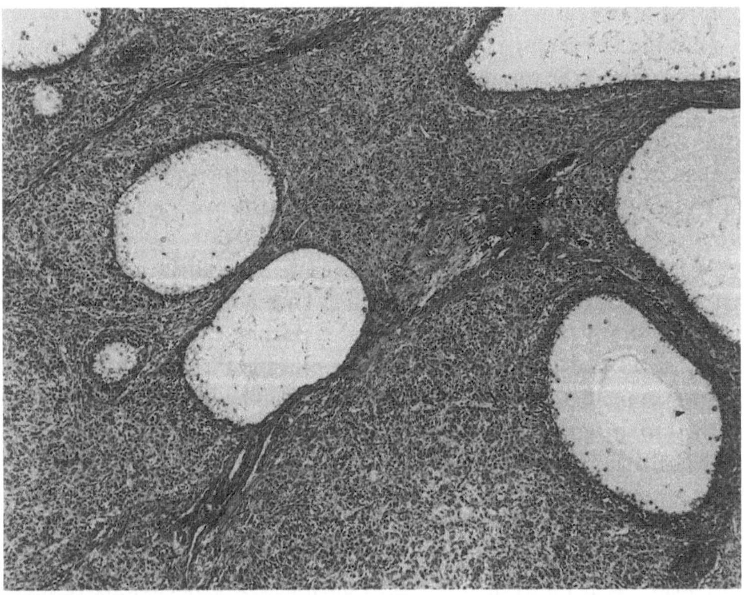

**Fig. 3.** Juvenile granulosa cell tumor. Follicles are present in an otherwise solid tumor. H&E, × 64

cells usually predominate over theca cells but in some areas the latter may predominate. Occasionally the two cells types are admixed in a haphazard fashion; in such areas the reticulin fibril distribution may aid in their differentiation. Foci resembling typical thecoma with hyaline bands are encountered rarely, but are usually minor in extent. Areas of sclerosis and calcification may also be seen.

The follicles typically vary in size and shape but may be regular and round to oval (Fig. 3); microfollicles (Call–Exner bodies) are rarely encountered, and the follicles rarely reach the large size of those in the macrofollicular adult granulosa cell tumor. The follicular lumens in the juvenile tumor contain eosinophilic or basophilic fluid, which stains with mucicarmine in approximately two-thirds of the cases. Layers of granulosa cells of varying thickness line the follicles and may be surrounded by mantles of theca cells; more often, however, the follicular granulosa cells blend with those in the intervening diffusely cellular areas. Rarely, the lining cells resemble hobnail cells.

The two characteristic cytologic features of the neoplastic granulosa cells that distinguish them from those of the adult granulosa cell tumor are their generally rounded, hyperchromatic nuclei, which almost always lack grooves (Fig. 4), and their almost invariable moderate to abundant eosinophilic or vacuolated (luteinized) cytoplasm. The theca cell component of the tumors is also usually luteinized, and lipid stains typically disclose moderate to large amounts of lipid within the cytoplasm of both cell types. The theca cells are more often spindle shaped than the granulosa cells, and, like the latter, usually contain hyperchromatic nuclei.

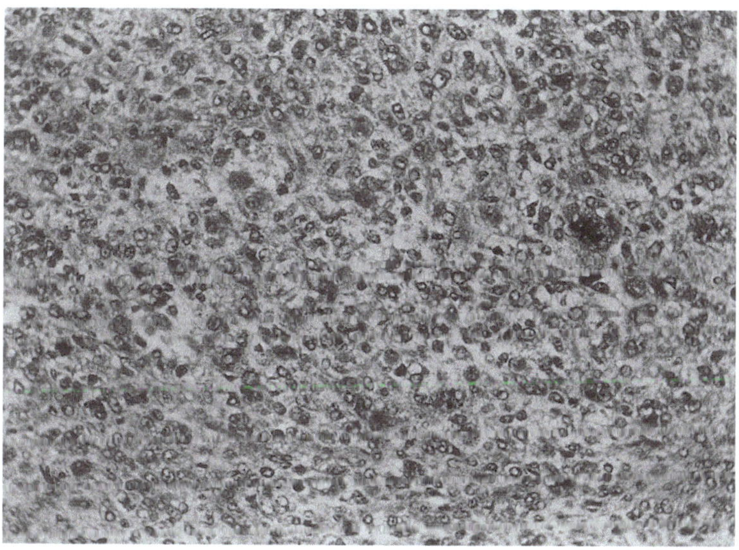

**Fig. 4.** Juvenile granulosa cell tumor. The neoplastic cells have immature nuclei without grooves. Two mitotic figures, one of them atypical, are present. H&E, × 200

Nuclear atypicality in juvenile granulosa cell tumors varies from minimal to marked; in approximately 13% of the cases severe degrees are present. The mitotic rate also varies greatly but is generally higher than that seen in adult granulosa cell tumors, often being 5 or more per 10 high power fields (Young et al. 1984a; Zaloudek and Norris 1982).

The differential diagnosis of the juvenile granulosa cell tumor includes the adult granulosa cell tumor and a wide variety of other ovarian neoplasms. The distinctive appearance of the follicles and the rarity of Call–Exner bodies in juvenile granulosa cell tumors, their cytologic features, i.e., dark, round, ungrooved nuclei and luteinized cytoplasm, and their usual content of mucin in the follicular lumens almost always enable one to distinguish these tumors from the adult granulosa cell tumor. A tumor of one type, however, occasionally has minor foci more characteristic of the other type and an extremely rare specimen contains sizable components of both tumor types. When the juvenile granulosa cell tumor is characterized by moderate to severe nuclear atypicality it may be mistaken for a yolk sac tumor or the exceptionally rare embryonal carcinoma, which may also cause isosexual pseudoprecocity by producing chorionic gonadotropin (hCG). Rarely, the diagnosis of yolk sac tumor is further suggested by the presence of hyaline bodies in a juvenile granulosa cell tumor. The variety of patterns seen in yolk sac tumors, i.e., reticular, endodermal sinus with Schiller–Duval bodies, papillary, and polyvesicular, and embryonal carcinomas, i.e., glandular and papillary, is not enountered in juvenile granulosa cell tumors, nor are the follicular patterns of the latter present in the germ cell tumors. The nuclei of a juvenile granulosa cell tumor, although occasionally having highly malignant characteristics, generally lack the primitive appearance of those of a yolk sac tumor or embryonal carcinoma. Also, very large, hyperchromatic, pleomorphic nuclei, although uncommon, are observed more frequently in juvenile granulosa cell tumors than in malignant germ cell tumors. Hyaline bodies, although a common feature of yolk sac tumors, are not specific and have been observed rarely to frequently in a wide variety of other ovarian tumors of diverse types. Finally, the characteristic immunohistochemical staining of yolk sac tumors for α-fetoprotein and of embryonal carcinomas for hCG has not been demonstrated in juvenile granulosa cell tumors.

The young age at which the small cell carcinoma occurs and its content of follicle-like structures often leads to a misdiagnosis of juvenile granulosa cell tumor. The follicles of the former, however, are typically round and contain eosinophilic fluid that does not stain for mucicarmine. The solid areas of the tumor are usually characterized by a monotonous proliferation of uniformly small cells that typically have scanty cytoplasm; in a minority of the tumors, there are similarly monotonous foci of cells with abundant eosinophilic cytoplasm. Finally, two-thirds of small cell carcinomas are associated with paraendocrine hypercalcemia, which has not been a feature of juvenile granulosa cell tumors.

The juvenile granulosa cell tumor is sometimes misinterpreted as a thecoma because of the occasional absence or rarity of follicles, the typically abundant cytoplasm of the neoplastic cells, and the occasional predominance of theca cells. Thorough sampling to demonstrate follicles and the performance of reticulum stains to help identify granulosa cells are important in establishing the correct diagnosis. Also, thecomas almost always lack significant mitotic activity, occur before 30 years of age in less than 10% of the cases, and rarely, if ever, occur in children. Focal nodular sclerosis is present in occasional juvenile granulosa cell tumors but the diagnosis of a sclerosing stromal tumor is rarely a serious consideration in differential diagnosis. Rarely a diffuse juvenile granulosa cell tumor with marked luteinization suggests the diagnosis of a steroid cell tumor but the former lacks the monotonous proliferation of uniform cells with central nuclei and generally single, prominent nucleoli of the latter.

The only surface epithelial tumors with which juvenile granulosa cell tumors might be confused are the clear cell carcinoma and the undifferentiated carcinoma. The tubulocystic variant of the clear cell carcinoma may be suggested by the occasional lining of follicles of a juvenile granulosa cell tumor by hobnail cells. The young age of the patient, the presence of follicles, and focal presence of more characteristic areas of juvenile granulosa cell tumors as well as the absence of other features of clear cell carcinoma should facilitate the differential diagnosis. Similar features of the juvenile granulosa cell tumor should also eliminate the possibility of undifferentiated carcinoma.

The granulosa cell tumor that is characterized by considerable nuclear atypicality may be confused with malignant melanoma involving the ovary, particularly when the latter is characterized by cells with abundant cytoplasm and the formation of spaces simulating follicles (Young and Scully 1991). The presence of melanin granules and intranuclear cytoplasmic inclusions suggests melanoma and staining for melanin granules or HMB-45 confirm the diagnosis. Staining for S-100 protein is not decisive since one-third of juvenile granulosa cell tumors are positive for this antigen (Aguirre et al. 1989b).

## 2.2 Thecomas and Related Tumors

### *2.2.1 Typical Thecoma*

Thecomas are approximately one-third as common as granulosa cell tumors and occur at an older average age, rarely if ever appearing prior to puberty. In one large series 84% of the patients were postmenopausal, with a mean age of 59 years; only 10% of the patients were under 30 years of age (Bjorkholm and Silfverswärd 1980). In the same series 60% of the postmenopausal women presented because of uterine bleeding and 21% of the patients had endometrial carcinoma.

Thecomas range from small, impalpable tumors to large, solid masses; most of them are 5–10 cm in diameter. Sectioning typically discloses a solid yellow mass, but in some cases the tumor is white with only focal tinges of yellow; cysts and foci of hemorrhage and necrosis are uncommon. Microscopic examination reveals masses of cells, most of which are ill-defined and oval or rounded; the cytoplasm is pale and vacuolated, containing moderate to large amounts of lipid. The nuclei vary from round to spindle-shaped and exhibit little or no atypia; mitotic figures are generally absent or infrequent. Hyaline plaques are often conspicuous. Thecomas have an excellent prognosis, but exceptionally a tumor that exhibits conspicuous mitotic activity and nuclear atypicality pursues a malignant course (WAXMAN et al. 1979). Very rare thecomas contain a minor component of sex cord cells in which case the designation "thecoma with minor sex cord elements" is recommended (YOUNG and SCULLY 1983c).

The differentiation of a thecoma from a fibroma is necessarily arbitrary since the ovarian stromal cell, which gives rise to both tumors, has the potential to form fibroblasts, and by metaplasia, myofibroblasts, smooth muscle cells, and fat cells, as well as hormone-secreting theca internal cells. It would be surprising, therefore, if stromal neoplasms in addition to including pure fibromas or pure thecomas did not also include a category of tumors with intermediate or mixed features. We arbitrarily include in the category of thecoma those tumors that are composed to a large extent of cells with moderate to large amounts of cytoplasmic lipid as well as those associated with clinical or laboratory evidence of steroid hormone secretion, and we diagnose fibroma when the tumor is composed exclusively or almost exclusively of spindle cells producing collagen and containing no more than small amounts of cytoplasmic lipid. Tumors with intermediate or combined features are categorized as tumors in the thecoma–fibroma group, unclassified. In the future hormonal enzyme immunohistochemistry may prove a valuable aid in differential diagnosis, but sections stained routinely and for lipid will probably remain the basis for differential diagnosis for some time.

### *2.2.2 Luteinized Thecoma*

Tumors that are predominantly fibromatous or thecomatous but also contain collections of steroid-type cells (Fig. 5) resembling luteinized theca and stromal cells are called luteinized thecomas (ZHANG et al. 1982; ROTH and STERNBERG 1983). When luteinization is extensive, areas of the tumor may resemble a steroid cell tumor (HUGHESDON 1983). In one series of 46 luteinized thecomas, half of them were estrogenic, 39% were nonfunctioning, and 11% were androgenic (ZHANG et al. 1982). This relatively high frequency of masculinization contrasts with its great rarity in association with nonluteinized thecomas. Luteinized thecomas also occur in a younger age group than typical thecomas; although they are most frequent in postmenopausal women 30% of them have been enountered in patients under 30 years of age. When, on rare occasions, crystals of Reinke are identified in the steroid-type cells, the term "stromal Leydig cell tumor" is appropriate. Only seven such tumors have been reported; three of them caused virilization (STERNBERG and ROTH 1973; ZHANG et al. 1982;

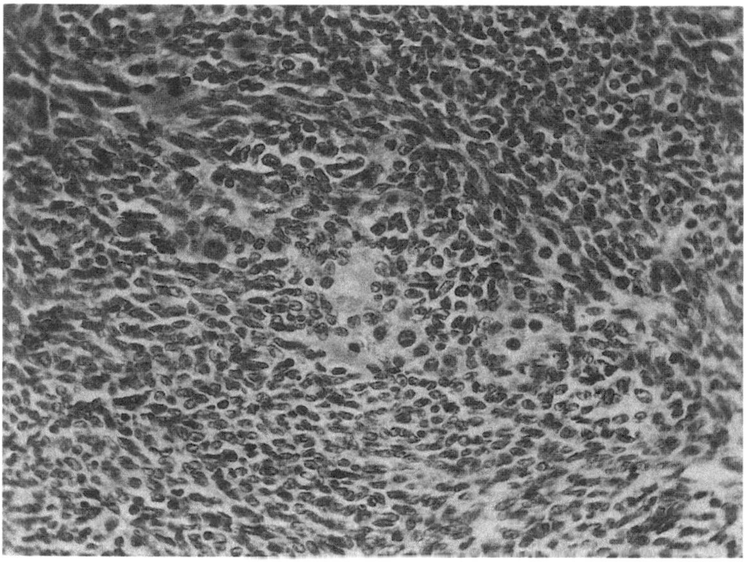

**Fig. 5.** Cellular luteinzed thecoma. Several nests of lutein cells are present on the background of a cellular fibroma. H&E, × 313

PAOLETTI et al. 1987). Rare luteinized thecomas have been malignant (ZHANG et al. 1982).

### *2.2.3 Sclerosing Stromal Tumor*

Sclerosing stromal tumor was included within the unclassified category of stromal tumors in the 1973 WHO classification (SEROV et al. 1973), but has subsequently been established as a distinct entity (CHALVARDJIAN and SCULLY 1973). Over 80% of these tumors have been encountered during the second and third decades, with an average age of 27 years (YOUNG and SCULLY 1982). In contrast to the thecoma, the sclerosing stromal tumor has been associated with evidence of estrogen secretion in only a few cases; androgenic manifestations have been present rarely. All the sclerosing stromal tumors encountered to date have been unilateral and benign.

Gross examination reveals a well-demarcated mass ranging from 1.5 to 17 cm in diameter. Its sectioned surface is basically solid and white but often shows areas of edema and cyst formation and contains yellow foci of varying extents (Fig. 6). A rare tumor is a unilocular cyst. Microscopic examination discloses a number of distinctive features: a pseudolobular pattern (Fig. 7) in which cellular nodules are separated by less cellular areas of densely collagenous or edematous connective tissue; sclerosis within the nodules; prominent thin-walled vessels in some of the nodules, the presence of which has occasionally

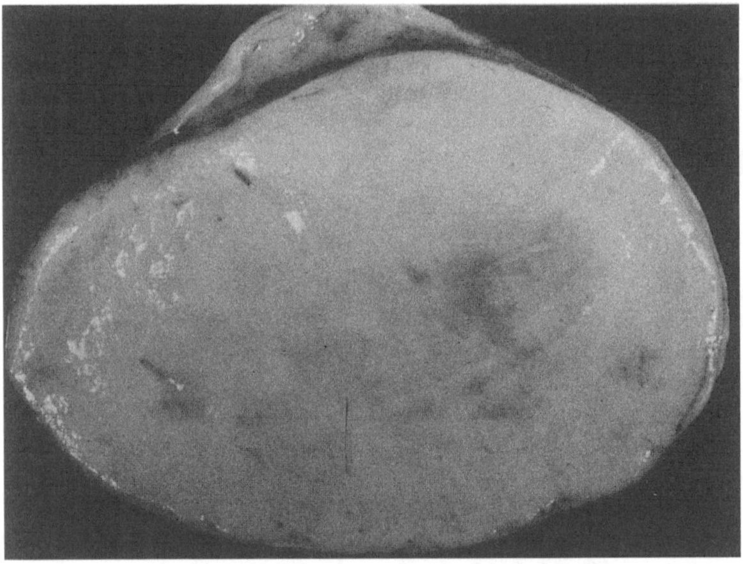

**Fig. 6.** Sclerosing stromal tumor. The sectioned surface of the neoplasm is solid; irregular, gray foci of edema are present

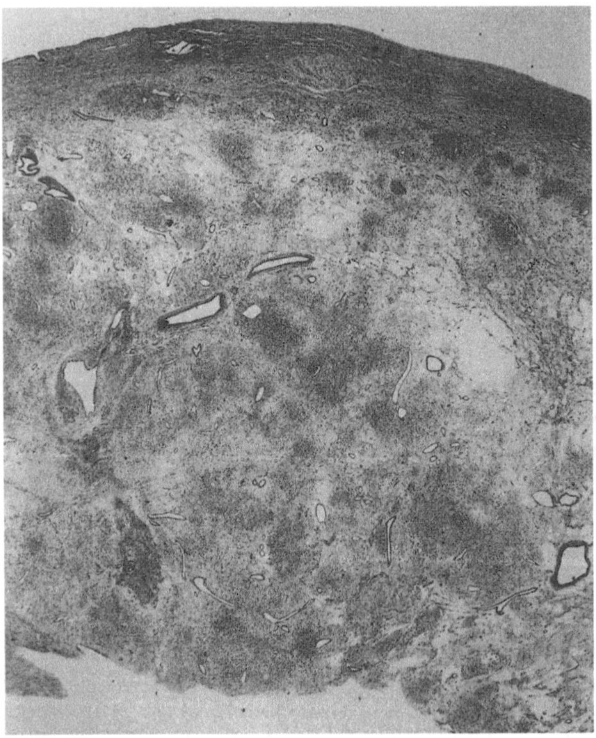

**Fig. 7.** Sclerosing stromal tumor. Cellular pseudolobules are separated by edematous hypocellular tissue. (CHALVARDJIAN and SCULLY 1973). H&E, × 13

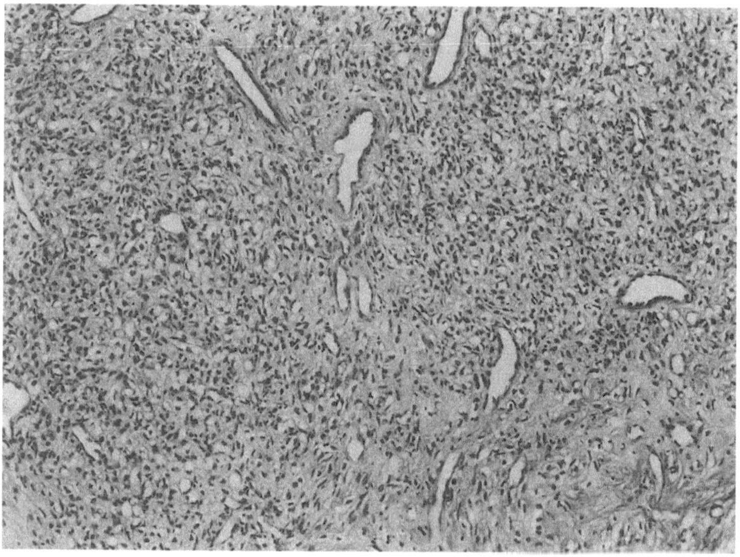

**Fig. 8.** Sclerosing stromal tumor. Characteristic features are sclerosis, ectatic blood vessels, and a dual cell population of fibroblasts and luteinized cells. H&E, × 125

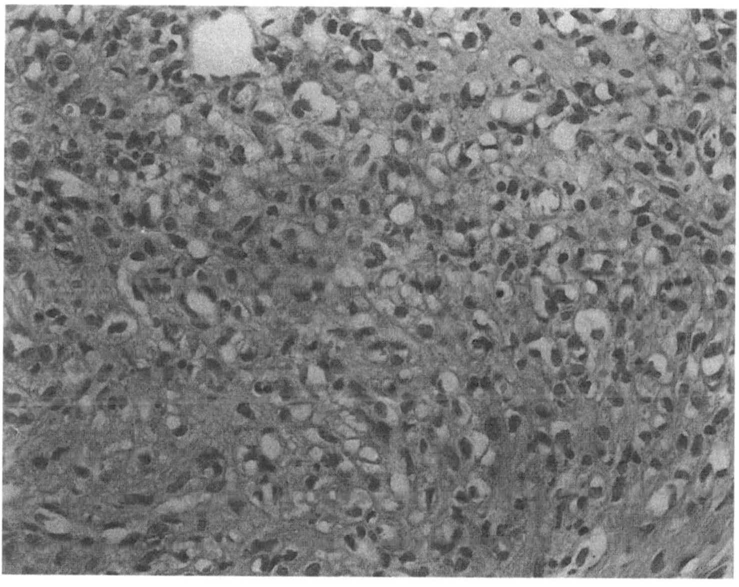

**Fig. 9.** Sclerosing stromal tumor. Luteinized cells are prominently vacuolated and some of them simulate signet ring cells. H&E, × 313

led to a misdiagnosis of hemangiopericytoma; and a disorganized admixture of fibroblasts and rounded, vacuolated cells with shrunken nuclei within the nodules (Fig. 8). Occasionally, the vacuolated cells have a signet cell appearance (Fig. 9), creating some confusion with the signet cells of a Krukenberg tumor, but the former cells contain lipid instead of mucin. The lipid-laden cells appear to be inactive or weakly active lutein cells; in the rare functioning tumors the lutein cells resemble more closely those encountered in a luteinized thecoma.

## 2.3 Sertoli–Stromal Cell Tumors

### *2.3.1 Sertoli Cell Tumors*

Sertoli cell tumors account for approximately 4% of Sertoli–stromal cell tumors (YOUNG and SCULLY 1984b). Seven of them, most or all of which appear to have been of the lipid-rich type, have resulted in isosexual pseudoprecocity. Two of these tumors were from patients with the Peutz-Jeghers syndrome (SOLH et al. 1983). One Sertoli cell tumor was associated with progesterone as well as estrogen production (TRACY et al. 1985). All the Sertoli cell tumors encountered to date have been stage IA. They have averaged 9 cm in diameter and typically formed lobulated, solid, yellow or brown masses. Microscopic examination discloses a predominant pattern of hollow or solid tubules, usually dispersed within a fibrous stroma that contains no Leydig cells or very few of them. When the Sertoli cells contain abundant cytoplasmic lipid the term lipid-rich Sertoli cell tumor has been used. Tumors of this type may have areas with a diffuse pattern resembling that of a lipid-rich steroid cell tumor, but the other areas of solid tubular differentiation establish the diagnosis. There is usually little, if any, nuclear atypia or mitotic activity, and the prognosis is usually excellent. Rare tumors exhibiting moderate nuclear atypicality have been reported, however, and one tumor in a sexually precocious child was focally poorly differentiated, metastasized distantly, and was rapidly fatal (YOUNG and SCULLY 1984b).

### *2.3.2 Sertoli–Leydig Cell Tumors*

Sertoli–Leydig cell tumors account for almost all Sertoli–stromal cell tumors, but for less than 0.5% of all ovarian tumors. They are now divided into five categories: well-differentiated, of intermediate differentiation, poorly differentiated, with heterologous elements, and retiform, but admixtures of these patterns also occur. Sertoli–Leydig cell tumors are found in all age groups but are encountered most often in young women, with an average age of 25 years; 75% of the patients are 30 years of age or younger and only approximately 10% are over 50 years of age (YOUNG and SCULLY 1985). The well-differentiated tumors occur on average a decade later than Sertoli–Leydig cell tumors in general and tumors with a retiform pattern are encountered on average a decade earlier, occurring more commonly in the first decade than any other subtype.

Although the most striking mode of presentation of Sertoli–Leydig cell tumors is virilization, it develops in only about one-third of the cases. In such cases a patient who has been having normal periods typically begins to have oligomenorrhea, followed within a few months by amenorrhea. There is a concomitant loss of female secondary sex characteristics, with atrophy of the breasts and disappearance of female bodily contours. Progressive masculinization is heralded by acne, with hirsutism, temporal balding, deepening of the voice, and enlargement of the clitoris following in its wake. The androgen secretion by the tumor may also result in erythrocytosis. There was no significant difference in the frequency of androgenic manifestations among the various subtypes in one large series except that it was lower in patients with tumors containing heterologous elements and lowest in those with tumors having a prominent retiform component (Young and Scully 1985). After the removal of a virilizing Sertoli–Leydig cell tumor, normal menses characteristically resume in about 4 weeks. The excessive hair almost always diminishes to some extent, but clitoromegaly and deepening of the voice are less apt to regress.

Most patients with Sertoli–Leydig cell tumors have no endocrine manifestations, and usually complain of abdominal swelling or pain. Occasional tumors have been associated with various estrogenic syndromes, including irregular menses, menorrhagia, or menometrorrhagia in women in the reproductive age group, and postmenopausal bleeding in older women. No well-documented case of a Sertoli–Leydig cell tumors associated with isosexual pseudoprecocity has been reported.

Virilizing Sertoli–Leydig cell tumors are typically associated with increased levels in the plasma of testosterone but weaker androgens may also be present in increased amounts. Twenty-one Sertoli–Leydig cell tumors have been associated with elevated plasma levels of α-fetoprotein, but values as high as those accompanying yolk sac tumors are rare (Gagnon et al. 1989).

Sertoli–Leydig cell tumors are stage Iai in about 80% of the cases; in 12% the tumor has either ruptured or involved the external surface of the ovary and 1%–2% are bilateral. Ascites is present in 4% of the cases. Only 2%–3% of the tumors have spread beyond the ovary at the time of operation, usually within the pelvis and rarely in the upper abdomen. All the well-differentiated tumors in one large series were stage Iai; the poorly differentiated tumors were more often ruptured or presented at a higher stage than the tumors of intermediate differentiation (Young and Scully 1985).

Sertoli–Leydig cell tumors vary as greatly in their gross appearance as granulosa cell tumors but contain cysts filled with blood less often, and almost never have the appearance of a unilocular thin-walled cyst. They vary in size from microscopic to huge masses but most of them are between 5 and 15 cm in diameter. Poorly differentiated tumors tend to be larger than those of better differentiation and contain areas of hemorrhage and necrosis more frequently.

Tumors with heterologous or retiform components are more often cystic than other tumors in this category. The heterologous tumors occasionally simulate mucinous cystic tumors on gross examination and retiform tumors may contain large, edematous intracystic papillae, resembling serous papillary tumors or may be soft and spongy with interspersed cysts (YOUNG and SCULLY 1983a).

Well-differentiated Sertoli–Leydig cell tumors are characterized by a predominantly tubular pattern (YOUNG and SCULLY 1984d). On low-power examination a nodular architecture is often conspicuous, with fibrous bands intersecting lobules composed of hollow or less often solid tubules; in some tumors tubules of both types are present. The hollow tubules are typically round to oval and small, but are occasionally large, resembling the tubular glands of a well-differentiated endometrioid adenocarcinoma (DARDI et al. 1982), and rarely are cystically dilated. The lumens are usually devoid of conspicuous secretion but in some cases eosinophilic fluid, which is occasionally mucicarminophilic, is present. The solid tubules are typically elongated but may be round or oval, and may resemble prepubertal or atrophic testicular tubules. The Sertoli cells are cuboidal to columnar and contain round or oblong nuclei without prominent nucleoli. Nuclear atypicality is usually absent or minimal and mitotic figures are rare. The cells lining the hollow tubules and filling the solid tubules typically contain moderate amounts of dense cytoplasm, but in some cases varying numbers of them have abundant pale cytoplasm rich in lipid. The stroma consists of nests or diffuse masses of Leydig cells, which may contain abundant fat or lipochrome pigment; crystals of Reinke are identified in some of the Leydig cells in approximately 20% of the cases (YOUNG and SCULLY 1984d).

Sertoli–Leydig cell tumors of intermediate and poor differentiation form a continuum characterized by a variety of patterns and combinations of cell types (YOUNG and SCULLY 1985). Some tumors exhibit intermediate differentiation in some areas and poor differentiation in others, and less commonly tumors of intermediate differentiation contain well-differentiated foci. Both the Sertoli cells and the Leydig cells may exhibit varying degrees of immaturity. In the tumors of intermediate differentiation, immature Sertoli cells have small, round, oval, or angular nuclei and generally scanty cytoplasm and are arranged typically in ill-defined masses, often creating a lobulated appearance on low power; solid and hollow tubules, nests, thin cords resembling the sex cords of the embryonic testis, and broad columns of Sertoli cells are often present. These structures are separated by stroma, which ranges from fibromatous to densely cellular to edematous, and typically contains clusters of well-differentiated Leydig cells. Cysts containing eosinophilic secretion may be present and create a thyroid-like appearance, and follicle-like spaces are encountered rarely. The Sertoli and Leydig cell elements, singly or in combination, may contain varying and sometimes large amounts of lipid in the form or small of large droplets. When a significant amount of the stromal component is made up of immature, cellular mesenchymal tissue with high mitotic activity resembling a nonspecific sarcoma, the tumor is considered poorly differentiated.

Fifteen percent of Sertoli–Leydig cell tumors have a retiform component (Fig. 10), and are so designated because they contain tubules and cysts, both of which may contain papillae, arranged in a pattern resembling that of the rete testis (YOUNG and SCULLY 1983a; ROTH et al. 1985; TALERMAN 1987). This pattern is usually accompanied by other patterns of Sertoli–Leydig cell tumor but sometimes an entire tumor has a retiform pattern. To date the retiform pattern has been encountered only in tumors that are otherwise intermediate, poorly differentiated, or heterologous. Microscopic examination reveals a network of irregularly branching, elongated, narrow, often slit-like tubules (Figs. 11–12) and cysts, into which papillae (Fig. 13) or polypoid structures may project. The tubules and cysts may contain eosinophilic secretion. They are lined by epithelial cells that exhibit varying degrees of stratification and nuclear atypicality. The papillae and polyps are of three types. Most commonly they are small and rounded, sometimes containing hyalinized cores (Fig. 13); sometimes they are large and bulbous, containing edematous cores; and finally, in some cases they are delicate and branch extensively and may be lined by stratified cells. The stroma within a retiform area is most commonly edematous but may be hyalinized, moderately cellular, or densely cellular and immature. Broad columns of epithelial cells, which are rare in other forms of Sertoli–Leydig cell tumor, are commonly encountered.

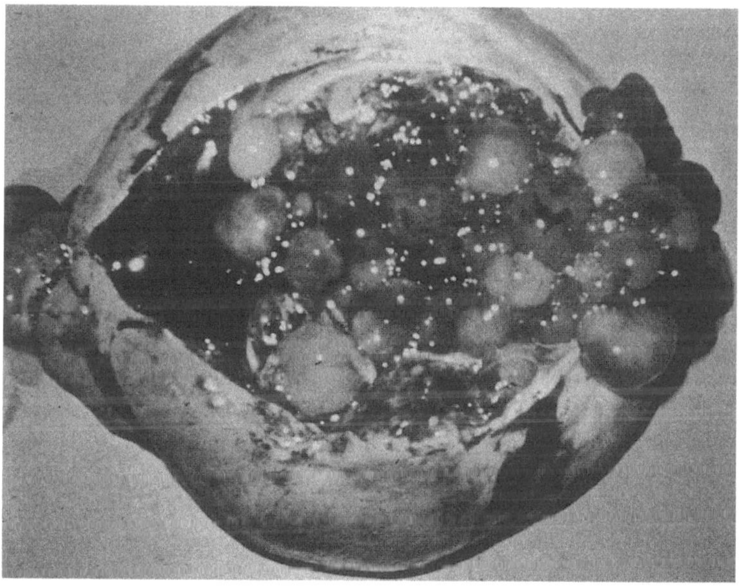

**Fig. 10.** Retiform Sertoli–Leydig cell tumor. The opened cyst contains numerous edematous polypoid structures projecting into its lumen. (YOUNG and SCULLY 1983a)

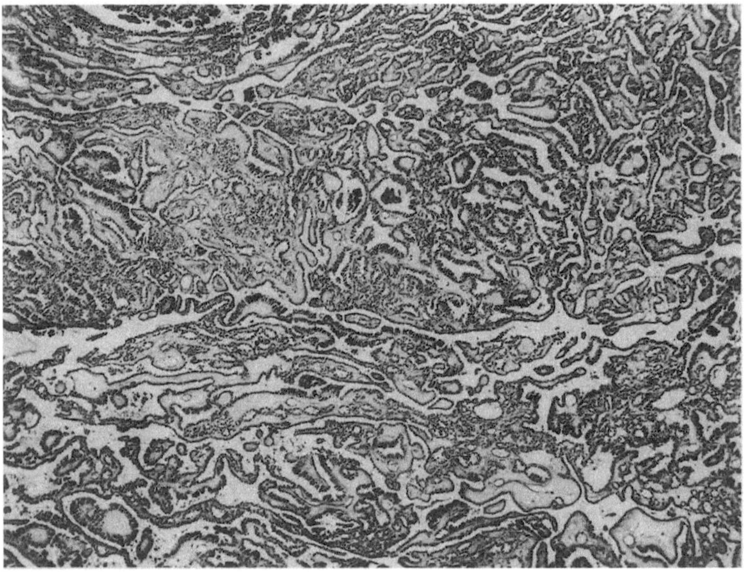

**Fig. 11.** Retiform Sertoli–Leydig cell tumor. There is a complex pattern of elongated tubules and papillae. H&E, × 64

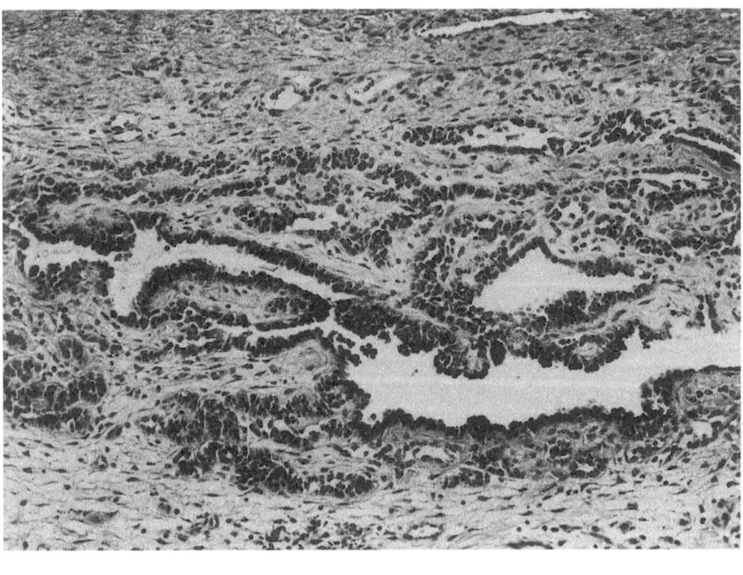

**Fig. 12.** Retiform Sertoli–Leydig cell tumor. Elongated retiform tubules are present adjacent to cords of immature Sertoli cells. H&E, × 160

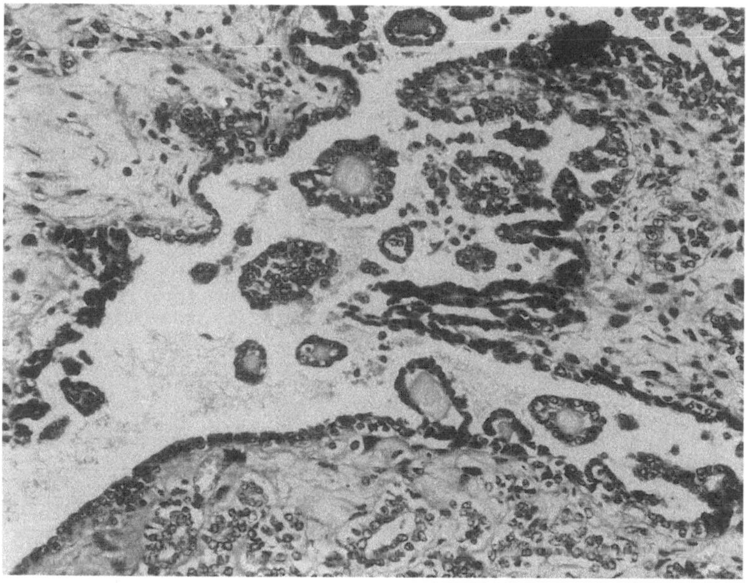

**Fig. 13.** Retiform Sertoli–Leydig cell tumor. Small papillae, some with hyalinized cores, project into a cyst lumen. H&E, × 256

Heterologous elements occur in approximately 20% of Sertoli–Leydig cell tumors (Fig. 14) (YOUNG et al. 1982b; WAXMAN et al. 1981; PRAT et al. 1982), most of which are otherwise of intermediate differentiation, but some of which are poorly differentiated or have a retiform pattern. In one large series of Sertoli–Leydig cell tumors, 18% contained glands and cysts lined by moderately to well-differentiated intestinal-type epithelium (Fig. 15), which included goblet cells, argentaffin cells, and rarely Paneth cells (YOUNG and SCULLY 1985). Sixteen percent of the heterologous Sertoli–Leydig cell tumors had one or a few microscopic foci of carcinoid. Mesenchymal heterologous elements, encountered in 5% of Sertoli–Leydig cell tumors, include islands of cartilage arising on a sarcomatous background, areas of embryonal rhabdomyosarcoma, or both (PRAT et al. 1982). One heterologous tumor contained cells resembling hepatocytes (YOUNG et al. 1984c), one has contained retinal tissue, and another had neuroblastoma in recurrent tumor (PRAT et al. 1982).

Because of their many patterns, Sertoli–Leydig cell tumors are often difficult to differentiate from tumors outside the sex cord–stromal category as well as from granulosa cell tumors (YOUNG and SCULLY 1982). The small hollow tubular structures and solid tubular aggregates, both of which may be lipid-rich, and cords that are occasionally seen in endometrioid carcinomas may closely mimic similar structures in Sertoli–Leydig cell tumors (ROTH et al. 1982; YOUNG et al. 1982a). The endometrioid tumors may also contain luteinized stromal cells

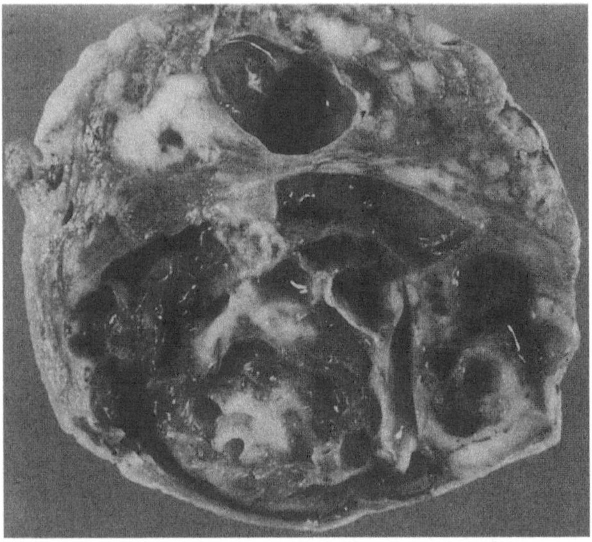

**Fig. 14.** Sertoli–Leydig cell tumor with heterologous elements. The sectioned surface has many cysts which were filled with mucinous fluid

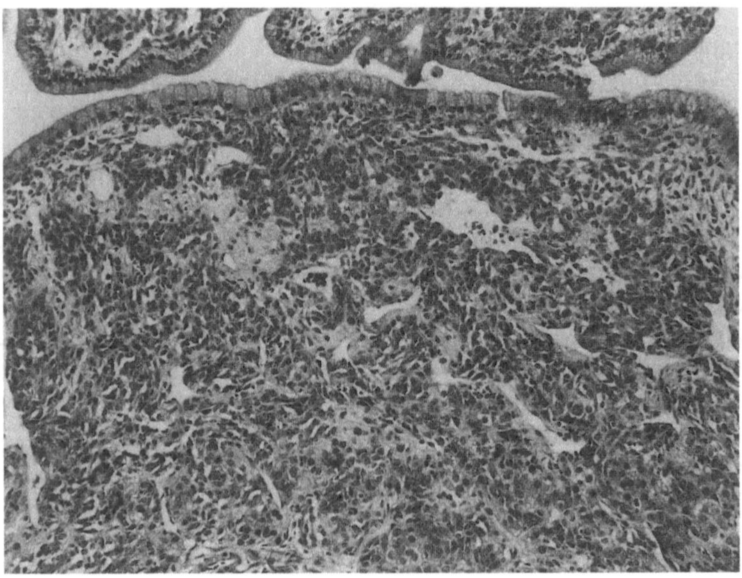

**Fig. 15.** Sertoli–Leydig cell tumor with heterologous elements. Two strips of benign-appearing mucinous epithelium line a cyst; the solid tissue is composed of immature Sertoli cell and Leydig cells. H&E, $\times$ 160

that resemble Leydig cells and be associated with androgenic or estrogenic manifestations, creating an even greater problem in differentiation. At least some of the glands of endometrioid carcinomas, however, are usually larger than the tubules of Sertoli–Leydig cell tumors and are lined by epithelium that is often less well differentiated. In addition, mucin secretion, areas of squamous differentiation that range from nests of uniform immature spindle-shaped epithelial cells to morules to keratinizing foci, and an adenofibromatous component of common epithelial type are present in many endometrioid carcinomas, facilitating their diagnosis. In rare cases immunohistochemistry may provide information that is of significant help diagnostically (AGUIRRE et al. 1989a). The cells of endometrioid adenocarcinomas are positive for epithelial membrane antigen and usually stain with a monoclonal antibody raised against an ovarian serous carcinoma, OM-1. Sertoli–Leydig cell tumors, in contrast, react only focally or weakly with these antibodies in occasional cases. Clinical features, such as the much older age of the patient and the almost invariable absence of androgenic manifestations, support the diagnosis of endometrioid carcinoma.

The tubular Krukenberg tumor (BULLON et al. 1981) may mimic a Sertoli–Leydig cell tumor especially if luteinization of the stroma is present; further confusion arises in the rare case in which the tumor is associated with virilization. Tubular Krukenberg tumors have been reported to be bilateral, however, in 50% of the cases and contain markedly atypical cells, including signet-ring cells that contain mucin, easily demonstrable by special stains.

Carcinoid tumors, especially those of the trabecular type, may be confused with intermediate Sertoli–Leydig cell tumors. The ribbons of the former, however, are longer, thicker, and more uniformly distributed than the sex cord-like formations of the latter. Also, rare carcinoid tumors with a solid tubular pattern can be difficult to distinguish from well-differentiated Sertoli cell tumors. Examination of the stroma of carcinoid tumors may be helpful in the differential diagnosis. It is typically less cellular and more fibromatous than that of Sertoli–Leydig cell tumors and does not contain Leydig cells. The most specific diagnostic criterion is the presence of argyrophil granules in almost all carcinoid tumors and of argentaffin granules in many of them; in contrast, only heterologous Sertoli–Leydig cell tumors with glands and cysts lined by gastrointestinal-type epithelium contain such granules. Finally, primary carcinoid tumors are associated with teratomatous elements in 70% of the cases, and metastatic carcinoids are almost always bilateral and are usually associated with a primary tumor of the intestine and metastases elsewhere in the abdomen.

The retiform variety of Sertoli–Leydig cell tumor causes specific problems in differential diagnosis. The most common misdiagnosis is yolk sac tumor, which is suggested clinically by the young age of the patient and pathologically by the presence of papillae within cystic spaces, which are mistaken for Schiller–Duval bodies. The association of androgenic manifestations with about one-quarter of retiform Sertoli–Leydig cell tumors, however, contrasts with their very rare association with yolk sac tumors that have a functioning stroma. On gross examination, the retiform tumors generally appear less malignant than yolk sac tumors and microscopic examination reveals less primitive appearing cells. The presence of other distinctive patterns of either tumor and immunohistochemical staining for α-fetoprotein in the yolk sac tumor almost always facilitate the diagnosis. A greater problem in differential diagnosis arises because of the characteristic papillary pattern and the frequent presence of cellular stratification on the papillae in retiform tumors, particularly if these features predominate in the specimen. Under such circumstances a misdiagnosis of a serous cystadenoma of borderline malignancy of a serous or endometrioid carcinoma may be made. A variety of clinical and pathologic features, including the young age of the patient, the occasional association with virilization, and the presence of other more easily recognizable patterns of Sertoli–Leydig cell tumor are helpful clues to the correct diagnosis. Finally, the juxtaposition of epithelial and immature mesenchymal elements in some retiform tumors has caused confusion with a malignant mesodermal mixed tumor, but the features outlined above also serve to exclude the latter diagnosis.

The prognosis of Sertoli–Leydig cell tumors is closely related to their stage and degree of differentiation. The rare tumors that present at a stage higher than I have a poor prognosis. The survival rates of patients with stage I tumors correlate with the degree of differentiation. In one large series of cases none of the well-differentiated tumors, 11% of those of intermediate differentiation, 59% of the poorly differentiated tumors, and 19% of those with heterologous elements were clinically malignant (YOUNG and SCULLY 1985). The homologous component of the tumor was poorly differentiated in all eight clinically malignant tumors in the heterologous category and in seven of them the heterologous elements included skeletal muscle, cartilage, or both. Other investigations have supported the findings in this series. The only clinically malignant tumor in the series of ROTH et al. (1981) was poorly differentiated, and 4 of the 20 poorly differentiated tumors reported by ZALOUDEK and NORRIS were malignant, in contrast to only one of the 44 tumors of intermediate differentiation and none of the seven well-differentiated tumors (ZALOUDEK and NORRIS 1984). In our experience the presence of a retiform pattern also had an adverse effect on the prognosis; 25% of stage I retiform tumors were malignant as opposed to only 10% of tumors of similar grade without a retiform component (YOUNG and SCULLY 1983a). In two other recent reports of retiform Sertoli–Leydig cell tumors metastases occurred in four of 15 patients and three of them died of their disease, suggesting a somewhat more aggressive behavior than nonretiform Sertoli–Leydig cell tumors (ROTH et al. 1985; TALERMAN 1987).

## 2.4 Sex Cord Tumor with Annular Tubules

This tumor is characterized by the presence of simple and complex annular tubules (SCULLY 1970; YOUNG et al. 1982c). The simple tubules have the shape of a ring, with the nuclei oriented around the periphery and around a central hyalinized body composed of basement membrane material; an intervening anuclear cytoplasmic zone forms the major component of the ring. The much more numerous complex tubules are rounded structures made up of intercommunicating rings revolving around multiple hyaline bodies (Fig. 16). Tumors containing annular tubules have been interpreted as Sertoli cell tumors by some observers and granulosa cell tumors by others (HART et al. 1980) but the pattern of growth has features intermediate between these two tumors and focal differentiation into both typical Sertoli cell tumor with elongated tubules and typical granulosa cell tumor with Call–Exner bodies in seen in some cases. Cells of Sertoli type have been identified ultrastructurally in some cases by the demonstration of Charcot–Bottcher filament bundles (TAVASSOLI and NORRIS 1980), which are considered specific cytoplasmic inclusions of Sertoli cells.

Sex cord tumors with annular tubules vary both clinically and pathologically depending on whether or not the patient has the Peutz–Jeghers syndrome (SCULLY 1970; YOUNG et al. 1982c). Almost all female patients with this syndrome whose ovaries have been examined microscopically have had sex cord tumorlets with annular tubules, which have been multifocal and bilateral in at least two-thirds of the cases; the largest reported lesion in a patient with this syndrome was 3 cm in diameter. Focal calcification has been seen in over half the cases. In almost all the patients the lesions have been incidental findings in

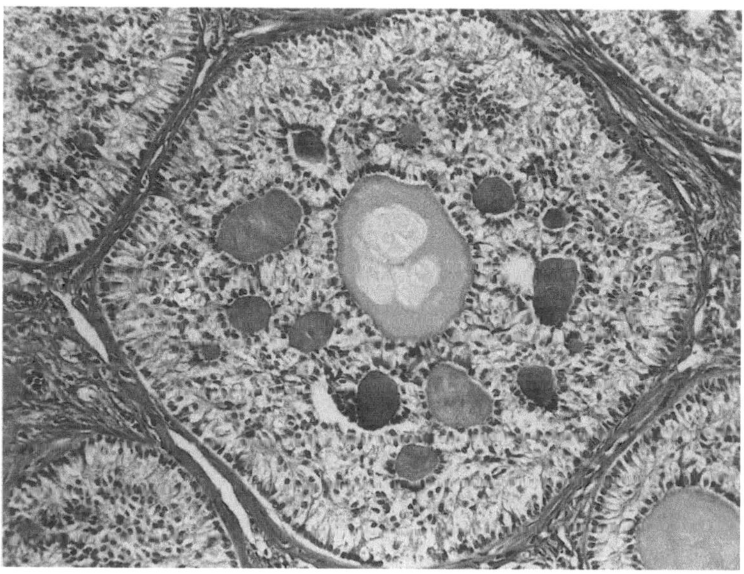

**Fig. 16.** Sex cord tumor with annular tubules. Complex annular tubules encircle rounded hyaline masses of basement membrane-like material. H&E, × 140

ovaries removed for other reasons. All the tumorlets associated with the Peutz–Jeghers syndrome have been benign, warranting conservative treatment.

In patients without the Peutz–Jeghers syndrome in contrast, the tumors are almost always unilateral and usually form palpable masses. Transitions to typical granulosa cell tumor and typical Sertoli cell tumor are much more common than in the lesions associated with the Peutz–Jeghers syndrome. Forty percent of the patients have had manifestations of estrogen secretion, and several have secreted progesterone. At least one-fifth of the tumors have been clinically malignant.

Four other ovarian tumors from girls with the Peutz–Jeghers syndrome have caused sexual precocity. Two of them, occurring in sisters, had the features of Sertoli cell tumor with lipid storage (SOLH et al. 1983), whereas the other two had unique microscopic features including diffuse areas, tubular differentiation, microcysts, and papillae, and the presence of two distinctive cell types, one containing abundant eosinophilic cytoplasm, and the other, scanty cytoplasm (YOUNG et al. 1983a). All four tumors appears to be clinically benign.

## 2.5 Sex Cord–Stromal Tumors, Unclassified

This ill-defined group of tumors, which accounts for less than 10% of those in the sex cord–stromal category, includes those in which a predominant pattern of testicular or ovarian differentiation is not clearly recognizable. The boundary lines between these tumors and those of ovarian and testicular cell types are vague because interpretations of intermediate patterns of growth and closely similar cell types are inevitably subjective. As discussed below, tumors from pregnant patients are particularly likely to be placed in this category.

TALERMAN and his associates (1982) segregated from within this category a group of tumors for which they proposed the designation "diffuse nonlobular androblastoma." The six ovarian tumors they reported were mostly estrogenic and had a predominant diffuse proliferation of cells resembling theca cells, granulosa cells, or both but also contained steroid cells in all the cases and tubules typical of Sertolic cell neoplasia in five of the six cases. Where to place these tumors in the schema of sex cord–stromal tumors is to a considerable extent subjective. The tumors we have seen that appear to be similar to those described by TALERMAN and his associates have looked significantly different from typical Sertoli–Leydig or granulosa cell tumors and we have usually placed them in the sex cord–stromal, unclassified category.

## 2.6 Sex Cord–Stromal Tumors During Pregnancy

Sex cord–stromal tumors may be particularly difficult to subclassify when they occur in pregnant patients because of alterations in their usual clinical and pathologic features (YOUNG et al. 1984b). Their nature is rarely suggested

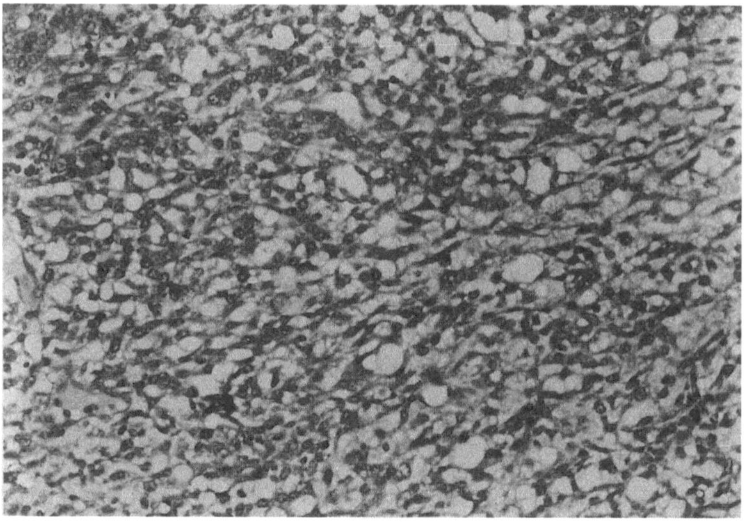

**Fig. 17.** Sex cord–stromal tumor, unclassified. This tumor from a pregnant patient has marked edema resulting in a reticular pattern. This pattern can be confused with that of a yolk sac tumor. H&E, ×200

clinically because during pregnancy estrogenic manifestations are not recognizable, and androgenic manifestations are rare, possibly because of the ability of the placenta to aromatize androgens to estrogens. Indeed, virilization of a pregnant patient is much more likely to be due to a nonneoplastic lesion such as a pregnancy luteoma or hyperreactio luteinalis or to a tumor with functioning stroma than to a sex cord–stromal tumor. In one study 17% of 36 sex cord–stromal tumors that were removed during pregnancy were placed in the unclassified group, and many of those that were classified in the granulosa cell or Sertoli–Leydig cell category had large areas with an indifferent appearance (YOUNG et al. 1984b). The features that led to difficulty in classification were the presence of prominent intercellular edema (Fig. 17), increased luteinization in the granulosa cell tumors, and marked degrees of Leydig cell maturation in one-third of the Sertoli–Leydig cell tumors. All of these changes, which were most common in tumors removed during the third trimester, tended to obscure the underlying architecture.

## 2.7 Immunohistochemistry of Sex Cord–Stromal Tumors

Relatively small numbers of sex cord–stromal tumors have been examined by immunohistochemical techniques. In one study 16 fibromas, 2 thecomas, and 12 granulosa cell tumors were positive for vimentin (Fig. 18) and negative for cytokeratin (MIETTINEN et al. 1985). A small number of tumors in these categories that were stained for desmin were negative. Subsequently, BENJAMIN and her colleagues showed that granulosa cell tumor express cytokeratins (Fig. 19) as well as vimentin (BENJAMIN et al. 1987). AGUIRRE et al. (1989b) have shown that Sertoli cell tumors and the Sertoli cell component of Sertoli–Leydig cell tumors as well as one-third to one-half of both adult and juvenile granulosa cell tumors are positive for one or more cytokeratins. Both types of granulosa cell tumor, however, are negative for epithelial membrane antigen and the serous carcinoma antigen OM-1, and Sertoli cell tumors are typically negative for these antigens or positive for them in only rare foci. Immunohistochemical staining for these two antigens may be helpful, therefore, in the differential diagnosis of sex cord–stromal tumors from surface epithelial stromal tumors since the latter are almost always positive for these antigens.

S-100 protein can be demonstrated immunohistochemically in approximately one-third of adult and juvenile granulosa cell tumors, and neuron-specific enolase in the majority of juvenile granulosa cell tumors (AGUIRRE et al. 1989b). Neither antigen has been identified in a small series of Sertoli cell tumor. Staining for these antigens, therefore, may not be helpful in the distinction of granulosa cell tumors from malignant melanoma or so-called neuroendocrine tumors, respectively.

The argyrophil cells of mucinous and carcinoid components of heterologous Sertoli–Leydig cell tumors have reacted for serotonin and one or more polypeptide hormones on immunohistochemical examination (AGUIRRE et al. 1986). In one Sertoli–Leydig cell tumor associated with elevated levels of α-fetoprotein in the serum, immunohistochemical staining for this antigen was localized in cells resembling liver cells within a heterologous tumor (YOUNG et al. 1984c); in other cases there has been staining of the Sertoli cell or the Leydig cell component of the neoplasm (YOUNG and SCULLY 1987a).

Two immunohistochemical approaches have been used to investigate the endocrine function of sex cord–stromal tumors and other steroid-hormone-producing tumors and nonneoplastic lesions of the ovary. The first technique was the usage of antibodies prepared against a variety of specific steroid hormones for immunohistochemical staining (KURMAN et al. 1978, 1979). Investigations of gonadal steroid-hormone-producing tumors with the use of this approach have yielded positive results (KURMAN et al. 1978, 1979; GAFFNEY et al. 1983) but have not been successful in identifying the cellular source of individual hormones for two main reasons: (a) cross-reactivity among the antibodies to the various hormones exists, and (b) a positive result does not differentiate between synthesis of the hormone by the cell and the existence of a receptor for the hormone within the cell. Thus, some of the results obtained have not been in keeping with modern concepts of cellular synthesis of various steroid hormones.

A much more promising approach to investigating the physiology of the normal ovary and the pathophysiology of steriod-hormone-producing tumors and nonneoplastic disorders of the ovary has been the immunohistochemical

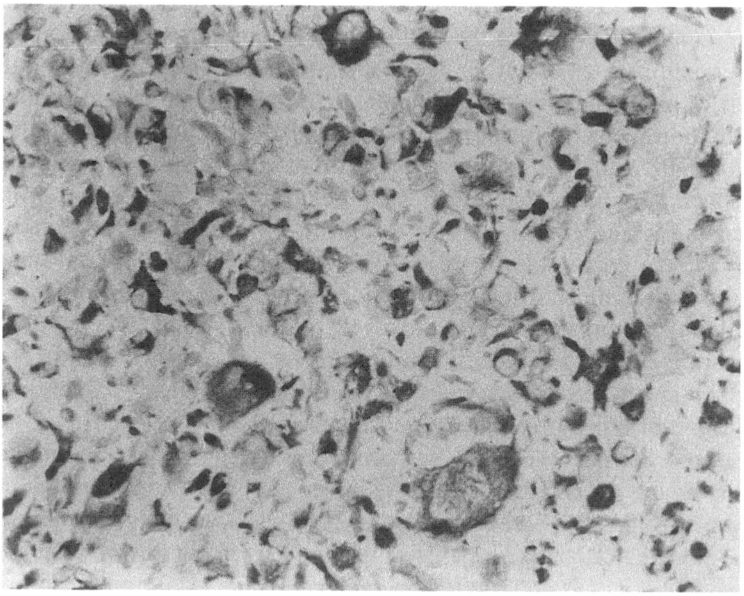

**Fig. 18.** Juvenile granulosa cell tumor. This tumor, which exhibited marked nuclear pleomorphism, has been stained by the immunohistochemical technique for vimentin. × 313

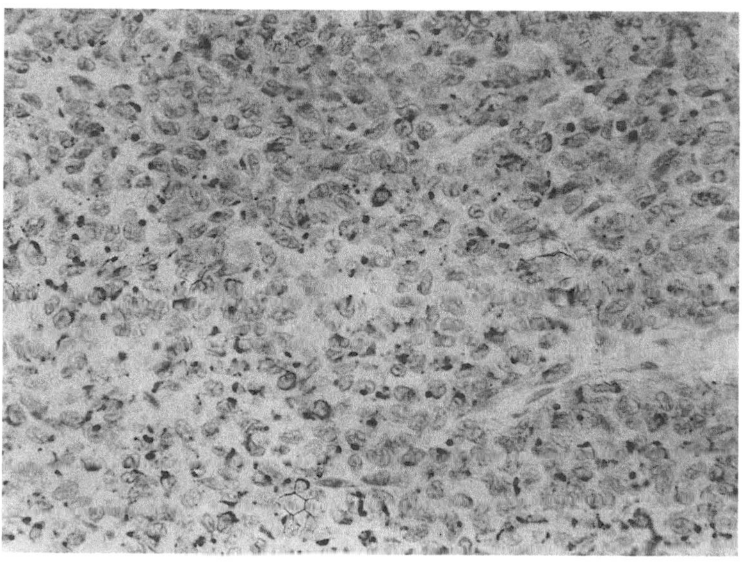

**Fig. 19.** Adult granulosa cell tumor. This tumor has been stained by the immunohistochemical technique for cytokeratin and shows the characteristic punctate pattern of cytoplasmic staining which one sees in this neoplasm. × 313

demonstration of the enzymes that convert cholesterol to pregnenolone and carry out interconversions among the various steroid hormones (SASANO et al. 1989). Using combinations of antibodies prepared against these enzymes, one can theoretically probe the range of enzymatic activity involved in the production of specific hormones by various ovarian cells. SASANO and SASANO (1989) and others have investigated a wide variety of ovarian lesions by enzyme immunohistochemistry with results that have been generally consonant with current concepts of the cellular sites of origin of various steroid hormones. Unfortunately, in the great majority of the cases studied, the findings have not been correlated with clinical or laboratory evidence of a hormonal disturbance. Such correlations may enhance the validity of the staining results; it is possible that quantification as well as identification of the various enzymes will prove necessary to obtain a close correlation between the immunohistochemical findings and those of clinical and laboratory investigation.

Neither steroid hormone nor enzyme immunohistochemical investigations have been carried out extensively on lesions other than those associated with steroid hormone production, and neoplastic cells of a variety of types contain steroid hormone receptors or are capable of limited enzymatic interconversion of various steroid hormones and, therefore, such cells may exhibit immunohistochemical staining similar to that of steroid-hormone-producing cells. Nevertheless, it appears highly probable that immunohistochemical staining for steroid hormones and their associated enzymes will prove of value in the differential diagnosis of various steroid-hormone-producing ovarian tumors and ovarian neoplasms without a functional potential.

## 3 Steroid Cell Tumors

The term "steroid cell tumor" is now applied to neoplasms that were formerly designated "adrenal rest tumor," "adrenal-like tumor," "masculinovoblastoma," "lipoid cell tumor," and "lipid cell tumor" (TAYLOR and NORRIS 1967). These neoplasms are composed entirely, or almost entirely, of cells resembling typical steroid-hormone-secreting cells, i.e., lutein cells, Leydig cells, and adrenocortical cells. The terms "lipoid cell tumor" and "lipid cell tumor" are inappropriate for these neoplasms since special staining has shown that 25% of them contain no intracellular fat.

Steroid cell tumors account for only 0.1% of all ovarian neoplasms. They are subclassified into three major categories: stromal luteoma, Leydig cell tumor (hilus cell tumor and Leydig cell tumor, nonhilar type), and steroid cell tumor, not otherwise specified (NOS) (HAYES and SCULLY 1987a).

### 3.1 Stromal Luteoma

Stromal luteomas account for approximately 25% of steroid cell tumors (HAYES and SCULLY 1987b). They are characterized by a location within the ovarian stroma and an absence of crystals of Reinke, which by definition would place the tumor in the Leydig cell group. Stromal luteomas are considered to arise from luteinized stromal cells or their precursors, the spindle cells of the ovarian stroma. This derivation is supported by the identification of luteinized stromal cells elsewhere in the same or contralateral ovary (stromal hyperthecosis) in 90% of the cases and the occurrence of a lesion intermediate between stromal hyperthecosis and the stromal luteoma, nodular hyperthecosis.

Eighty percent of stromal luteomas occur in postmenopausal women. Approximately two-thirds of these patients present with uterine bleeding presumably related to estrogen production by the tumor. About 10% of stromal luteomas are androgenic and the remainder are nonfunctioning, at least at a clinically detectable level.

On gross examination, the tumors are located within the ovarian stroma, and are almost always under 3 cm in diameter and unilateral. They are well circumscribed, solid, and usually gray-white or yellow, but they may have red or brown areas. Microscopic examination reveals an unencapsulated, rounded nodule composed of polyhedral cells arranged diffusely or in nests and cords. In 20% of the cases, foci of degeneration within aggregates of neoplastic cells result in the formation of spaces that may be elongated and slit-like or rounded; these

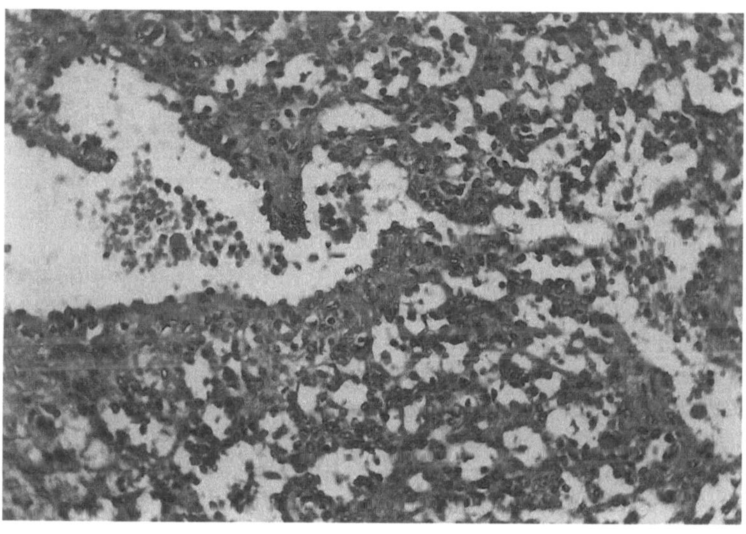

**Fig. 20.** Leydig cell tumor. This neoplasm shows extensive degeneration and simulates an adenocarcinoma or hemangiosarcoma. H&E, × 200

spaces, which may also be seen in other categories of steroid cell tumor (Fig. 20), are often misinterpreted as the acini of an epithelial tumor or the vascular lumens of a vascular neoplasm, but careful examination reveals their degenerative nature. The cytoplasm of the neoplastic cells is abundant and usually eosinophilic and slightly granular but occasionally it is pale or foamy; lipochrome granules are commonly present. The nuclei are typically small and round and contain single prominent nucleoli; mitotic figures are almost always absent or rare. The stroma is typically sparse, but in about 20% of the cases is more prominent and occasionally hyalinized. As noted above, stromal hyperthecosis is present in the stroma of one or both ovaries in 90% of the cases, and hilus cell hyperplasia is also seen in 25% of the cases (HAYES and SCULLY 1987b). All the reported cases have had a benign behavior, possibly related to their small size.

## 3.2 Leydig Cell Tumors

The Leydig cell nature of a steroid cell tumor is proven only by the finding of Reinke crystals on either light microscopic or electron microscopic examination. Almost all ovarian Leydig cell tumors arise in the hilus from hilar Leydig cells (hilus cells), which can be identified in over 80% of normal adult ovaries. Very rare Leydig cell tumors that are located within the ovarian stroma are referred to as Leydig cell tumors, non-hilar type.

Hilus cell tumors account for approximately 15% of steroid cell tumors and are usually encountered in postmenopausal patients (PARASKEVAS and SCULLY 1989). They are only rarely palpable. Androgenic manifestations are present in about 80% of the cases and sometimes have existed for many years prior to presentation; the androgenic changes are typically less abrupt in onset and milder than those associated with Sertoli–Leydig cell tumors. Estrogenic changes may also be present and can be attributed to: direct secretion of estrogen by the tumor, peripheral conversion to estrogen of androgen secreted by the tumor, associated stromal hyperthecosis, or a combination of these mechanisms. No convincing example of malignant hilus cell tumor has been reported.

Hilus cell tumors are typically reddish-brown to yellow but may be dark brown and almost black. They are characteristically small (mean diameter, 2.4 cm), circumscribed nodules centered in the ovarian hilus but many extend for varying distances into the ovarian stroma; very rare tumors are bilateral. Microscopic examination reveals an unencapsulated nodule composed of steroid cells usually growing diffusely but occasionally as nests or nodules separated by fibrous stroma. The tumor cells typically contain abundant granular eosinophilic cytoplasm; occasional cells have foamy cytoplasm suggesting the presence of lipid. Varying amounts of cytoplasmic lipochrome pigment are present in most cases. Perivascular nuclear clustering with abvascular pooling of cytoplasm or hyalinized stroma is present in half the cases. The round or angular nuclei are often hyperchromatic and contain single small nucleoli. The nuclei may exhibit some variation in size and shape but this feature is usually not marked; occasional multinucleated cells may be observed. Invagination of the cytoplasm into the nuclei may given them a hollow appearance. Rare mitotic figures are present in an occasional case. Elongated eosinophilic Reinke crystals of varying sizes are present in varying numbers but may require prolonged search for their identification. Special stains such as iron hematoxylin and trichrome stains may make these inclusions more conspicuous. On electron microscopic examination crystals of Reinke typically appear needle shaped when cut longitudinally and hexagonal when cut in cross-section. Intracytoplasmic spheres, which may be crystal precursors, are also typically present, but are not specific for the diagnosis of hilus cell tumor. Degenerative spaces similar to those seen in stromal luteomas may be present; sometimes the spaces contain cells with abundant spongy cytoplasm, and the stroma between the spaces may be prominent and fibrous. An unusual feature in one-third of the cases is fibrinoid change of vessel walls unassociated with an inflammatory infiltrate (Fig. 21). Stromal hyperthecosis, hilus cell hyperplasia, or both, are associated findings in occasional cases.

A diagnosis of crystal-negative or probable hilus cell tumor is made if a crystal-free hilar steroid cell tumor has one or more of the following features: a juxtaposition to nonmedullated nerve fibers like that of normal hilus cells, a background of hilus cell hyperplasia, perivascular nuclear clustering with

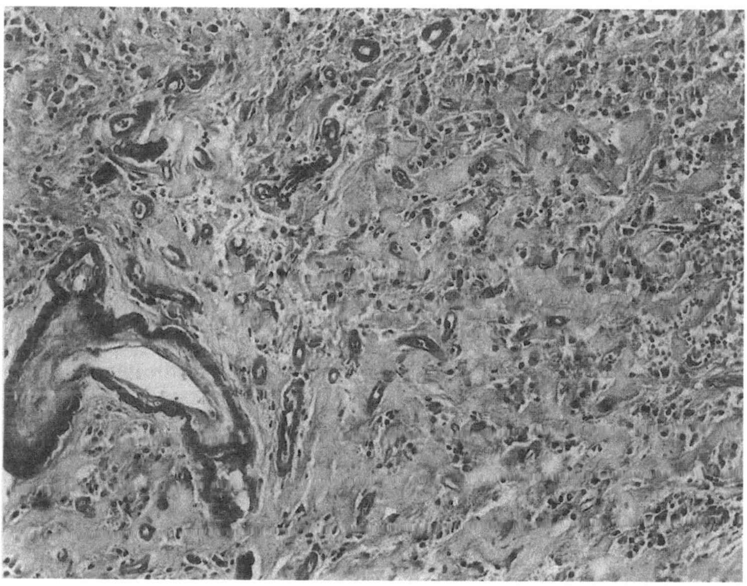

**Fig. 21.** Leydig cell tumor. Several blood vessels show fibrinoid change of their walls. H&E, × 125

intervening anuclear zones, and fibrinoid change of vessel walls (PARASKEVAS and SCULLY 1989).

Only four nonhilar Leydig cell tumors have been reported, and their features are similar to those of hilus cell tumors except for their location (ROTH and STERNBERG 1973). An ovarian stromal derivation of these tumors is supported by the finding of stromal Leydig cells with crystals of Reinke in rare otherwise typical cases of stromal hyperthecosis (STERNBERG and ROTH 1973).

### 3.3 Steroid Cell Tumor, Not Otherwise Specified

This neoplasm accounts for approximately 60% of steroid cell tumors. The patients are typically younger (mean age 43 years) than those with other forms of steroid cell tumor and occasional tumors occur in children, in whom they may cause heterosexual pseudoprecocity or less commonly isosexual pseudoprecocity (HAYES and SCULLY 1987a). Steroid cell tumors NOS are androgenic in about half of the cases. Eight percent of them are estrogenic and occasional examples are progestagenic. Four tumors have caused Cushing's syndrome, and three others have been accompanied by elevated cortisol levels without clinical manifestations of the syndrome (MARIEB et al. 1983; YOUNG and SCULLY 1987b). One tumor secreted aldosterone (KULKARNI et al. 1990). Hormone studies performed in patients with androgenic changes, Cushing's syndrome, or both typically show elevated urinary levels of 17-ketosteroids and 17-hydroxycorticosteroids as well as increased serum levels of testosterone and androstenedione. In 20% of the cases, extraovarian spread of tumor is apparent at the time of operation.

The tumors are typically solid, well circumscribed, and occasionally lobulated, and average 8.4 cm in diameter; approximately 5% of them are bilateral. They are typically yellow of orange but are occasionally red to brown or black. Necrosis, hemorrhage, and cystic degeneration are occasionally observed. On microscopic examination, the cells are typically arranged diffusely (Fig. 22) but occasionally they grow in nests, irregular clusters, thin cords (Fig. 23) and columns; a rich vascular network is usually evident. The stroma is inconspicuous in most cases but in approximately 15% of them it is relatively prominent. A minor fibromatous component or stromal hyalinization may be seen. Rarely, the stroma is edematous or myxoid (Fig. 23) with the tumor cells loosely dispersed within it. Necrosis and hemorrhage may be prominent, particularly in tumors that have significant cytologic atypia.

The polygonal to rounded tumor cells have distinct cell borders, central nuclei, and moderate to abundant amounts of cytoplasm that varies from eosinophilic and granular (lipid-free or lipid-poor) to vacuolated and spongy (lipid-rich) (Fig. 22). Rarely, cells with large fat droplets have a signet-ring appearance. Intracytoplasmic lipochrome pigment is present in 40% of the cases. In approximately 60% nuclear atypia is absent or minimal, and mitotic activity is low [less than 2 mitotic figures (MFs)/10 high power fields (HPFs)].

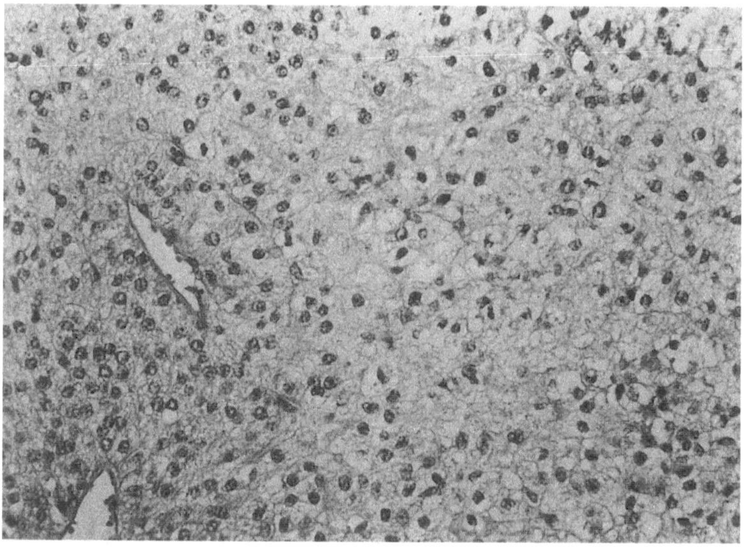

**Fig. 22.** Steroid cell tumor, not otherwise specified. The tumor cells have abundant pale vacuolated cytoplasm. This tumor was associated with Cushing's syndrome and was clinically malignant. H&E, × 200

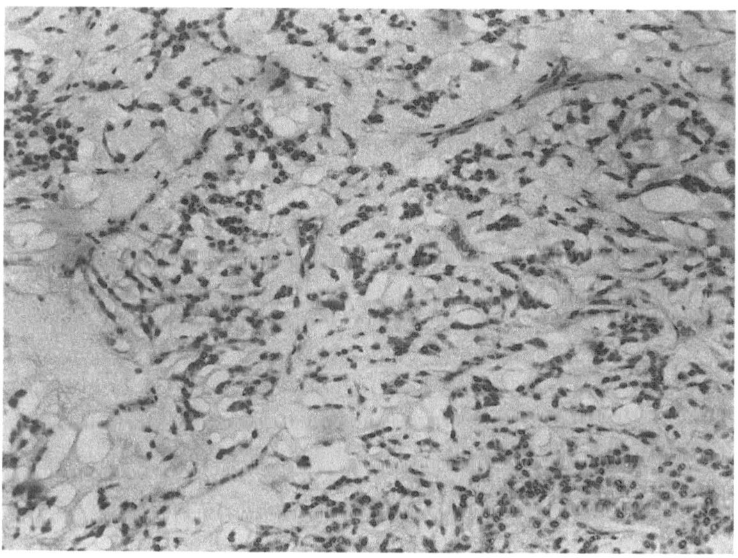

**Fig. 23.** Steroid cell tumor, not otherwise specified. The tumor cells are growing in cords separated by an abundant stroma that was basophilic. H&E, × 125

In the remaining cases, grades 1–3 nuclear atypia, usually associated with an increase in mitotic activity (up to 15 MFs/10 HPFs), is present.

Between 25% and 40% of these tumors are clinically malignant. Such a behavior is more frequent in older patients and all the reported tumors from patients in the first two decades have been benign. The best pathologic correlates with a malignant behavior in one series (HAYES and SCULLY 1987a) were: 2 or more MFs per 10 HPFs (92% malignant); necrosis (86% malignant); a diameter of 7 cm or greater (78% malignant); hemorrhage (77% malignant); and grade 2 or 3 nuclear atypia (64% malignant); occasional tumors that appear cytologically benign, however, are clinically malignant.

Steroid cell tumors, particularly those in the NOS category, may be confused with numerous other neoplasms—in particular extensively luteinized granulosa cell tumors and thecomas, lipid-rich Sertoli cell tumors, clear cell carcinomas (especially those of the oxyphil type) (YOUNG and SCULLY 1987c), hepatoid yolk sac tumors, hepatoid carcinomas (ISHIKURA and SCULLY 1987), metastatic renal cell, adrenocortical, and hepatocellular carcinomas, primary and metastatic melanomas, oxyphilic struma ovarii, the rare pheochromocytoma, and the pregnancy luteoma. The focal presence of nonluteinized areas in luteinized granulosa cell tumors and luteinized thecomas, as well as the characteristic cytologic features and patterns of these neoplasms, and the finding of abundant reticulum in thecomas facilitate the identification of these tumors. The distinction of lipid-rich Sertoli cell tumor with a prominent diffuse pattern from a steroid cell tumor rests on identifying areas with a solid tubular pattern in the former. The clear cells of the clear cell carcinoma and metastatic renal cell carcinomas, unlike those of steroid cell tumors, have glycogen-rich cytoplasm and eccentric nuclei. Also, other patterns of clear cell carcinoma such as tubulocystic, glandular, and papillary are inconsistent with a steroid cell tumor. Oxyphilic clear cell carcinomas, hepatoid yolk sac tumors, and hepatoid carcinomas all have neoplastic cells with abundant eosinophilic cytoplasm. These tumors generally exhibit epithelial patterns and may contain glandular lumens incompatible with the diagnosis of a steroid cell tumor. Both types of hepatoid tumor are also characterized by immunohistochemical staining for α-fetoprotein. Primary and metastatic melanomas can simulate steroid cell tumors if amelanotic, and if they are pigmented, the pigment granules may be confused with the lipochrome granules of a steroid cell tumor. Melanomas generally have more malignant nuclear features than steroid cell tumors and may have a sarcomatoid pattern not seen in the latter. Special staining, including immunohistochemical staining, may be helpful in difficult cases. Rare examples of struma ovarii have a focal solid oxyphil (Hürthle cell) pattern in some cases resembling a steroid cell tumor but we have not seen a struma in which that pattern was uniform throughout the specimen. Therefore, the presence of the more common patterns of struma, an association with other teratomatous elements, the presence of colloid, and immunostaining for thyroglobulin should enable one to make the correct diagnosis. Degenerative spaces in some steroid cell tumors may cause confusion with an adenocarcinoma and more often a vascular tumor. Awareness of this phenomenon, as well as the finding of typical steroid cell tumor elsewhere in the specimen, facilitates the diagnosis. Very rarely a primary pheochromocytoma and potentially a metastatic pheochromocytoma involve the ovary. In addition to clinical distinctions, staining for chromogranin and the finding of dense core granules on electron microscopic examination enable one to distinguish this tumor from a steroid cell tumor.

A pregnancy luteoma can closely resemble a steroid cell tumor and may also be androgenic. Unlke steroid cell tumors, however, pregnancy luteomas are bilateral in about one-third of the cases and multiple in almost half of them. On microscopic examination, the cells have abundant eosinophilic cytoplasm with little or no cytoplasmic lipid, and the nuclei often show brisk mitotic activity. In contrast, a steroid cell tumor with minimal cytologic atypicality that resembles a pregnancy luteoma usually shows no mitotic activity or minimal degrees of it. An ovarian mass composed of steroid cells that is encountered during the third trimester is usually presumed to be a pregnancy luteoma unless clearly proven otherwise.

## 4 Ovarian Tumors with Functioning Stroma

A wide variety of ovarian tumors other than those in the sex cord–stromal and steroid cell categories may be hormonally active as a result of steroid hormone production by their stromal cells. These tumors, which have been designated ovarian tumors with functioning stroma (Scully 1987), may be benign or malignant and, if the latter, primary or metastatic. Almost every ovarian tumor has been reported to be associated with stromal hormone production but, as discussed below, this phenomenon is seen much more often with some neoplasms than others.

Ovarian tumors with functioning stroma are infrequently associated with overt endocrine manifestations but commonly accompanied by subclinical elevations of steroid hormone values (Rome et al. 1973). In one early investigation (Rubin and Frost 1963) 39% of postmenopausal women with ovarian cancer were reported to have increased cornification of their cervical and vaginal squamous cells on cytologic smears. In another study (Rome et al. 1981) an elevation of total urinary estrogens was found in 50% of a series of patients with common epithelial tumors or metastatic carcinomas in the ovary. The stromal cells responsible for the hormone secretion in many ovarian tumors with functioning stroma typically resemble steroid cells and are referred to as luteinized stromal cells; in other cases only densely cellular stroma is observed. The steroid type cells almost always lie within the tumor diffusely or in clusters, but on rare occasions they are mainly distributed just outside the tumor, as discussed below.

Ovarian tumors with functioning stroma can be divided into three major categories. In the first two, germ cell tumors that contain syncytiotrophoblast cells and tumors in pregnant patients, the luteinized stromal cells probably develop as a result of stimulation by hCG (HERRINGTON and SCULLY 1983). The cause of the stromal alteration in the third (idiopathic) group, which accounts for the majority of the cases, is unclear, but ectopic production of hCG or some other stromal stimulant by the neoplastic cells may be responsible.

### 4.1 Germ Cell Tumors Containing Syncytiotrophoblast Cells

Dysgerminomas with syncytiotrophoblast cells (ZALOUDEK et al. 1981) have rarely been associated with luteinization of the stroma and endocrine manifestations such as isosexual precocity or postpubertal virilization (SCULLY 1987). Other germ cell tumors that produce hCG, such as choriocarcinomas and embryonal carcinomas, may also be responsible for manifestations of steroid hormone secretion by stimulating the follicular apparatus of the contralateral uninvolved ovary in the absence of recognized stromal luteinization.

### 4.2 Tumors with Functioning Stroma Occurring During Pregnancy

Although ovarian tumors with functioning stroma in pregnant patients may secrete estrogens, this possibility has not been proven by hormone assay, and clinical manifestations of estrogen excess are not manifest during gestation. In contrast, 19 examples of virilization caused by ovarian tumors with functioning stroma during pregnancy have been reported. These tumors have included nine Krukenberg tumors, five mucinous cystic tumors, two Brenner tumors, and single examples of serous cystadenoma, endodermal sinus tumor, and dermoid cyst (SCULLY 1987). The onset of the virilization in these patients has ranged from the 3rd to the 9th month of gestation. The endocrine status of the offspring is known in ten cases; five of the seven females were virilized.

### 4.3 Idiopathic Group of Tumors with Functioning Stroma

Whereas ovarian tumors with functioning stroma in the first two categories are encountered in young females, patients with tumors in the idiopathic group are usually postmenopausal, reflecting the higher prevalence of ovarian tumors, both primary and metastatic, and possibly the higher levels of circulating pituitary luteinizing hormone in this age group. A wide variety of ovarian tumors have been associated with an idiopathic functioning stroma but its frequency has varied from one type of neoplasm to another.

Mucinous tumors often contain functioning stroma, resulting in either estrogenic or androgenic manifestations. In one series (EDDIE 1967) approximately one-quarter of both mucinous cystadenomas and cystadenocarcinomas were accompanied by evidence of an "active endometrium" in postmenopausal women. In another study (ROME et al. 1981) approximately two-thirds of patients with mucinous tumors of various types had elevated total estrogen levels in the urine. Three mucinous tumors have been responsible for virilization of nonpregnant patients.

Occasional cases of endometrioid carcinoma have been reported to be associated with endometrial hyperplasia in postmenopausal women, and in one case virilization and breast secretion developed. We have seen one well-differentiated endometrioid carcinoma from a patient with an elevated serum testosterone level and hirsutism. ROME et al. found that urinary estrogen levels were elevated in five of six patients with endometrioid carcinoma, indicating that this type of tumor may be associated with function more often than has been realized. Clear cell carcinomas have been accompanied only exceptionally by endometrial hyperplasia, and ROME et al. found that the urinary estrogens were normal in all four of their patients with tumors of this type. Serous tumors have also been associated only rarely with evidence of hyperestrinism. Two of three patients with undifferentiated carcinoma of the ovary studied by ROME et al. had elevated urinary total estrogen excretion. Brenner tumors have been accompanied by endometrial hyperplasia in 10%–16% of the cases. In one case Leydig cells were identified in the stroma (HAMEED 1972). These studies indicate that all types of common epithelial tumor may be associated with stromal activation but that endocrine manifestations are seen with significant frequency only in patients with mucinous tumors.

Germ cell tumors of various types lacking trophoblastic cells have rarely been associated with stromal luteinization and evidence of steroid hormone secretion in the absence of pregnancy. The germ cell tumors within the idiopathic category that have been accompanied by androgenic or estrogenic manifestations have included a variety of subtypes such as: dermoid cyst, struma ovarii, carcinoid tumors, and yolk sac tumor. The steroid cells that are stimulated in cases of germ cell tumor are peripheral rather than within the tumor in many, if not most, of the cases (RUTGERS and SCULLY 1986). In such cases, the steroid cells form a band of variable width at the edge of tumor, sometimes recognizable grossly as a yellow rim. Occasionally the steroid cells in these cases contain crystals of Reinke and are, therefore, Leydig cells of stromal origin, or hilus cells if they are restricted to the hilar border of the tumor. Solid mature teratomas and immature teratomas have not been accompanied by evidence of steroid hormone production to the best of our knowledge.

Metastatic carcinomas that contain mucinous cells, like primary mucinous tumors of the ovary, are frequently associated with luteinization of the stroma and in a significant proportion of cases are accompanied by clinical or laboratory evidence of elevated steroid hormone levels. SCULLY and RICHARDSON found clinical evidence of excess estrogens as manifested by irregular premenopausal bleeding or postmenopausal bleeding in one-quarter of patients with metastatic adenocarcinoma from the large intestine and stomach. One metastatic adenocarcinoma from the colon was responsible for masculinization and another for both virilizing and estrogenic changes. Seven Krukenberg tumors from non-pregnant patients have been associated with virilization. The majority of these tumors were of gastric origin but one arose in the breast and another in the appendix. One Krukenberg tumor of gastric origin and a metastatic adenocarcinoma of colonic origin have been associated with decidual changes in the endometrium in addition to virilization.

Several theories have been proposed to explain the stromal function of tumors in the idiopathic group. One theory evokes a simple mechanical effect of the expansion of tumor nests, likening the process of stromal luteinization to the development of luteinized theca cells from stroma around an expanding follicle. A second theory, which is most pertinent for tumors with functioning stroma that occur in postmenopausal women, implicates a high level of pituitary luteinizing hormone in this age group. The most widely accepted theory is that the tumor cells produce hCG or hCG-like substances that stimulate the stroma. The possible role of hCG is discussed further later in this review.

## 5 Thyroid Hyperfunction Associated with Ovarian Tumors

Although struma ovarii has been demonstrated by immunohistochemical staining to contain triiodothyronine and thyroxine and, therefore, probably produces thyroid hormones at subclinical levels in many cases, clinical evidence suggestive of hyperthyroidism has rarely been confirmed by modern laboratory tests. Rare strumal carcinoids have been accompanied by evidence of hypersecretion of thyroid hormone in the form of postoperative thyroid storm or hypothyroidism, and thyroglobulin has been demonstrated in the colloid within tumors of this type.

## 6 Carcinoid Syndrome Associated with Ovarian Tumors

Of the three major categories of primary carcinoid tumor of the ovary, insular, trabecular, and strumal, one-third of the insular tumors and a single example of strumal carcinoid have been associated with the carcinoid syndrome. This disorder occurs in the absence of hepatic or other metastases in cases of ovarian carcinoid because the hormonal effluent of the tumor enters the systemic circulation directly, bypassing the portal venous system and avoiding inactivation in the liver. Since almost all primary insular carcinoids of the ovary are clinically benign, it is almost always possible to cure the associated syndrome by removal of the ovarian tumor.

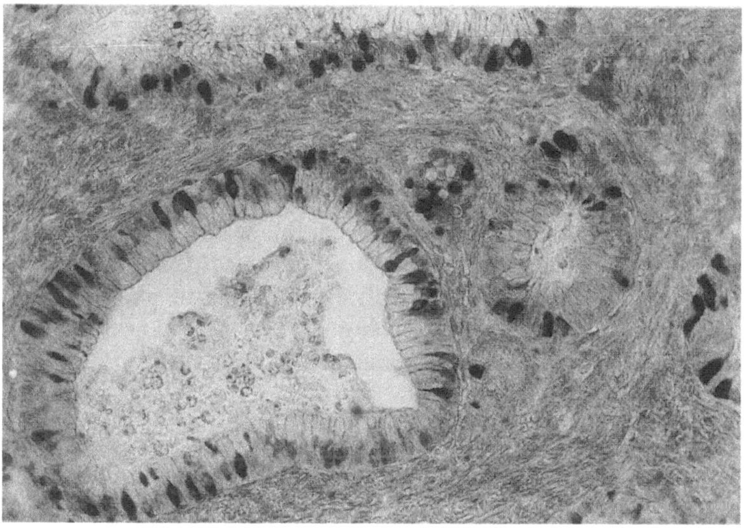

**Fig. 24.** Mucinous cystadenoma associated with Zollinger–Ellison syndrome. Numerous cells lining mucinous glands are stained by the immunohistochemical technique for gastrin. × 200

## 7 Zollinger–Ellison Syndrome Associated with Ovarian Tumors

Mucinous tumors of the ovary contain argyrophil cells in the linings of their glands and cysts in over one-third of the cases, and serotonin and a wide variety of peptide hormones have been demonstrated in these cells immunohistochemically (SCULLY et al. 1984). Eight mucinous tumors, four cystadenomas (Fig. 24), one cystadenoma of borderline malignancy, and three cystadenocarcinomas, have caused the Zollinger–Ellison syndrome (COCCO and CONWAY 1975; LONG et al. 1980; MORGAN et al. 1985; PRIMROSE et al. 1988; HEYD et al. 1989; MATON et al. 1989; GARCIA-VILLANEUVA et al. 1990). In seven of these cases gastrin-containing cells were identified immunohistochemically in argyrophil cells within the cyst linings (Fig. 24).

## 8 Ovarian Tumors Associated with Production of Hormones of Anterior Pituitary Type

Pituitary tissue is present rarely in the walls of ovarian dermoid cysts and a variety of anterior pituitary hormones have been demonstrated in its cells immunohistochemically. Hyperplasia or neoplasia of the pituitary tissue has rarely resulted in syndromes of pituitary hormone excess.

### 8.1 Cushing's Syndrome

In one remarkable case, a pituitary adenoma composed of cells that stained immunohistochemically for adrenocorticotropic hormone (ACTH) arose within a dermoid cyst, secreted ACTH, and caused Cushing's syndrome (Axiotis et al. 1987). A similar case in which either hyperplastic or neoplastic pituitary tissue in a dermoid cyst was associated with Cushing's syndrome had been reported much earlier in the German literature (Kronke and Parade 1938).

### 8.2 Hyperprolactinemia

Two dermoid cysts that contained pituitary tissue and were responsible for hyperprolactinemia have recently been reported Kallenberg et al. 1990; Palmer et al. 1990). In one of them the pituitary tissue formed a 2.5 cm neoplastic nodule but in the other it only formed a 1 mm questionably neoplastic nest of cells. In each case the lesional cells stained immunohistochemically for prolactin.

## 9 Paraendocrine Disorders with Ovarian Tumors

A variety of paraendocrine disorders have been described in association with numerous types of ovarian tumor, some manifested by signs and symptoms of a well-known endocrine disease and others by subclinical laboratory abnormalities, indicating ectopic production of hormones or hormone-like substances by the tumor cells. In some of these cases the hormone being produced has been identified while in others, such as in cases of hypercalcemia, the mechanism of the disorder remains unclear. In all the cases included within this category of neoplasms successful therapy of the tumor has led to disappearance of the paraendocrine state.

### 9.1 ACTH Production and Cushing's Syndrome

As more commonly encountered with tumors of other organs, rare ovarian tumors have secreted ACTH ectopically and resulted in Cushing's syndrome. These tumors have included an adenocarcinoma, a small cell carcinoma presumably primary in the ovary, and a tumor interpreted as a Sertoli cell tumor

(YOUNG and SCULLY 1987b). Immunohistochemical staining for ACTH has revealed its frequent presence in a variety of ovarian tumors, which helps to explain the occasional clinically evident production of ACTH by these neoplasms. As mentioned earlier, several cases of Cushing's syndrome have resulted from cortisol production by a steroid cell tumor as well as from secretion of ACTH by pituitary tissue in a teratoma.

## 9.2 Hypercalcemia

Approximately 50 ovarian tumors have been reported to be associated with paraendocrine hypercalcemia, which has not been accompanied by recognizable clinical manifestations in most of the cases. Approximately half the tumors have been a distinctive type of small cell carcinoma; the next most common type has been the clear cell carcinoma, followed by serous and undifferentiated carcinomas.

The small cell carcinoma, which is associated with hypercalcemia in two-thirds of the cases, was first described in 1981. This tumor, of which we have now seen over 100 examples, is, in our experience, the most common form of undifferentiated carcinoma of the ovary in females under 40 years of age. The age of the patients has ranged from 10 to 44 (average 22) years. The presenting symptoms, abdominal pain and swelling, have been those associated with ovarian tumors in general. Rarely, a patient has had symptoms related to hypercalcemia and in at least one patient a negative parathyroid exploration had been performed before an adnexal mass was appreciated.

At laparotomy the tumors have been unilateral with one exception. Spread beyond the ovary occurred in approximately one-quarter of the cases. Gross examination reveals a fleshy white to pale tan mass, often containing large areas of hemorrhage and necrosis (Fig. 25). The most common microscopic pattern is a diffuse arrangement of closely packed generally small epithelial cells. The tumor cells also grow in nests, cords, and irregular groups. Distinctive follicle-like structures containing eosinophilic fluid and lined by tumor cells are present in almost all the cases (Fig. 26). The most commonly encountered tumor cells have scanty cytoplasm and small nuclei, which typically contain single small nucleoli (Fig. 27); mitotic figures are usually numerous. In about 30% of the tumors large cells with abundant eosinophilic cytoplasm resembling luteinized cells have been present focally (Fig. 28); rarely, these cells have predominated. Mucin-rich cells ranging from well-differentiated cells lining glands and cysts (Fig. 29) to atypical cells containing variable amounts of mucin to signet-ring cells are also present in minor amounts in about 10% of the cases. The stroma is generally scanty and consists of nonspecific fibrous tissue.

Special staining and ultrastructural examination (MCMAHON and HART 1988) have not revealed any features that identify the cell type of this tumor; although it is composed of relatively small cells, convincing dense core granules have not been found in our opinion (ABELER et al. 1988; SCULLY and DICKERSIN 1989).

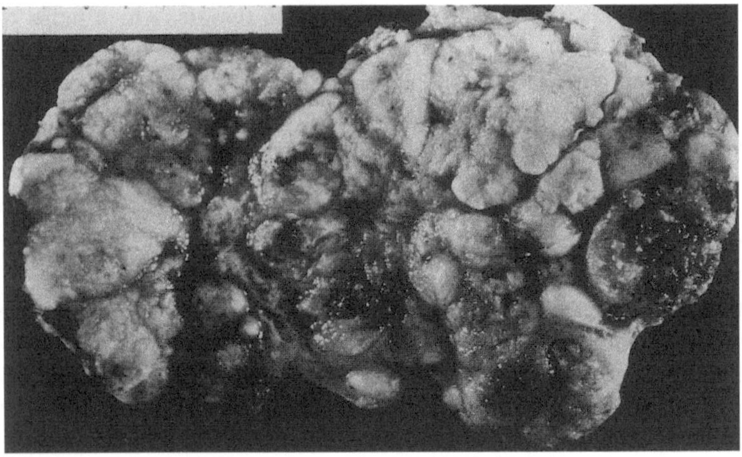

**Fig. 25.** Small cell carcinoma. The sectioned surface of the tumor is lobulated and contains foci of necrosis and hemorrhage

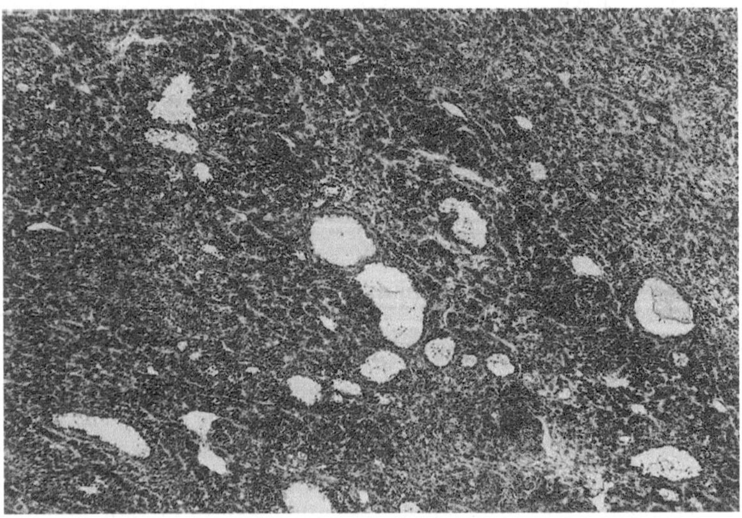

**Fig. 26.** Small cell carcinoma. Many follicle-like spaces are present. H&E, × 50

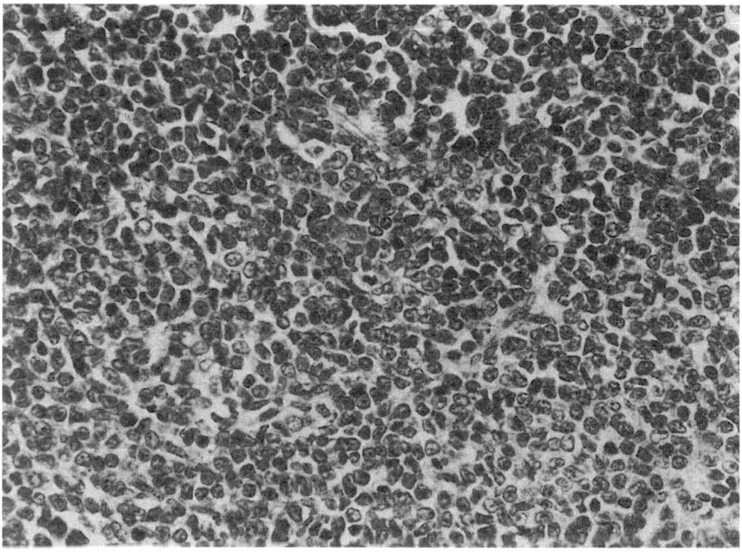

**Fig. 27.** Small cell carcinoma. The tumor cells are small with scanty cytoplasm and the nuclei lack grooves. Several mitotic figures are visible. H&E, × 313

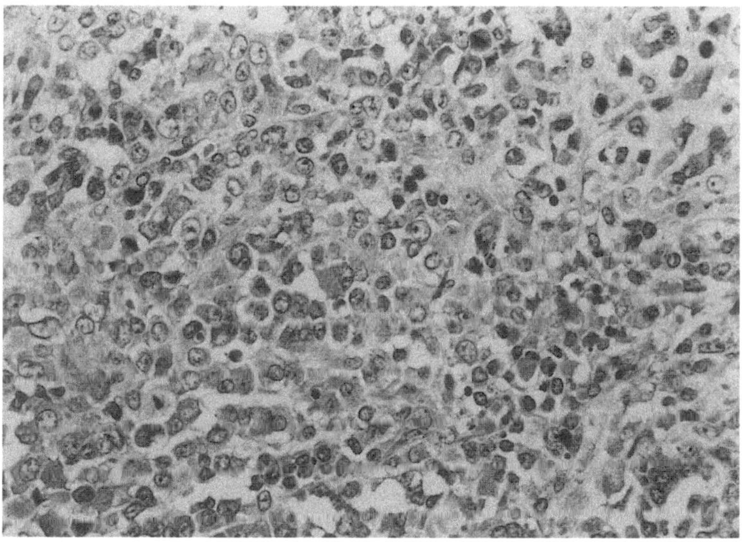

**Fig. 28.** Small cell carcinoma. The tumor cells have abundant cytoplasm that was eosinophilic. H&E, × 313

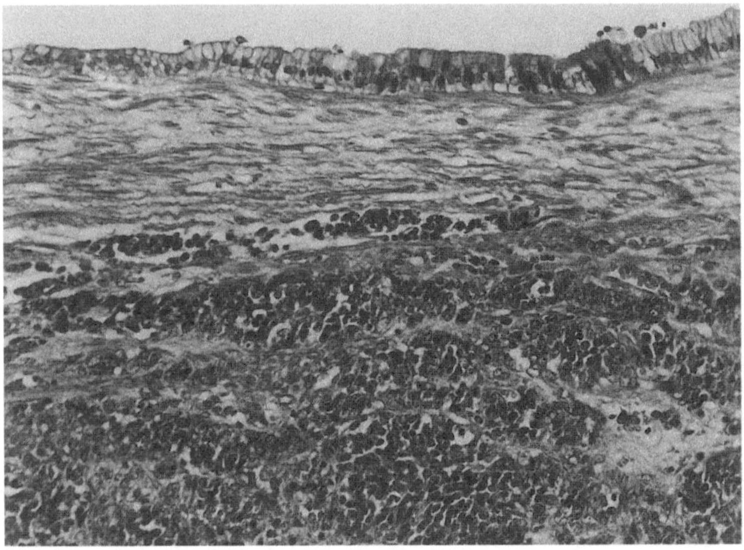

**Fig. 29.** Small cell carcinoma. A strip of mucinous epithelium is present adjacent to characteristic foci of small cell carcinoma. H&E, × 200

We are not impressed with arguments in favor of a germ cell origin (ULBRIGHT et al. 1987). The age distribution and the characteristic presence of uniform small cells and follicle formation suggest a sex cord derivation, but transitions to recognizable forms of sex cord tumors have not been reported.

The small cell carcinoma is often confused with a granulosa cell tumor of either adult or juvenile type, as discussed under those headings. Diffuse small cell carcinomas may also resemble malignant lymphomas, particularly on low-power examination, but adequate sampling reveals patterns of growth that indicate the epithelial nature of the tumor; also, the cytologic features of the neoplastic cells are incompatible with any form of malignant lymphoma. Immunohistochemical staining may be positive for various cytokeratins, vimentin, and epithelial membrane antigen, unlike the typical staining of lymphomas. The differential diagnosis of the small cell carcinomas also includes other small cell malignant tumors of the ovary, including neuroendocrine forms of small cell carcinoma, primitive neuroectodermal tumors, various small cell sarcomas, and malignant melanoma, as discussed in detail elsewhere (YOUNG and SCULLY 1989). The mechanism of the hypercalcemia associated with the small cell carcinoma and other ovarian cancers remains unknown.

## 9.3 hCG Production

Ectopic hCG production was reported by CIVANTOS and RYWLIN (1972) in three women with serous papillary or mucinous adenocarcinomas of the ovary. All of them had elevated urinary hCG levels ranging from 1000 to 25000 IU per 24 hrs. Each of the tumors contained poorly differentiated areas with cells resembling syncytiotrophoblast cells; these cells were positive for hCG on immunofluorescence staining. In one of these cases the contralateral ovary contained numerous lutein cells, and a decidual reaction was present in the endometrium; the patient in this case had vaginal bleeding but no endocrine effects were evident in the other two patients. VAITUKAITIS reported that 10 of 28 ovarian tumors of various types were associated with the presence of immunoreactive hCG in the plasma and SAMAAN and associates found the β subunit of hCG in the plasma of 41% of women with carcinomas of surface epithelial derivation. Immunohistochemical staining of common epithelial tumors for hCG has yielded varying results. One group found an approximately 40% frequency of staining, with no significant differences among benign, borderline, and invasive tumors, whereas another group found only a 10% frequency of staining of carcinomas and no staining of benign tumors. Because of its presence in a wide variety of tumors, including one granulosa cell tumor, immunohistochemical identification of hCG is of relatively little help in differential diagnosis. The subject of ectopic hCG production by ovarian tumors overlaps with that of ovarian tumors with idiopathic functioning stroma. MATIAS-GUIU and PRAT (1990) used two polyclonal antibodies and four monoclonal antibodies to hCG in an investigation of 100 ovarian tumors with variable results; staining of the neoplastic cells with both polyclonal and monoclonal antibodies was much more common in tumors with condensation or luteinization of their stroma than in those without either of these features. As yet, however, there has been no clear-cut correlation among plasma hCG elevations, immunohistochemical demonstration of hCG in ovarian tumors, luteinization of the stroma of the tumors, and clinical manifestations of steroid hormone excess.

## 9.4 Hypoglycemia

Four cases have been reported in which an ovarian neoplasm has been associated with hypoglycemia (YOUNG and SCULLY 1987c). The tumors have been a serous cystadenocarcinoma, a dysgerminoma, a fibroma, and a malignant schwannoma. In the case of the malignant schwannoma insulin and proinsulin were recovered from the tumor tissue (SHETTY et al. 1982).

## 9.5 Renin Production

KORZETS et al. (1986) have reported a case of renin-producing Sertoli cell tumor of the ovary with secondary hyperaldosteronism. These authors interpreted a Sertoli cell tumor previously reported as an aldosterone-secreting tumor as probably belonging in the category of a renin-producing tumor. Another Sertoli cell tumor associated with renin production has recently been reported

(AIBA et al. 1990). Finally an aldosterone-secreting neoplasm interpreted as a sex cord–stromal tumor (JACKSON et al. 1986) with low renin values in the serum has been reported, as has a single case of steroid cell tumor as noted earlier (KULKARNI et al. 1990).

## References


Abeler V, Kjorstad KE, Nesland JM (1988) Small cell carcinoma of the ovary. A report of six cases. Int J Gynecol Pathol 7:315–329

Aguirre P, Scully RE, Delellis RA (1986) Ovarian heterologous Sertoli–Leydig cell tumors with gastrointestinal-type epithelium. An immunohistochemical analysis. Arch Pathol Lab Med 110:528–533

Aguirre P, Thor AD, Scully RE (1989a). Ovarian endometrioid carcinomas resembling sex cord-stromal tumors: an immunohistological study. Int J Gynecol Pathol 8:364–373

Aguirre P, Thor AD, Scully RE (1989b) Ovarian small cell carcinoma—histogenetic considerations based on immunohistochemical and other findings. Am J Clin Pathol 92:140–149

Aiba M, Hirayama A, Sakurada M, Naruse K, Ishikawa C, Aiba S (1990) Spironolactone rod-like structure in renin-producing Sertoli cell tumor of the ovary. Surg Pathol 3:143–149

Axiotis CA, Lippes HA, Merino MJ, deLanerolle NC, Stewart AF, Kinder B (1987) Corticotroph cell pituitary adenoma within an ovarian teratoma: a new cause of Cushing's syndrome. Am J Surg Pathol 11:218–224

Benjamin E, Law S, Bobrow LG (1987) Intermediate filament cytokeratin and vimentin in ovarian sex cord–stromal tumors with correlative studies in adult and fetal ovaries. J Pathol 152:253–263

Bjorkholm E, Pettersson F (1980) Granulosa-cell and theca-cell tumors. The clinical picture and long term outcome for the Radiumhemmet series. Acta Obstet Gynecol Scand 59:361–365

Bjorkholm E, Silfversward C (1980) Theca-cell tumors. Clinical features and prognosis. Acta Radiol Oncol Radiat Phys Biol 19:241–244

Bjorkholm E, Silfversward C (1981) Prognostic factors in granulosa cell tumors. Gynecol Oncol 11:261–274

Bullon A, Arseneau J, Prat J, Young RH, Scully RE (1981) Tubular Krukenberg tumor. A problem in histopathologic diagnosis. Am J Surg Pathol 5:225–232

Chadha S, van der Kwast TH (1989) Immunohistochemistry of ovarian granulosa cell tumors. The value of tissue specific proteins and tumor markers. Virchows Arch [A] 414:439–445

Ghalvardjian A, Scully RE (1973) Sclerosing stromal tumors of the ovary. Cancer 31:664–670

Civantos F, Rywlin AM (1972) Carcinomas with trophoblastic differentiation and secretion of chorionic gonadotrophins. Cancer 29:789–798

Clement PB, Scully RE (1980) Large solitary luteinized follicle cyst of pregnancy and puerperium. A clinicopathological analysis of eight cases. Am J Surg Pathol 4:431–438

Cocco AE, Conway SJ (1975) Zollinger–Ellison syndrome associated with ovarian mucinous cystadenocarcinoma. N Engl J Med 293:485–486

Dardi LE, Miller AW, Gould VE(1982) Sertoli–Leydig cell tumor with endometrioid differentiation. Case report and discussion of histogenesis. Diagn Gynecol Obstet 4:227–234

Dickersin GR, Kline IW, Scully RE (1982) Small cell carcinoma of the ovary with hypercalcemia. A report of eleven cases. Cancer 49:188–197

Eddie DAS (1967) Hormonal activity with ovarian tumors. J Obstet Gynecol Br Commonw 74:283–285

Fathalla MF (1967) The occurrence of granulosa and theca tumors in clinically normal ovaries. A study of 25 cases. J Obstet Gynecol Br Commonw 74:279–282

Fox H, Agrawal K, Langley FA (1975) A clinicopathologic study of 92 cases of granulosa cell tumor of the ovary with special reference to the factors influencing prognosis. Cancer 35:231–241

Gaffney EF, Majmudar B, Hertzler GL, Zane R, Furlong B, Breding E (1983). Ovarian granulosa cell tumors—immunohistochemical localization of estradiol and ultrastructure, with functional correlations. Obstet Gynecol 61:311–318

Gagnon S, Tetu B, Silva EG, McCaughey WTE (1989). Frequency of α-fetoprotein production by Sertoli–Leydig cell tumors of the ovary: an immunohistochemical study of eight cases. Mod Pathol 2:63–67

Garcia-Villaneuva M, Figuerola NB, del Arbol LR, Ortiz MJH (1990) Zollinger–Ellison syndrome due to a borderline mucinous cystadenoma of the ovary. Obstet Gynecol 75:549–551

Hameed H (1972) Brenner tumor of the ovary with Leydig cell hyperplasia. A histologic and ultrastructural study. Cancer 30:945–952

Hart WR, Kumar N, Crissman JD (1980) Ovarian neoplasms resembling sex cord tumors with annular tubules. Cancer 45:2352–2363

Hayes MC, Scully RE (1987a) Ovarian steroid cell tumor (not otherwise specified): a clinicopathological analysis of 63 cases. Am J Surg Pathol 11:835–845

Hayes MC, Scully RE, (1987b) Stromal luteoma of the ovary: a clinicopathological analysis of 25 cases. Int J Gynecol Pathol 6:313–321

Herrington JB, Scully RE (1983) Endocrine aspects of germ cell tumors. In: Damjanov I, Knowles B, Solter D (eds) The human teratomas. Humana, Clifton, New Jersey, pp 215–229

Heyd J, Livni N, Herbert D, Mor-Yosef S, Glaser B (1989) Gastrin-producing ovarian cystadenocarcinoma: sensitivity to secretin and SMS 201–995. Gastroenterology 97: 464–467

Hughesdon PE (1983) Lipid cell thecomas of the ovary. Histopathology 7:681–692

Ishikura H, Scully RE (1987) Hepatoid carcinoma of the ovary. A newly described tumor. Cancer 60:2775–2784

Jackson B, Valentine R, Wagner G (1986) Primary aldosteronism due to a malignant ovarian tumor. Aust NZ J Med 16:69–71

Kallenberg GA, Pesce CM, Norman B, Ratner RE, Silverberg SG (1990) Ectopic hyperprolactinemia resulting from an ovarian teratoma. JAMA 263:2472–2474

Korzets A, Nouriel H, Steiner Z, Griffel B, Kraus L, Freund U, Klajman A (1986) Resistant hypertension associated with a renin-producing ovarian Sertoli cell tumor. Am J Clin Pathol 85:242–247

Kronke E, Parade GW (1938) Morbus Cushing bei ovarial Teratoma. Z Klin Med 134:698–718

Kulkarni JN, Mistry RC, Kamat MR, Chinoy R, Lotlikar RG (1990) Autonomous aldosterone-secreting ovarian tumor. Gynecol Oncol 37:284–289

Kurman RJ, Andrade D, Goebelsmann U, Taylor CR (1978) An immunohistological study of steroid localization in Sertoli–Leydig tumors of the ovary and testis. Cancer 42:1772–1783

Kurman RJ, Goebelsmann U, Taylor CR (1979) Steroid localization in granulosa–theca tumors of the ovary. Cancer 43:2377–2384

Lack EE, Perez-Atayde AR, Murthy ASK, Goldstein DP, Grigler JF, Vawter GF (1981) Granulosa theca cell tumors in premenarchal girls. A clinical and pathologic study of ten cases. Cancer 48:1846–1854

Long TT, Barton TK, Draffin R, Reeves WJ, McCarty KS (1980) Conservative management of the Zollinger–Ellison Syndrome. Ectopic gastrin production by an ovarian cystadenoma. JAMA 243:1837–1839

Marieb HJ, Spangler S, Kashgarian M, Heiman A, Schwartz ML, Schwartz PE (1983) Cushing's syndrome secondary to ectopic cortisol production by an ovarian carcinoma. J Clin Endocrinol Metab 57:737–740

Matias-Guiu X, Prat J (1990) Ovarian tumors with functioning stroma. An immunohistochemical study of 100 cases with human chorionic gonadotropin monoclonal and polyclonal antibodies. Cancer 65:2001–2005

Maton PN, Mackem SM, Norton JA, Gardner JD, O'Dorisio TM, Jensen RT (1989) Ovarian carcinoma as a cause of Zollinger–Ellison syndrome. Gastroenterology 97:468–471

McMahon JT, Hart WR (1988) Ultrastructural analysis of small cell carcinomas of the ovary. Am J Clin Pathol 90:523–529

Miettinen M, Talerman A, Wahlstrom T, Astengo-Osuna C, Virtanen I (1985) Cellular differentiation in ovarian sex-cord–stromal and germ-cell tumors studied with antibodies to intermediate-filament proteins. Am J Surg Pathol 9:640–651

Morgan DR, Wells A, MacDonald RC, Johnston D (1985) Zollinger–Ellison syndrome due to a gastrin secreting ovarian mucinous cystadenoma. Case report. Br J Obstet Gynecol 92:867–869

Nakashima N, Young RH, Scully RE (1984) Androgenic granulosa cell tumors of the ovary. A clinicopathological analysis of seventeen cases and review of the literature. Arch Pathol Lab Med 108:786–791

Palmer PE, Bogojavlensky S, Bhan AK, Scully RE (1990) Prolactinoma in wall of ovarian dermoid cyst with hyperprolactinemia. Obstet Gynecol 75:540–543
Paoletti M, Pridjian G, Okagaki T, Talerman A (1987) A stromal Leydig cell tumor of the ovary occurring in a pregnant 15-year-old girl. Ultrastructural findings. Cancer 60:2806–2810
Paraskevas M, Scully RE (1989) Hilus cell tumor of the ovary: a clinicopathological analysis of 12 Reinke-crystal-positive and 9 crystal-negative cases. Int J Gynecol Pathol 8:299–310
Prat J, Young RH, Scully RE (1982) Ovarian Sertoli–Leydig cell tumors with heterologous elements (ii) cartilage and skeletal muscle. A clinicopathologic analysis of twelve cases. Cancer 50:2465–2475
Primrose JN, Maloney M, Wells M, Bulgim O, Johnston D (1988) Gastrin-producing ovarian mucinous cystadenomas: a cause of the Zollinger–Ellison syndrome. Surgery 104:830–833
Rome RM, Laverty CR, Brown JB (1973) Ovarian tumors in postmenopausal women. Clinicopathological features and hormonal studies. J Obstet Gynecol Br Commonw 80:984–991
Rome RM, Fortune DW, Quinn MA, Brown JB (1981) Functioning ovarian tumors in postmenopausal women. Obstet Gynecol 57:705–710
Roth LM, Sternberg WH (1973) Ovarian stromal tumors containing Leydig cells. II. Pure Leydig cell tumor, non-hilar type. Cancer 32:952–960
Roth LM, Sternberg WH (1983) Partly luteinized theca cell tumor of the ovary. Cancer 51:1697–1704
Roth LM, Anderson MC, Govan ADT, Langley FA, Gowing NFC, Woodcock AS (1981) Sertoli–Leydig cell tumors. A clinicopathologic study of 34 cases. Cancer 48:187–197
Roth LM, Liban E, Czernobilsky B (1982) Ovarian endometrioid tumors mimicking Sertoli and Sertoli–Leydig cell tumors. Sertoliform variant of endometrioid carcinoma. Cancer 50:1322–1331
Roth LM, Slayton RE, Brady LW, Blessing JA, Johnson G (1985) Retiform differentiation in ovarian Sertoli–Leydig cell tumors. A clinicopathologic study of six cases from a gynecologic oncology study group. Cancer 55:1093–1098
Rubin DK, Frost JK (1963) The cytologic detection of ovarian cancer. Acta Cytol 7:191–195
Rutgers J, Scully RE (1986) Functioning ovarian tumors with peripheral steroid cell proliferation: a report of twenty-four cases. Int J Gynecol Pathol 5:319–337
Samaan NA, Smith JP, Rutledge FN, Schultz PN (1976) The significance of measurement of human placental lactogen, human chorionic gonadotropin, and carcinoembryonic antigen in patients with ovarian carcinoma. Am J Obstet Gynecol 126:186–189
Sasano H, Sasano N (1989) What's new in the localization of sex steroids in the human ovary and its tumors? Pathol Res Pract 185:942–948
Sasano H, Okamoto M, Mason JI, Simpson ER, Mendelson CR, Sasano N, Silverberg SG (1989) Immunohistochemical studies of steroidogenic enzymes (aromatase, 17-hydroxylase and cholesterol side-chain cleavage cytochromes P-450) in sex cord–stromal tumors of the ovary. Hum Pathol 20:452–457
Scully RE (1970) Sex cord tumor with annular tubules. A distinctive ovarian tumor of the Peutz–Jeghers syndrome. Cancer 25:1107–1121
Scully RE (1979) Tumors of the ovary and maldeveloped gonads. Atlas of tumor pathology; 2nd series, fascicle No. 16. Armed Forces Institute of Pathology, Washington, D.C.
Scully RE (1987). Ovarian tumors with functioning stroma. In: Fox H (ed) Haines and Taylor's gynaecological and obstetrical pathology, 3rd edn. Churchill Livingstone, Edinburgh, pp 724–736
Scully RE, Richardson GS (1961) Luteinization of the stroma of metastatic cancer involving the ovary and its endocrine significance. Cancer 14:827–840
Scully RE, Dickersin GR (1989) Letter to the editor. Int J Gynecol Pathol 8:196
Scully RE, Aguirre P, DeLellis RA (1984) Argyrophilia, serotonin, and peptide hormones in the female genital tract and its tumors. Int J Gynecol Pathol 3:51–70
Serov SF, Scully RE, Sobin LH (1973) International histological classification of tumors, No. 9. Histological typing of ovarian tumors. World Health Organization, Geneva
Shetty MR, Boghossian HM, Duffell D, Freel R, Gonzales JC (1982) Tumor-induced hypoglycemia: a result of ectopic insulin production. Cancer 49:1920–1923
Solh HM, Azoury RS, Najjar SS (1983) Peutz–Jeghers syndrome associated with precocious puberty. J Pediatr 103:593–595
Stenwig JT, Hazekamp JT, Beecham JB (1979) Granulosa cell tumors of the ovary. A clinicopathological study of 118 cases with long-term follow-up. Gynecol Oncol 7:136–152

Sternberg WH, Roth LM (1973) Ovarian stromal tumors containing Leydig cells. 1. Stromal–Leydig cell tumor and non-neoplastic transformation of ovarian stroma to Leydig cells. Cancer 32:940–951

Susil BJ, Sumithran E (1987) Sarcomatous change in granulosa cell tumor. Hum Pathol 18:397–399

Talerman A (1987) Ovarian Sertoli–Leydig cell tumor (androblastoma) with retiform pattern: a clinicopathologic study. Cancer 60:3056–3064

Talerman A, Hughesdon PE, Anderson MC (1982) Diffuse nonlobular ovarian androblastoma usually associated with feminization. Int J Gynecol Pathol 1:155–171

Tavassoli FA, Norris HJ (1980) Sertoli tumors of the ovary. A clinicopathologic study of 28 cases with ultrastructural observations. Cancer 46:2281–2297

Taylor HB, Norris HJ (1967) Lipid cell tumors of the ovary. Cancer 20:1953–1962

Tracy SL, Askin FB, Reddick RL, Jackson B, Kurman RJ (1985) Progesterone secreting Sertoli cell tumor of the ovary. Gynecol Oncol 22:85–96

Ulbright TM, Roth LM, Stehman FB, Talerman A, Senekjian EK (1987) Poorly differentiated (small cell) carcinoma of the ovary in young women: evidence supporting a germ cell origin. Hum Pathol 18:175–184

Vaitukaitis JL (1974) Human chorionic gonadotropin as a tumor marker. Ann Clin Lab Sci 4:276–280

Waxman M, Vuletin JC, Urcuyo R, Belling CG (1979) Ovarian low-grade stromal sarcoma with thecomatous features: a critical reappraisal of the so-called "malignant thecoma." Cancer 44:2206–2217

Waxman M, Damjanov I, Alpert L, Sardinsky T (1981) Composite mucinous ovarian neoplasms associated with Sertoli–Leydig and carcinoid tumors. Cancer 47:2044–2052

Young RH, Scully RE (1982) Ovarian sex cord–stromal tumors. Recent progress. Int J Gynecol Pathol 1:101–123

Young RH, Scully RE (1983a) Ovarian Sertoli–Leydig cell tumors with a retiform pattern: a problem in histopathologic diagnosis. A report of 25 cases. Am J Surg Pathol 7:755–771

Young RH, Scully RE (1983b) Ovarian sex cord–stromal tumors with bizarre nuclei. A clinicopathologic analysis of seventeen cases. Int J Gynecol Pathol 1:325–335

Young RH, Scully RE (1983c) Ovarian stromal tumors with minor sex cord elements: a report of seven cases. Int J Gynecol Pathol 2:227–234

Young RH, Scully RE (1984a) Fibromatosis and massive edema of the ovary, possibly related entities. A report of 14 cases of fibromatosis and 11 cases of massive edema. Int J Gynecol Pathol 3:153–178

Young RH, Scully RE (1984b) Ovarian Sertoli cell tumors. A report of ten cases. Int J Gynecol Pathol 2:349–363

Young RH, Scully RE (1984c) Ovarian sex cord–stromal tumors: recent advances and current status. Clin Obstet Gynecol 11:93–134

Young RH, Scully RE (1984d) Well-differentiated ovarian Sertoli–Leydig cell tumors. A clinicopathological analysis of 23 cases. Int J Gynecol Pathol 3:277–290

Young RH, Scully RE (1985) Ovarian Sertoli–Leydig cell tumors. A clinicopathological analysis of 207 cases. Am J Surg Pathol 9:543–569

Young RH, Scully RE (1987a) Sex cord–stromal tumors, steroid cell tumors and other ovarian tumors with endocrine, paraendocrine and paraneoplastic manifestations. In: Kurman RJ (ed) Balustein's pathology of the female genital tract. Springer, New York, pp 607–658

Young RH, Scully (1987b) Ovarian steroid cell tumors associated with Cushing's syndrome. A report of three cases. Int J Gynecol Pathol 6:40–48

Young RH, Scully RE (1987c) Oxyphilic clear cell carcinoma of the ovary. A report of nine cases. Am J Surg Pathol 11:661–667

Young RH, Scully RE (1989) Alveolar rhabdomyosarcoma metastatic to the ovary. A report of two cases and discussion of the differential diagnosis of small cell malignant tumors of the ovary. Cancer 64:899–904

Young RH, Scully RE (1990) Sarcomas metastatic to the ovary. A report of 21 cases. Int J Gynecol Pathol 9:231–252

Young RH, Scully RE (1991) Malignant melanoma metastatic to the ovary: A clinicopathologic analysis of 20 cases. Am J Surg Pathol, 15:849–860

Young RH, Prat J, Scully RE (1982) Ovarian endometrioid carcinomas resembling sex cord–stromal tumors. A clinicopathological analysis of 13 cases. Am J Surg Pathol 6:513–522

Young RH, Part J, Scully RE (1982b) Ovarian Sertoli–Leydig cell tumors with heterologous elements. (i) Gastrointestinal epithelium and carcinoid: a clinicopathologic analysis of thirty-six cases. Cancer 50:2448–2456
Young RH, Welch WR, Dickersin GR, Scully RE (1982c) Ovarian sex cord tumor with annular tubules: review of 74 cases including 27 with Peutz–Jeghers syndrome and 4 with adenoma malignum of the cervix. Cancer 50:1384–1402
Young RH, Dickersin GR, Scully RE (1983a) A distinctive ovarian sex cord–stromal tumor causing sexual precocity in the Peutz–Jeghers syndrome. Am J Surg Pathol 7:223–243
Young RH, Prat J, Scully RE (1983b) Endometrioid stromal sarcomas of the ovary. A clinicopathological analysis of twenty-three cases. Cancer 53:1143–1155
Young RH, Dickersin GR, Scully RE (1984a) Juvenile granulosa cell tumor of the ovary. A clinicopathologic analysis of 125 cases. Am J Surg Pathol 8:575–596
Young RH, Dudley AG, Scully RE (1984b) Granulosa cell, Sertoli–Leydig cell and unclassified sex cord–stromal tumors associated with pregnancy. A clinicopathological analysis of thirty-six cases. Gynecol Oncol 18:181–205
Young RH, Perez–Atayde AR, Scully RE (1984c) Ovarian Sertoli-Leydig cell tumor with retiform and heterologous components. Report of a case with hepatocytic differentiation and elevated serum α-fetoprotein. Am J Surg Pathol 8:709–718
Zaloudek C, Norris HJ (1982) Granulosa tumors of the ovary in children. A clinical and pathologic study of 32 cases. Am J Surg Pathol 6:503–512
Zaloudek C, Norris HJ (1984) Sertoli–Leydig tumors of the ovary. A clinicopathologic study of 64 intermediate and poorly differentiated neoplasms. Am J Surg Pathol 8:405–418
Zaloudek CJ, Tavassoli FA, Norris HJ (1981) Dysgerminoma with syncytiotrophoblastic giant cells. A histologically and clinically distinctive subtype of dysgerminoma. Am J Surg Pathol 5:361–367
Zhang J, Young RH, Arseneau J, Scully RE (1982) Ovarian stromal tumors containing lutein or Leydig cells (luteinized thecomas and stromal Leydig cell tumors). A clinicopathological analysis of fifty cases. Int J Gynecol Pathol 1:270–285

# Germ Cell Tumors

A. TALERMAN



## 1 Introduction

Although the remarkable progress in the pathology of ovarian germ cell tumors which was achieved during the preceding three decades did not proceed at the same rapid pace during the 1980s, the past decade not only witnessed the accumulation of new knowledge, but was also characterized by the consolidation, expansion, and wider application of the knowledge gained previously. These developments were accompanied by further advances in the therapy of this group of neoplasms. The use of efficacious combination chemotherapy has led to a spectacular improvement in the prognosis of patients with some of the most malignant types of ovarian germ cell neoplasms. In addition a number of substances which have proven themselves as tumor markers in some types of

Current Topics in Pathology
Volume 85, Ed. N. Sasano

germ cell neoplasms became an integral part in the investigation and follow-up of patients with malignant germ cell tumors.

This chapter will focus on the recent advances in the pathology of germ cell tumors of the ovary, as well as their impact on therapy and prognosis. Only a very brief discussion of genetic and chromosomal aspects is provided and recent studies on tumor differentiation are beyond the scope of this chapter. The subject of oncogenes in ovarian germ cell tumors is discussed in the chapter dealing with oncogenes in gynecological neoplasms. In common with general practice the different types of ovarian germ cell neoplasms will be discussed in turn using the World Health Organization (WHO) classification (SEROV et al. 1973) with some recent modifications (SCULLY et al. 1990). In addition to pure germ cell tumors, neoplasms composed of germ cells and sex cord stromal derivatives will also be included.

## 2 General Aspects

Germ cell neoplasms are the second most common group of ovarian tumors after the epithelial tumors. In Europe and North America germ cell neoplasms represent approximately 20% of all ovarian tumors, while the incidence is relatively higher in Asian and African countries due to paucity of epithelial tumors. The great majority of ovarian germ cell neoplasms are benign and consist of mature cystic teratomas. The latter make up more than 90% of ovarian germ cell tumors, while all the malignant germ cell neoplasms account for the remaining 5%–8%. Germ cell tumors are encountered at all ages from birth to very old age, but are seen most frequently from the first to the sixth decade. Thus unlike the epithelial tumors, germ cell tumors have a predilection for the young. Sixty percent of all ovarian neoplasms in children and adolescents are of germ cell origin and one-third of these are malignant. Apart from mature cystic teratoma with malignant transformation, which normally occurs in perimenopausal and postmenopausal women, malignant germ cell tumors with rare exceptions occur from birth to the menopause and the great majority are seen in patients aged less than 35 years (TALERMAN 1987a).

Unlike testicular teratomas, which are always aneuploid, have higher than normal chromosome complement (ATKIN 1973), and are considered to originate before the first meiotic division (PARRINGTON et al. 1986), mature ovarian teratomas are diploid, have normal 46, XX karyotype, and have been considered to originate from germ cells after the first meiotic division (LINDER et al. 1975). Recent studies (NOMURA et al. 1983; PARRINGTON et al. 1984) using new and more advanced banding techniques have demonstrated diverse modes of origin of mature cystic teratoma. Although the majority of ovarian cystic teratomas originate from germ cells after the first meiotic division, it has been demonstrated that some originate before this event (PARRINGTON et al. 1984). The recent finding of a small isochromosome i (12 p) as a specific chromosome abnormality, and thus a possible chromosomal marker for testicular germ cell tumors (Atkin and Baker 1983; Gibas et al. 1984) has been extended to some ovarian germ cell neoplasms. The presence of this marker chromosome has been noted in two dysgerminomas (Atkin and Baker 1987; Jenkyn and McCartney 1987). Neither mature cystic teratomas (Parrington et al. 1984) nor immature teratomas (King et al.1990a) have shown this abnormality.

## 3 Classification

The classification of ovarian tumors which will be followed is the original widely accepted World Health Organization (WHO) classification published almost 20 years ago (Serov et al. 1973) with a few modifications, which are going to be included in its updated version to be published shortly (Scully et al. 1990). Thus ovarian germ cell tumors are classified as follows:

I. Germ Cell tumors
  A. Dysgerminoma
  B. Yolk sac tumor (endodermal sinus tumor)
  C. Embryonal carcinoma
  D. Polyembryoma
  E. Choriocarcinoma
  F. Teratomas
    1. Immature (solid, cystic, or both)
    2. Mature
      a) Solid
      b) Cystic
        i) Mature cystic teratoma (dermoid cyst)
        ii) Mature cystic teratoma (dermoid cyst) with malignant transformation
    3. Monodermal or highly specialized
      a) Struma ovarii
      b) Carcinoid
      c) Strumal carcinoid
      d) Others
  G. Mixed forms (tumors composed of types A through F in any possible combination)
II. Tumors composed of germ cells and sex cord-stroma derivatives
  A. Gonadoblastoma
  B. Mixed germ cell–sex cord-stroma tumor

This classification differs from the original WHO classification by the acceptance of the more embracing term "yolk sac tumor" for the more specific "endodermal sinus tumor," although retaining the latter as an alternative term. It also includes the more correct term "mature cystic teratoma" for "dermoid cyst," retaining the latter as an alternative term due to its widespread use. The category "monodermal or highly specialized teratoma" includes various newly described or unusual entities. The tumors composed of germ cells and sex cord-stroma derivatives have been divided into "gonadoblastoma" and "mixed germ cell–sex cord-stroma tumor." The category "gonadoblastoma with dysgerminoma" has been deleted, and this entity has been included under "gonadoblastoma."

## 4 Histogenesis

It is now fully accepted that germ cell tumors are ultimately derived from primitive germ cells. The most widely accepted view of the histogenesis of germ cell tumors and the interrelationships of the various types is best illustrated by a scheme proposed by TEILUM (1965) and depicted in Fig. 1. TEILUM (1965, 1976) regarded dysgerminoma (seminoma) as a primitive germ cell neoplasm which has not acquired the potential for further differentiation. Embryonal carcinoma was considered as a morphologic as well as conceptual entity, and as a germ cell tumor composed of totipotential cells capable of further differentiation. The view that dysgerminoma is incapable of further differentiation has been chal-

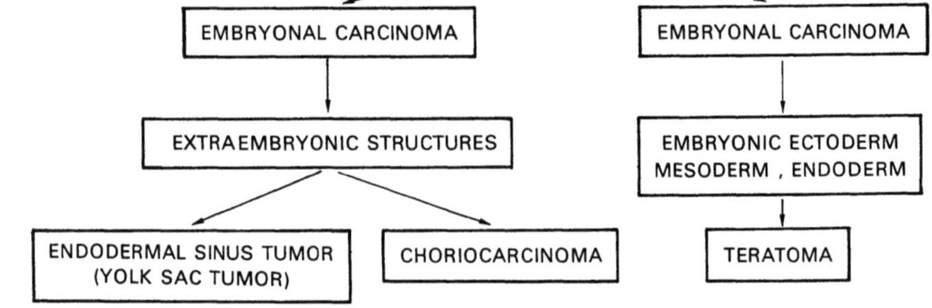


**Fig. 1.** The histogenesis and interrelationships of germ cell neoplasms (modified from TEILUM (1965)

lenged by recent immunocytochemical studies which revealed the presence of occasional low molecular weight cytokeratin positive cells in some seminomas and dysgerminomas, suggesting that these tumors may have the capability to differentiate further (MIETTINEN et al. 1986). While the very great majority of dysgerminoma cells are cytokeratin negative, cells of embryonal carcinoma, yolk sac tumor, and choriocarcinoma are uniformly positive. The presence of occasional cytokeratin-positive cells in some dysgerminomas would suggest that these cells have undergone further differentiation. This view is also supported by the intimate admixture of dysgerminoma cells with other neoplastic germ cell elements seen in a considerable number of germ cells tumors.

## 5 Dysgerminoma

Dysgerminoma is the most common malignant ovarian germ cell neoplasm occurring in pure form (SCULLY 1979; TALERMAN 1987a; BJORKHOLM et al. 1990). Although at one time it was considered to be much more common than any other malignant ovarian germ cell tumor, it is now closely followed by yolk sac (endodermal sinus) tumor. Nowadays more dysgerminomas are found to be combined with other neoplastic germ cell elements than reported previously. This is mainly due to more extensive and careful sampling. These tumors are included in the category of malignant mixed germ cell tumors (TALERMAN et al. 1973; KURMAN and NORRIS 1976b ; GERSHENSON et al. 1984).

Recent studies (GORDON et al. 1981; BJORKHOLM et al. 1990) lend further support to previous observations as regards the age incidence of patients with dysgerminoma. They emphasize the fact that the majority of the affected subjects are adolescent or young adult females, that the peak incidence is found in the second and third decades, and that 80% of patients are younger than 30 years.

Although dysgerminoma is the most common germ cell tumor encountered in subjects with gonadal maldevelopment and chromosomal abnormalities, only 5%–10% of dysgerminomas occur in such subjects and the great majority of patients are normally developed young females with normal 46, XX chromosome complement (TALERMAN 1987a). Abdominal enlargement is the most frequent presenting symptom (GORDON et al. 1981; BJORKHOLM et al. 1990). Dysgerminoma may be found incidentally, or during the investigation of patients with primary amenorrhoca. In the latter case it is usually associated with gonadoblastoma. Due to its age incidence, dysgerminoma is one of the most common ovarian neoplasms occurring during pregnancy and puerperium. Occassionally patients present with acute abdominal emergency due to torsion of the tumor (TALERMAN 1987a).

Dysgerminoma is usually unilateral, but bilateral involvement is observed in approximately 10% of cases (GORDON et al. 1981; TALERMAN 1987a;

BJORKHOLM et al. 1990). In this respect it differs from other malignant ovarian germ cell neoplasms which are virtually never bilateral. Bilaterality must be distinguished from metastatic involvement. The finding of multiple tumor nodules scattered throughout the ovarian tissue, especially when well circumscribed, is strongly suggestive of metastatic spread from the contralateral ovary. The presence of similar findings microscopically, associated with well-documented vascular involvement, is diagnostic of metastatic disease. Sometimes bilateral involvement may only be observed microscopically on a wedge biopsy.

Pure dysgerminomas are gray-yellow, solid, round, oval, or lobulated, rapidly growing tumors, usually with smooth glistening capsule. The tumors can reach a considerable size within a few months. They grow even more rapidly during pregnancy. On cross-section pure dysgerminomas are solid, and vary in consistency from soft to rubbery depending on the amount of fibrous tissue present. In larger tumors hemorrhagic and necrotic areas are usually seen. Microscopically dysgerminoma is composed of aggregates, islands, or strands of large uniform cells which are separated by connective tissue containing lymphocytes, other inflammatory cells, and a granulomatous reaction with foreign body and Langhans' giant cells. The amount of connective tissue which varies from fine fibrovascular septa to large fibrous bands tends to determine the appearance of the tumor. The great majority of dysgerminoma cells do not react with any intermediate filament antibodies including low molecular weight cytokeratin. As cells of embryonal carcinoma, yolk sac tumor, and choriocarcinoma are uniformly cytokeratin-positive, staining for low molecular weight cytokeratin provides a useful diagnostic test (BATTIFORA et al. 1984; MIETTINEN et al. 1986). The presence of occasional low molecular weight cytokeratin-positive cells in some dysgerminomas suggests a possible differentiation of these cells towards embryonal carcinoma, yolk sac tumor, or choriocarcinoma (MIETTINEN et al. 1986).

Dysgerminoma cells contain double the amount of DNA present in normal somatic cells (ASADOURIAN and TAYLOR 1969; KOMMOSS et al. 1990). Ultrastructurally dysgerminoma cells are characterized by a cytoplasm showing paucity of organelles, and a large nucleus with prominent strand-like nucleolonema.

It has been suggested that dysgerminomas showing paucity of lymphocytic and granulomatous infiltration, scanty fibrous tissue, increased cellularity, and mitotic activity in common with the so-called anaplastic seminoma follow a more aggressive course and are associated with a worse prognosis. Recent studies describing therapeutic results in patients with dysgerminoma have failed to confirm these views, or to detect a group of patients with a worse prognosis (THOMAS et al. 1987; BJORKHOLM et al. 1990)

Between 8% and 10% of dysgerminomas contain syncytiotrophoblastic giant cells (Fig. 2), which have been conclusively shown to produce hCG and β-hCG (ZALOUDEK et al. 1981; TALERMAN 1987a). Cytotrophoblastic cells have not been observed in conjunction with the syncytiotrophoblastic giant cells. The

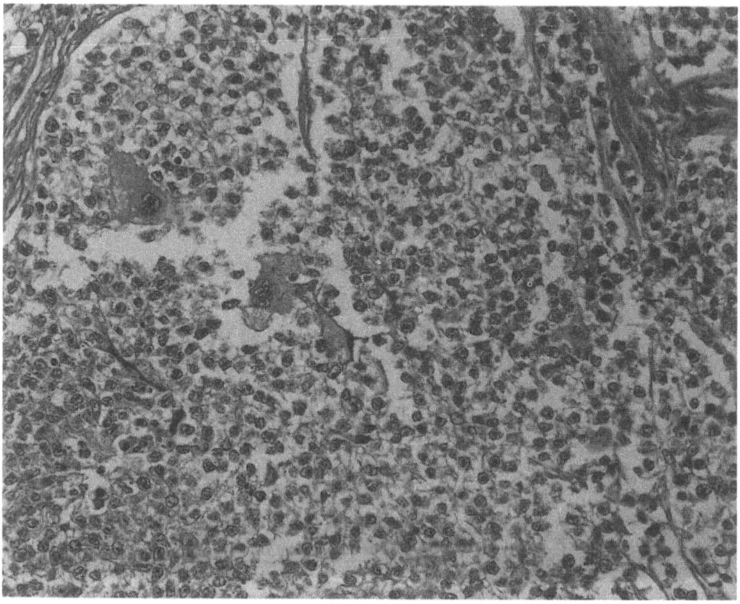

**Fig. 2.** Dysgerminoma with syncytiotrophoblastic giant cells. Note the irregular contour, voluminous slightly vacuolated cytoplasm, and large nuclei. H&E, × 235

latter must be differentiated from foreign body and Langhans' giant cells associated with granulomatous reaction.

Patients with dysgerminoma containing syncytiotrophoblastic giant cells usually show elevations of hCG or β-hCG in the serum, although the levels are usually much lower than in patients with tumors containing choriocarcinoma. There is no evidence that patients with dysgerminoma containing syncytiotrophoblastic giant cells have a worse prognosis (Zaloudek et al. 1981; Talerman 1987a). It is of utmost importance to recognize these cells as syncytiotrophoblastic giant cells and not to misinterpret them as choriocarcinoma. As dysgerminoma is frequently combined with other malignant neoplastic germ cell elements (Scully 1979; Talerman 1987a), and as the presence of these elements alters the therapeutic approach, as well as the prognosis, the importance of judicious and extensive sampling of the tumor and of careful histologic examination need no further emphasis.

Dysgerminoma is an aggressive neoplasm which grows rapidly. Direct invasion of the surrounding organs and structures is seen with larger tumors. It metastasizes first via the lymphatics to the parailiac and para-aortic lymph nodes. Hematogenous spread occurs later and metastases are found in the lungs, liver, bones and other sites. Although the metastases are usually composed of dysgerminoma, in approximately 10% of cases they contain other malignant neoplastic germ cell elements (Talerman 1987a).

Because of the very high cure rates of patients with dysgerminoma, in recent years in some quarters it has become regarded as a less malignant neoplasm. It must be emphasized that dysgerminoma is a highly malignant and aggressive neoplasm which fortunately responds very well to radiation therapy as well as to combination chemotherapy, resulting in high curability.

As dysgerminoma occurs in young females in whom preservation of fertility is desirable, it is now agreed that patients with unilateral tumors should be treated by excision of the affected adnexa and carefully followed up (Scully 1979; Talerman 1987a; Thomas et al. 1987). Although such therapy may be complicated by recurrences, due to the very good response to radiotherapy and combination chemotherapy, patients with recurrent disease can be treated successfully. When preservation of fertility is not desired, bilateral salpingooophorectomy and hysterectomy is performed, followed by radiation therapy to the lymph nodes draining the adnexa. Bilateral gonadectomy is also the mode of therapy used in patients with dysgerminoma associated with gonadal dysgenesis. Because metastases in this group of patients are less frequent than in patients with dysgerminoma arising de novo, radiotherapy may be withheld. Careful follow-up including the use of modern scanning techniques should be used to detect metastases and recurrences and appropriate therapy should be administered if necessary (Talerman 1987a; Thomas et al. 1987).

α-Fetoprotein (AFP) and hCG are not elevated in the serum of patients with pure dysgerminoma (Talerman et al. 1980). Elevated levels of serum lactic dehydrogenase (LDH) have been noted in patients with dysgerminoma (Awais 1983) and more recently even better correlation was noted when isoenzymes 1 and 2 of LDH have been estimated (Fujii et al. 1985; Schwartz and Morris 1988). It has been noted that there is a good correlation between the amount of tumor present and the serum enzyme levels (Awais 1983). Unfortunately, the amount of tumor tissue needed to produce elevated levels is relatively large, thus limiting the use of these substances as tumor markers. In cases with larger tumors the estimation of LDH and especially its isoenzymes 1 and 2 is of considerable diagnostic value (Awais 1983; Fujii et al. 1985; Schwartz and Morris 1988).

## 6 Yolk Sac Tumor (Endodermal Sinus Tumor)

Yolk sac tumor (YST) is the second most common ovarian malignant germ cell neoplasm occurring in pure form, and is also a frequent component of mixed or combined germ cell tumors (Talerman 1987a). Although originally YST was considered to be very rare, it is now being diagnosed with much greater frequency, and its incidence follows closely that of dysgerminoma. This increase in incidence is due to the much better recognition of YST as a specific pathologic entity, and to the fact that presence of perivascular formations (Schiller–Duval bodies) is not a prerequisite for the diagnosis of YST (Teilum 1976; Langley et al. 1981; Talerman 1987a).

Yolk sac tumor is encountered most frequently in the second and third decades, followed by first and fourth, and is rare in women in the fifth decade (Teilum 1976; Kurman and Norris 1976a; Scully 1979; Langley et al. 1981; Talerman 1987a). It is very rare after the menopause, with only a few well-documented cases recorded (Talerman 1987a). Recently two cases of ovarian epithelial tumor, associated with YST and occurring in elderly patients, have been reported (Rutgers et al. 1987; Mazur et al. 1988), and another well-documented case is known to the author. Although the histogenesis of such tumors is uncertain, the likely explanation is that they originate from the epithelial component by a process of neoplastic differentiation or transformation and therefore their histogenesis is totally different from that of germ cell neoplasms (Rutgers et al. 1987; Mazur et al. 1988).

Patients with ovarian YST usually present with abdominal enlargement, abdominal pain, or both. The tumors are rapidly growing. Occasionally YST may be discovered as an incidental finding. Due to its age incidence it may be encountered during pregnancy. It is unilateral, and to date no well-documented cases of bilateral ovarian YST have been recorded. Metastatic involvement of the contralateral ovary may be observed and must be differentiated from bilaterality, with which it has been confused (Talerman 1987a). YST, like any other malignant germ cell tumor, may be associated with mature cystic teratoma in the contralateral ovary. The tumor is round, oval, or lobulated and soft. When large it may be invading the surrounding structures. On cross-section it is solid, gray-white, often with hemorrhagic and necrotic areas, and its surface is mucoid (Teilum 1976; Scully 1979; Talerman 1987a).

Microscopically YST usually shows a variety of histologic patterns and appearances. One of the patterns may predominate, and occasionally tumors may exhibit only a single histologic pattern. The histologic appearances of YST have been described in detail (Teilum 1976; Kurman and Norris 1976a; Langley et al. 1981; Talerman 1987a; Jacobsen and Talerman 1989). Ten histologic patterns have been described (Talerman 1987a; Jacobsen and Talerman 1989) as follows:

1. Microcystic
2. Endodermal sinus
3. Papillary
4. Glandular–alveolar
5. Solid
6. Myxomatous
7. Macrocystic
8. Polyvesicular vitelline
9. Hepatoid
10. Primitive intestinal (enteric)

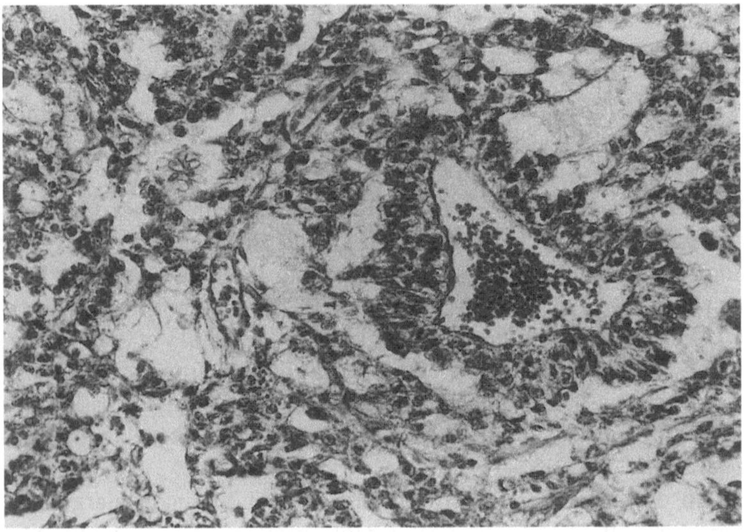

**Fig. 3.** The typical appearance of a preivascular formation (Schiller–Duval body), the hallmark of YST. H&E, × 235

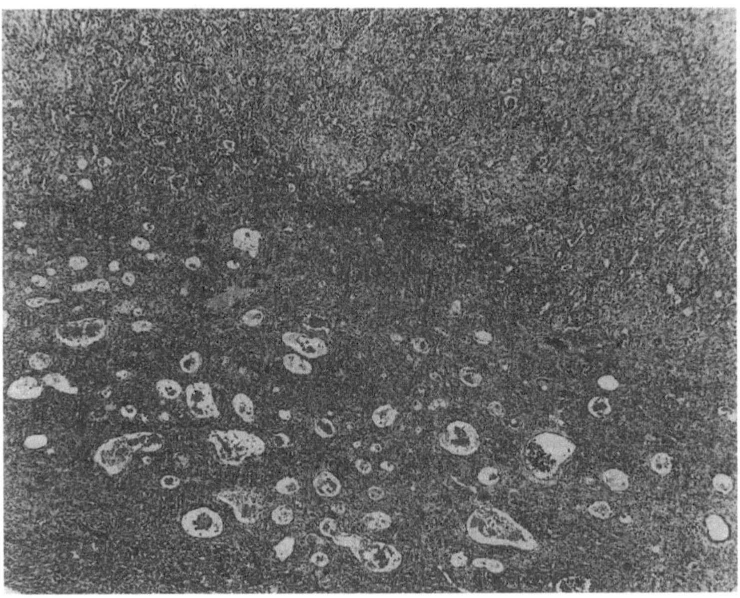

**Fig. 4.** Polyvesicular vitelline pattern of YST (*bottom*) associated with alveolar glandular pattern and marked stromal luteinization (*top*) in a YST excised from a 25-year-old pregnant woman. Note the numerous vesicles of different shape and size. H&E, × 40

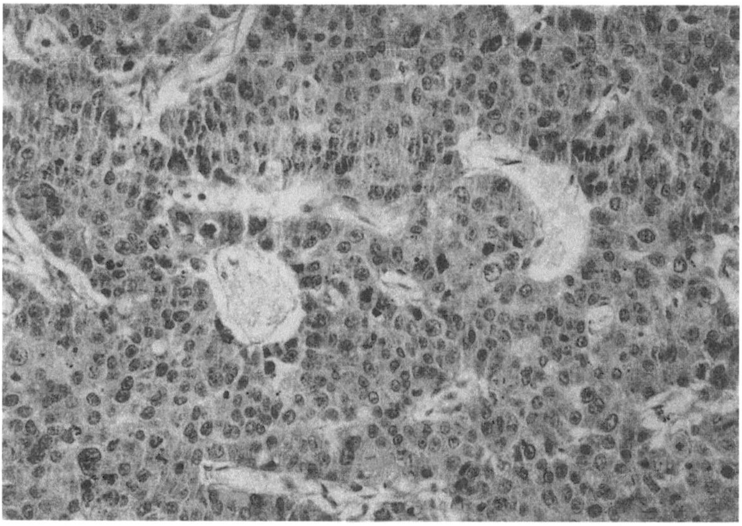

**Fig. 5.** Hepatoid pattern of YST. Note the solid pattern and the similarity to hepatocellular carcinoma. H&E, × 185

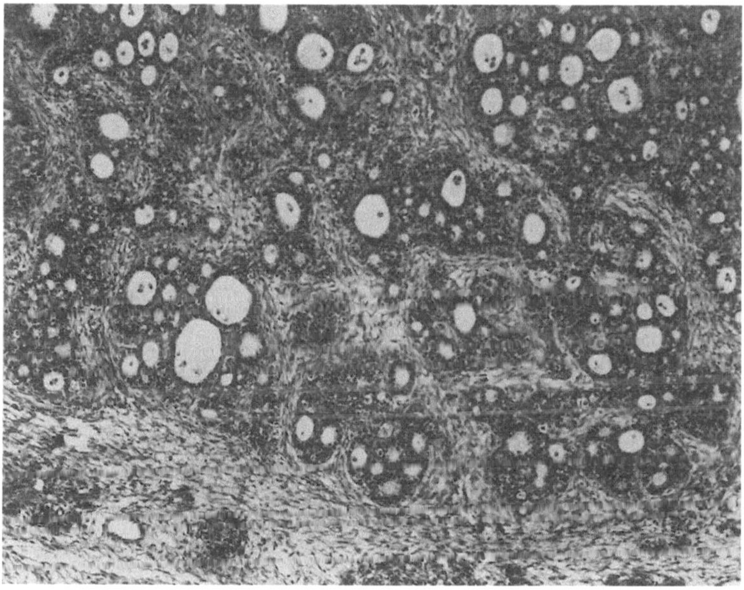

**Fig. 6.** Primitive intestinal pattern of YST composed of collections of small glands forming irregular nests surrounded by connective tissue. H&E, × 75

The presence of perivascular formations (Schiller–Duval bodies), a hallmark of YST (Fig.3), is no longer considered a prerequisite for the diagnosis. Although perivascular formations are seen in the majority of ovarian YSTs, in a number of tumors they may be undetectable (LANGLEY et al. 1981; TALERMAN 1987a).

While many of the histologic patterns of YST may be seen in a single tumor, occasionally a tumor may exhibit only one pattern and this may lead to diagnostic difficulties. Two of the three histologic patterns of YST which are most frequently seen in pure form, the hepatoid pattern (PRAT et al. 1982) and the primitive intestinal pattern (COHEN et al. 1986, 1987), have been described during the past decade. The third pattern, the polyvesicular vitelline, had been described in detail earlier (TEILUM 1965). It is characterized by the presence of numerous small vesicles and cysts, usually oval, sometimes with central constriction, and lined by columnar, cuboidal, or flattened epithelial cells. They are surrounded by connective tissue which may vary from dense cellular, composed of spindle-shaped cells, to loose and edematous. A tumor of this type associated with focal glandular–alveolar pattern markedly compressed by hyperplastic and highly luteinized ovarian stroma was seen in a 25-year-old pregnant patient (Fig. 4). The presence of the polyvesicular vitelline pattern provided the only clue to the correct diagnosis, and to successful therapy.

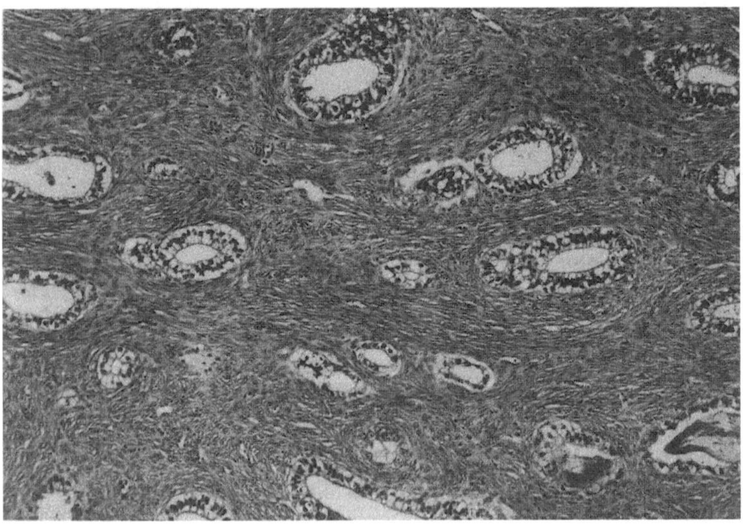

**Fig. 7.** Primitive intestinal pattern of YST composed of glands lined by tall columnar cells with clear cytoplasm and pleomorphic nuclei and surrounded by dense connective tissue. The glands show a superficial resemblance to secretory endometrial carcinoma. H&E, × 90

The hepatoid pattern (PRAT et al. 1982) resembles the appearance of hepatocellular carcinoma or primitive hepatic tissue. The tumor is composed of large polygonal cells with eosinophilic cytoplasm, which usually show a considerable degree of cellular and nuclear pleomorphism and brisk mitotic activity (Fig. 5).

The primitive intestinal pattern (COHEN et al. 1986, 1987) is characterized by collections of glands lined by pleomorphic cells with large hyperchromatic nuclei and showing brisk mitotic activity (Fig. 6). The glands contain mucin, which may be dense and inspissated. Hyaline globules may be numerous in places. The collections of glands are surrounded by connective tissue, the amount and appearance of which may vary (COHEN et al. 1986, 1987). Another variant of this pattern is characterized by primitive glands of various sizes lined by tall columnar or cuboid cells with clear cytoplasm (Fig. 7), and may resemble secretory endometrial carcinoma (CLEMENT et al. 1987).

The YSTs showing these histologic patterns in common with other YSTs produce and secrete AFP. Tumors exhibiting the primitive intestinal pattern are usually associated with very high levels of serum AFP (COHEN et al. 1987). The demonstration of AFP within the tumor tissue by immunocytochemistry or immunofluorescence and of elevated levels in the serum is helpful in making the diagnosis in these cases. The young age of the patient and evidence that the tumor is of primary ovarian origin are also helpful factors. Although during the past decade occasional patients with ovarian Sertoli–Leydig cell tumor, mostly with the retiform pattern (YOUNG and SCULLY 1983; TALERMAN 1987b), as well as occasional patients with mucinous cystadenocarcinoma of the ovary (KONISHI et al. 1988) have been noted to have elevated levels of serum AFP, the finding of considerably increased levels of serum AFP in a young female with an ovarian tumor is virtually diagnostic of YST. The serum AFP levels can be correlated with the amount of YST present within the tumor, and estimation of serum AFP can be used for evaluation of the results of primary surgical treatment, for follow-up of patients during chemotherapy, and for early detection of metastases and recurrences (TALERMAN et al. 1980; TALERMAN 1987a). YST, in addition to AFP synthesis, also produces $\alpha_1$-antitrypsin and a number of other serum proteins (TSUCHIDA et al. 1978). None of these substances can in any way equal the value of AFP as a tumor marker for YST. Recently the synthesis of a number of additional proteinaceous substances by YST, and the normal yolk sac, has been noted (NISHI, personal communication, 1990).

Yolk sac tumor is a highly malignant neoplasm which grows rapidly, invades the surrounding structures, and metastasizes early via the lymphatic route to the regional lymph nodes and by hematogenous spread to the lungs, liver, and other organs. YST is resistant to radiation therapy. Although prognosis has been very poor in the past, there has been a dramatic improvement due to the advent of combination chemotherapy first with vincristine, actinomycin D, and cyclophosphamide (VAC), and then with cis-diaminoplatinum, bleomycin, and vinblastine (PVB). Recently VP16 or etopoxide has been substituted for vinblastine with reduction in toxic side-effects. Although the VAC regimen is less toxic, it has been shown that it is less efficacious in the treatment of YST compared to the PVB or other combination chemotherapy regimens containing cis-diaminoplatinum (BRADOF et al. 1982; GERSHENSON et al. 1983; TAYLOR et al. 1985; SAWADA et al. 1985; SESSA et al. 1987). As a result of the new methods of treatment, patients with ovarian YST achieve a cure rate in excess of 80%. The occasional cases of YST composed of the newly described hepatoid and primitive intestinal types have a less satisfactory response to combination chemotherapy and are therefore associated with worse prognosis (PRAT et al. 1982; COHEN et al. 1987; CLEMENT et al. 1987).

Ovarian YST does not contain estrogen and progesterone receptors (KOMMOSS et al. 1989). It has also been shown recently that ovarian YST is virtually always aneuploid (Fig. 8). In a series of 20 ovarian YSTs, all but one were aneuploid. The only exception was a tumor of the rare pure primitive intestinal type, which was diploid (KOMMOSS et al. 1990).

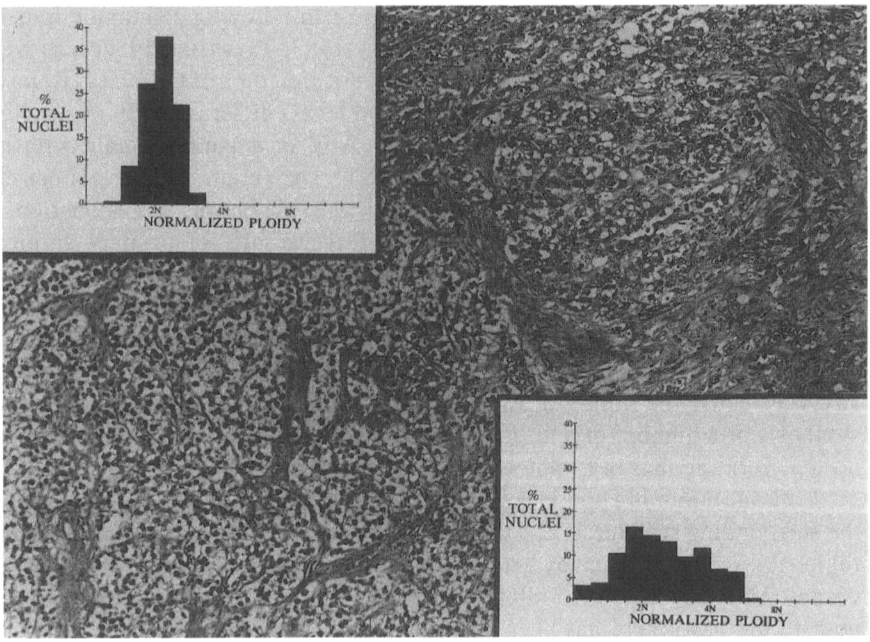


**Fig. 8.** Ovarian mixed germ cell tumor consisting of dysgerminoma (*bottom left*) and YST (*top right*). H&E, × 75. The dysgerminoma shows little variation in DNA values, which peak at 2N (*inset*), and the YST is aneuploid (*inset*). (KOMMOSS et al. 1990)

## 7 Embryonal Carcinoma

The term "embryonal carcinoma" is used here to describe ovarian germ cell neoplasms showing the same appearance as their more common testicular counterparts (MOSTOFI and SOBIN 1977), and strict diagnostic criteria should be followed when making this diagnosis. Ovarian tumors composed entirely of embryonal carcinoma are very rare, and embryonal carcinoma is more common in combination, especially with YST (TALERMAN 1987a).

Embryonal carcinoma is seen in the same age group as other malignant ovarian germ cell tumors, with which it has many features in common. The prognosis of patients with embryonal carcinoma has been considered to be somewhat more favourable than that of those with YST (KURMAN and NORRIS 1976c), but since the introduction of efficacious combination chemotherapy regimens, and due to the rarity of pure embryonal carcinoma, this can hardly be verified. Embryonal carcinoma frequently contains isolated syncytiotrophoblastic giant cells, and occasionally is combined with choriocarcinoma. Elevated levels of serum hCG or β-hCG are seen in either instance, but the levels tend to be higher when choriocarcinoma is present. Embryonal carcinoma may be associated with elevated levels of serum AFP. This may be due to partial differentiation to YST but is more frequently due to combination with YST, when the serum AFP levels are much higher (TALERMAN 1987a).

The behavior and treatment of embryonal carcinoma are similar to those of YST and the prognosis of patients with this tumor is now favorable due to the administration of efficacious combination chemotherapy regimens.

## 8 Polyembryoma

Polyembryoma is generally considered as a germ cell tumor composed entirely of embryoid bodies resembling morphologically presomite embryos, which do not develop beyond the 18-day stage. Polyembryoma in pure form has not been observed in the ovary, and in the few reported cases (SIMARD 1957; BECK et al. 1969; TAKEDA et al. 1982) the tumor, although largely or predominantly composed of polyembryoma, has been combined with other neoplastic germ cell elements. The presence of occasional isolated embryoid bodies which are sometimes seen in testicular germ cell tumors is less common in their ovarian counterparts (MARIN-PADILLA 1965). Tumors reported as polyembryoma have usually been large and have not differed materially from other malignant ovarian germ cell tumors. Microscopically, polyembryoma is composed of embryoid bodies which, when well formed, consist of an embryonic disk located in the center and surrounded on one side by an amniotic cavity and on the other by yolk sac. Atypical or malformed embryoid bodies may contain an embryonic

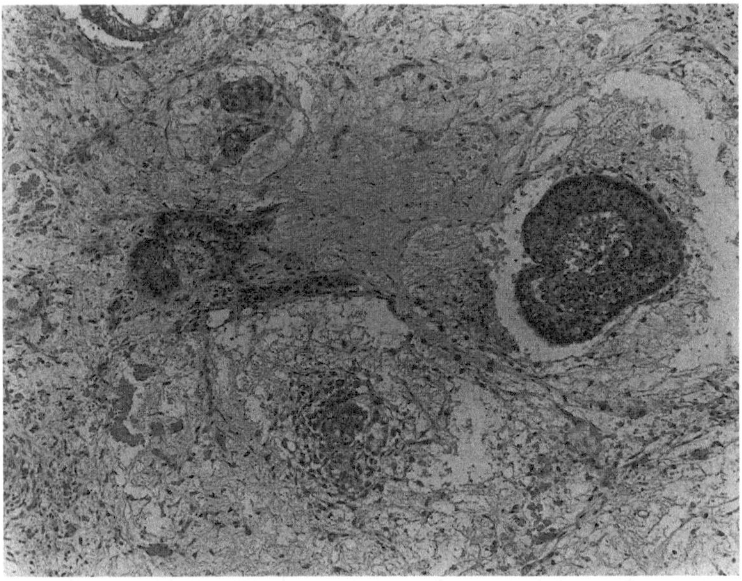

**Fig. 9.** Polyembryoma composed of blastocyst-like embryoid bodies and morula-like formations surrounded by myxomatous tissue. H&E, × 420

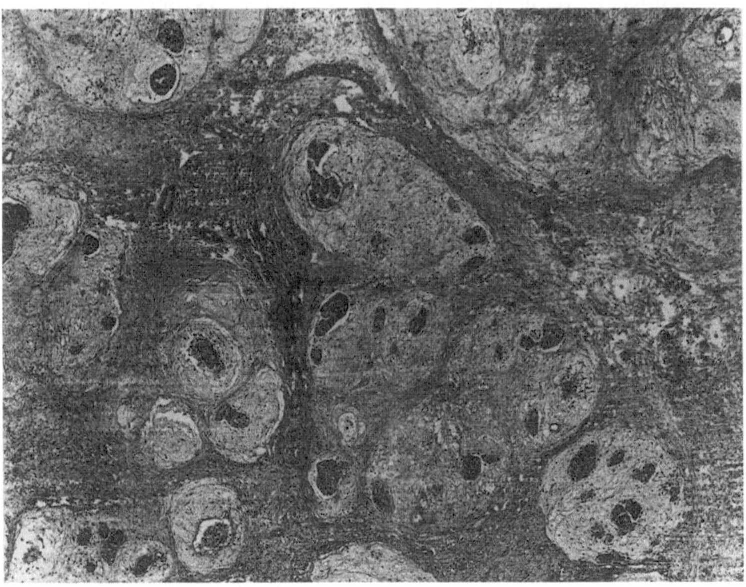

**Fig. 10.** General appearance of the tumor shown in Fig. 9, containing numerous round or oval nests composed of myxomatous tissue containing single or multiple embryoid bodies mainly in the blastocyst stage. H&E, × 60

disk, which may not be well formed, and two or more yolk sacs with a single amniotic cavity, or viceversa. The embryoid bodies are surrounded by myxomatous tissue or primitive mesenchymal tissue. Syncytiotrophoblastic giant cells are often seen in the vicinity of the embryoid bodies, and teratomatous elements may also be present (TALERMAN 1987a).

A recent report (KING et al. 1991) described an ovarian mixed germ cell tumor composed predominantly of polyembryoma, which although showing occasional fully developed embryoid bodies was composed of embryoid bodies in earlier developmental stages, mainly in the blastocyst and morula stage (Fig. 9). They were surrounded by myxomatous tissue forming numerous round or oval structures (Fig. 10). Although the presence of occasional structures of this type had been observed in testicular germ cell tumors containing embryoid bodies, this had not been noted in their ovarian counterparts (MARIN-PADILLA 1965). This further emphasizes the fact that polyembryoma may be composed of embryoid bodies in various stages of differentiation up to the 18-day stage. Tumors composed mainly of polyembryoma are malignant and should be treated in the same manner as YST or other malignant germ cell neoplasms.

## 9 Choriocarcinoma

The nongestational choriocarcinoma discussed here is a germ cell tumor which is indistinguishable from its more common gestational counterpart. It has the same age incidence as other malignant ovarian germ cell tumors, and therefore, when occurring in pure form during the reproductive years, primary pure non-gestational choriocarcinoma can only be diagnosed after very careful investigations, which must exclude the presence of its gestational counterpart (TALERMAN 1987a). Although occasional cases of well-documented pure nongestational choriocarcinoma have been reported (JACOBS et al. 1982; VANCE and GEISINGER 1985), these tumors are very rare (TALERMAN 1987a). On the other hand choriocarcinoma is now seen more frequently as a component of mixed germ cell tumors due to better and more extensive sampling.

Choriocarcinoma can only be diagnosed when both syncytiotrophoblast and cytotrophoblast are present within the tumor. The presence of scattered syncytiotrophoblastic giant cells, which may be seen within a number of germ cell tumors, does not constitute choriocarcinoma. The presentation of patients with this neoplasm is usually similar to that of other malignant germ cell tumors. Isosexual precocious pseudopuberty may be oberved in premenarchal children, while adults may complain of menorrhagia, menometrorrhagia, and pseudopregnancy. The tumor produces large amounts of hCG and elevated serum levels are present. hCG, and preferably its β-subunit (β-hCG), which does not cross-react with luteinizing hormone, is a valuable tumor marker for patients with ovarian germ cell tumors containing or composed of choriocarcinoma

(TALERMAN 1987a). Choriocarcinomas, or tumors containing choriocarcinoma, are usually large, solid, rapidly growing tumors which are invariably hemorrhagic. They are unilateral but may be associated with metastases or mature cystic teratoma in the contralateral ovary. Choriocarcinoma is composed of aggregates of centrally located cytotrophoblast and peripherally located syncytiotrophoblast, and is usually associated with hemorrhage. The importance of sampling tissue from the immediate vicinity of hemorrhagic areas within germ cell tumors has been emphasized (TALERMAN 1987a; JACOBSEN and TALERMAN 1989), as it may facilitate the diagnosis of choriocarcinoma elements affected by hemorrhage. The latter may completely obliterate foci of choriocarcinoma present within a tumor. Nongestational choriocarcinoma is an aggressive malignant germ cell tumor which metastasizes widely via hematogenous and lymphatic routes and invades locally. It is treated in the same manner as YST, and there has been marked improvement in the previously dismal prognosis. Like its gestational counterpart, nongestational choriocarcinoma is associated with the synthesis of a number of placental proteins. All of them, including pregnancy-specific $\beta_1$-glycoprotein (SP1), have been found to be inferior to β-hCG as tumor markers (JACOBSEN and TALERMAN 1989).

## 10 Teratoma

Teratomas are germ cell tumors composed of derivatives of the three primitive germ layers, ectoderm, mesoderm, and endoderm. They represent the result of further differentiation of embryonal carcinoma along the somatic or embryonic pathway, in contrast to YST and choriocarcinoma, which are the result of extraembryonal differentiation. As the process of differentiation of teratoma is dynamic they exhibit varying degrees of maturity. In the ovary the overwhelming majority (99%) of teratomas are mature and cystic. They are classified as mature cystic teratomas or dermoid cysts, and by virtue of complete maturity of the constituent tissues are benign.

### 10.1 Mature Cystic Teratoma (Dermoid Cyst)

Unlike the malignant germ cell neoplasms described above, which occur from birth to premenopause, mature cystic teratomas have a much wider age range and are encountered from birth to old age. They are more common in the first five decades of life and therefore have the same tendency as other germ cell tumors of the ovary to occur in the young. They have been encountered in stillborn fetuses (TALERMAN 1987a).

Mature cystic teratomas are usually unilateral, but they are bilateral in approximately 15% of cases, and in a number of cases may be associated with a malignant germ cell tumor in the contralateral ovary. Occasionally multiple tumors may be present in the same ovary. This is only seen in ovaries containing small tumors because when the tumors are large they usually coalesce and form a single mass. Occasionally mature cystic teratoma, like its solid mature or immature counterparts, may be associated with mature neural (glial) implants in the peritoneal cavity also known as gliomatosis peritonei (ROBBOY and SCULLY 1970). Because these implants are fully mature they are benign, and the only treatment required is the excision of the ovarian tumor (ROBBOY and SCULLY 1970; TRUAN et al. 1982; NIELSEN et al. 1985).

## 10.2 Mature Solid Teratoma

Mature solid teratoma is very rare (SCULLY 1979; TALERMAN 1987a). Since the great majority of solid teratomas contain immature elements and are malignant, the diagnosis of mature solid teratoma can only be made after extensive sampling and very careful histologic examination. Mature solid teratoma occurs in young subjects and has the same age range as malignant germ cell tumors like YST, choriocarcinoma, and immature teratoma. Because all its constituent tissues are mature, the tumor is benign and is treated by excision of the affected adnexa.

## 10.3 Immature Teratoma

Immature teratoma is an uncommon tumor and represents less than 1% of ovarian teratomas. It is unilateral but may be associated with mature cystic teratoma in the contralateral ovary (SCULLY 1979; TALERMAN 1987a). This is a not uncommon finding, which has been noted more frequently in recent years, and must be differentiated from a metastasis of the immature teratoma. The tumors are usually large (frequently larger than their mature counterparts), round, oval, and solid. They may contain cystic areas. Microscopically they are composed of immature tissues derived from the three primitive germ layers and show varying degrees of immaturity. Mature elements are frequently intermingled with the immature, which usually predominate. Immature teratoma may be combined with other germ cell elements, forming a malignant mixed germ cell tumor. In such cases the levels of serum AFP and B-hCG may be elevated, reflecting the presence of YST or choriocarcinoma. There is a strong correlation between the degree of immaturity of the tumor and its behavior. This has led to be formulation of grading systems, two of which tend to be used nowadays. One system is based predominantly on the degree of immaturity of the neural elements which frequently tend to form the predominant component in these tumors (NORRIS et al. 1976), while the other (THURLBECK and SCULLY 1960; TALERMAN 1987a) takes into consideration the degree of immaturity of all the elements present within the tumor. Although basically the two grading systems correspond to each other, in view of the fact that sometimes tissue elements other than neural are the most important in this context, the more general grading system shown below (THURLBECK and SCULLY 1960; TALERMAN 1987a) is advocated in preference to the one relying only on the neural elements (NORRIS et al. 1976).

This grading system is as follows :

*Grade 0*: All tissues mature; no mitotic activity.
*Grade 1*: Minor foci of abnormally cellular or embryonal tissue mixed with mature elements; slight mitotic activity.
*Grade 2*: Moderate quantities of embryonal tissue mixed with mature elements; moderate mitotic activity.
*Grade 3*: Large quantities of embryonal tissue present; high mitotic activity

Immature teratoma shows many features in common with other malignant germ cell neoplasms described above and behaves in a similar manner. It is not radiosensitive but responds well to the combination chemotherapy regimens used for other malignant germ cell neoplasms. The administration of such chemotherapy regimens has radically improved the prognosis of patients with immature teratoma, especially those with grade 2 or 3 tumors.

## 10.4 Mature Cystic Teratoma (Dermoid Cyst) with Malignant Transformation

Malignant transformation is an uncommon complication which occurs in approximately 2% of mature cystic teratomas (SCULLY 1979; TALERMAN 1987a). Unlike the vast majority of patients with malignant ovarian germ cell tumors, who are premenopausal, most of the patients with this tumor are postmenopausal (SCULLY 1979; STAMP and MCCONNELL 1983; TALERMAN 1987a). The tumors are unilateral but may be associated with mature cystic teratoma in the contralateral ovary. The tumors are usually large but generally are indistinguishable from a large mature cystic teratoma, except when they penetrate the ovarian surface, showing nodularity or an irregular outline. They may invade the surrounding structures and may be associated with extensive involvement of the peritoneal cavity by tumor deposits.

Microscopically the tumor at least in some areas shows appearances of typical mature cystic teratoma and malignant transformation of one of its components, usually squamous epithelium which forms a squamous cell carcinoma. The latter is often well-differentiated, but the degree of differentiation may vary. Any tissue within the tumor may undergo malignant change. Mature cystic teratoma with malignant transformation differs from other malignant germ cell tumors in other respects. It does not spread via the lymphatic and hematogenous routes, but spreads extensively throughout the abdominal cavity, and does not respond to the combination chemotherapy regimens which are used nowadays to treat successfully other malignant germ cell tumors. It does not respond to radiotherapy. In view of this, the treatment is primarily surgical and although patients with squamous cell carcinoma and tumors confined to the ovary have a 63% 5-year survival, those with disseminated disease have only a 15% 5-year survival. The prognosis is even worse when the malignant element is other than squamous cell carcinoma, and there are no 5-year survivors in this category. Early stage at diagnosis and complete excision of the tumor are at present the best prognostic features (Scully 1979; Talerman 1987a).

## 10.5 Monodermal or Highly Specialized Teratomas

The tumors that make up this group are composed entirely or predominantly of a single tissue and are considered to represent one-sided development of a teratoma. It is in this group that new entities became established and recognized during the past decade, and they will be discussed in some detail below.

### *10.5.1 Struma Ovarii*

Struma ovarii is the best known and most widely recognized member of this group of neoplasms. It is composed of thyroid tissue. Struma ovarii is uncommon, accounting for approximately 1% of ovarian teratomas (Scully 1979; Talerman 1987a). It must be distinguished from mature cystic teratoma containing thyroid tissue, which is much more common. The age incidence is the same as for mature cystic teratoma, and patients present in the same manner, except for occasional cases where thyroid enlargement has been noted and the rare case associated with thyrotoxicosis. The tumors vary in size; they are usually unilateral but in 15% of cases are associated with mature cystic teratoma in the contralateral ovary. The tumor is usually soft, smooth, round or oval, fleshy, and light tan. Microscopically it is composed of normal thyroid tissue, which may in parts exhibit evidence of hyperplastic, nodular, or adenomatous changes. Occasionally such changes may be extensive and marked, and it is important to distinguish them from malignant change, which is very rare (Talerman 1987a). Struma ovarii is treated by excision of the affected adnexa. When malignant change occurs, it manifests itself more frequently as papillary than as follicular carcinoma, and the tumor is indistinguishable from those occurring within the thyroid gland. The tumors are usually well-differentiated and metastasize first to the para-aortic lymph nodes. Treatment is surgical and therapies used in the treatment of thyroid malignancy may be administered if necessary (Talerman 1987a).

### *10.5.2 Carcinoid*

Ovarian carcinoid tumors have become better recognized during the past decade (Talerman 1984). They are the second most common type of monodermal teratoma after struma ovarii. The classification of carcinoid tumors of the ovary is as follows :

1. Primary
   (a) Insular carcinoid (carcinoid tumors of midgut derivation)
   (b) Trabecular carcinoid (carcinoid tumors of foregut and hindgut derivation)
   (c) Mucinous (goblet cell, adeno-) carcinoid
2. Metastatic

The strumal carcinoid tumor is classified according to the amended WHO classification (SCULLY et al. 1990) separately from other carcinoid tumors, because in addition to its carcinoid content it also contains thyroid tissue.

*10.5.2.1 Insular Carcinoid.* Insular carcinoid is the most common type of primary ovarian carcinoid tumor. It is usually found in association with mature cystic teratoma, but may be seen with other teratomatous tumors, and occasionally with Sertoli–Leydig cell tumor (SCULLY 1979; WAXMAN et al. 1981). In 40% of cases it is seen in pure form. More than 70 cases have been reported, and the number of unreported cases is probably as high (TALERMAN 1987a). The majority of patients with ovarian insular carcinoid are either postmenopausal or perimenopausal. Like patients with mature cystic teratoma, they present with an ovarian mass which may be associated with abdominal pain. One-third of patients exhibit stigmata of the carcinoid syndrome (ROBBOY et al. 1975). Because the venous drainage of the ovary enters the systemic circulation and bypasses the liver, which is capable of detoxifying the serotonin produced by the tumor, the carcinoid syndrome is seen in the absence of metastatic disease. There is a good correlation between the size of the tumor and the presence of the syndrome, which is virtually only seen in patients with tumors larger than 10 cm in the longest diameter (SCULLY 1979). Excision of the tumor results in remission of the symptoms and the disappearance of serotonin from the blood and 5-hydroxyindoleacetic acid (5-HIAA) from the urine. Serotonin and 5-HIAA can be used as tumor markers in patients with functioning ovarian insular carcinoid tumors.

Insular carcinoid forms a solid, yellow–gray tumor nodule within a mature cystic teratoma, or a similar nodule within an ovary when occurring in pure form. The tumor is nearly always unilateral but may be associated with mature cystic teratoma in the contralateral ovary. Microscopically it shows typical appearances of a midgut carcinoid tumor and is composed of solid nests and collections of small acini made up of uniform polygonal cells with an ample amount of cytoplasm and centrally located round or oval nuclei (Fig. 11). Mitotic activity is generally low. The cytoplasm contains orange, red, or brown granules which show the argyrophil and argentaffin reaction when stained with Grimelius and Masson–Fontana stains respectively. The cellular nests are surrounded by connective tissue, which may be dense and hyalinized (Fig. 11) (ROBBOY et al. 1975; SCULLY 1979; TALERMAN 1984).

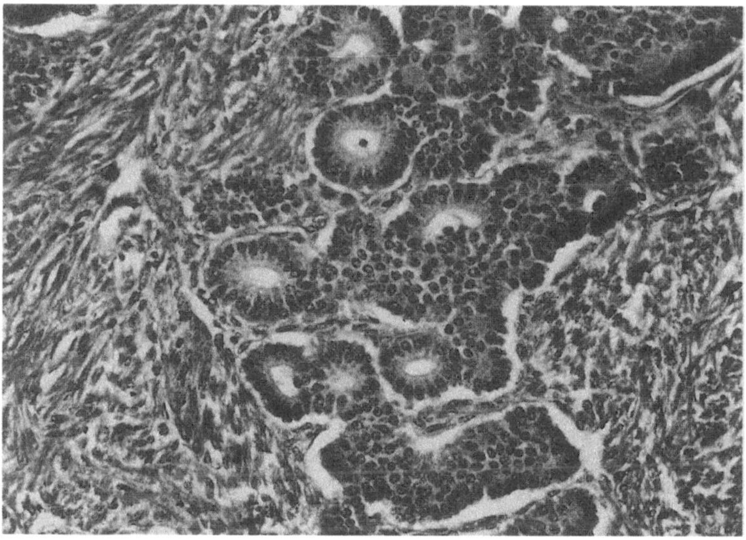

**Fig. 11.** Insular carcinoid tumor composed of solid cellular nests and small acini surrounded by dense connective tissue. H&E, × 140

Ultrastructural examination shows numerous neurosecretory granules which are very pleomorphic, varying in shape and size. Cytokeratin, chromogranin, serotonin, and gastrin can be demonstrated within the tumor cells by immunocytochemistry, but the range of the neurohormonal polypeptides which can be demonstrated is much more limited than in the case of trabecular or strumal carcinoids (SPORRONG et al. 1982).

Insular carcinoid behaves as a neoplasm of low-grade malignancy and only very occasionally has been associated with metastases (ROBBOY et al. 1975; SCULLY 1979; TALERMAN 1984). The treatment of choice is the excision of the tumor, and if the tumor is large a follow-up is recommended, including serum serotonin and urinary 5-HIAA estimations.

*10.5.2.2 Trabecular Carcinoid.* Trabecular carcinoid is far less common than its insular counterpart and only 21 cases have been reported (TALERMAN and EVANS 1982; TALERMAN 1984). It usually arises in association with mature cystic teratoma but also occurs in pure form. The age distribution is similar to insular carcinoid and the affected patients are mainly postmenopausal (TALERMAN 1984). The presenting symptoms are also similar, except that in common with other carcinoid tumors of foregut and hindgut derivation, trabecular carcinoid is not associated with the carcinoid syndrome (TALERMAN 1984). The macroscopic appearance is similar to insular carcinoid. Microscopically, trabecular carcinoid shows very distinctive appearances, being composed of long wavy cords or ribbons running in parallel and surrounded by narrow bands of connective tissue (Fig. 12). The cords or ribbons are composed of one or two cell layers.

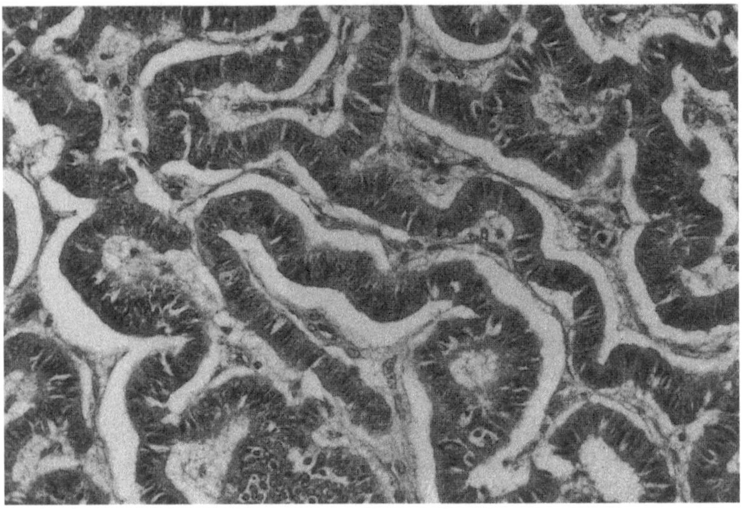

**Fig. 12.** Trabecular carcinoid tumor composed of long wavy cords or ribbons surrounded by fine fibrovascular septa. H&E, × 185

The cells are large columnar or polygonal and contain an ample amount of cytoplasm which may contain orange–red granules. The nuclei are ovoid with dispersed chromatin. Occasional mitoses are present. The orange–red granules stain with argyrophil and sometimes with argentaffin stains (TALERMAN and EVANS 1982; TALERMAN 1984). Ultrastructurally, neurosecretory granules are present which are uniformly round or oval but vary in size (Fig. 13), thus differing from those seen in insular carcinoid (TALERMAN and OKAGAKI 1985). Immunocytochemistry shows a much wider range of neurohormonal polypeptides compared with insular carcinoid, including serotonin, pancreatic polypeptide, glucagon, somatostatin, enkephalin, gastrin, vasoactive intestinal polypeptide and calcitonin (SPORRONG et al. 1982). Trabecular carcinoid to date has not been associated with metastases and therefore prognosis is excellent following excision of the tumor (TALERMAN 1984).

*10.5.2.3 Mucinous (Goblet Cell, Adeno-) Carcinoid.* Mucinous carcinoid is the least common type of primary ovarian carcinoid tumor (TALERMAN 1984). It seems to occur in slightly younger subjects than other types of carcinoid tumors. It is often seen in pure form but is also observed in association with teratomatous elements (TALERMAN et al., unpublished observations). It is usually unilateral but may be associated with mature cystic teratoma or with metastases in the contralateral ovary (ALENGHAT et al. 1986; TALERMAN et al., unpublished observations). The tumors are usually of medium to large size, solid, and gray–yellow, but may contain cystic areas. Microscopically, mucinous carcinoid is composed of numerous small glands or acini with very small lumina, lined by

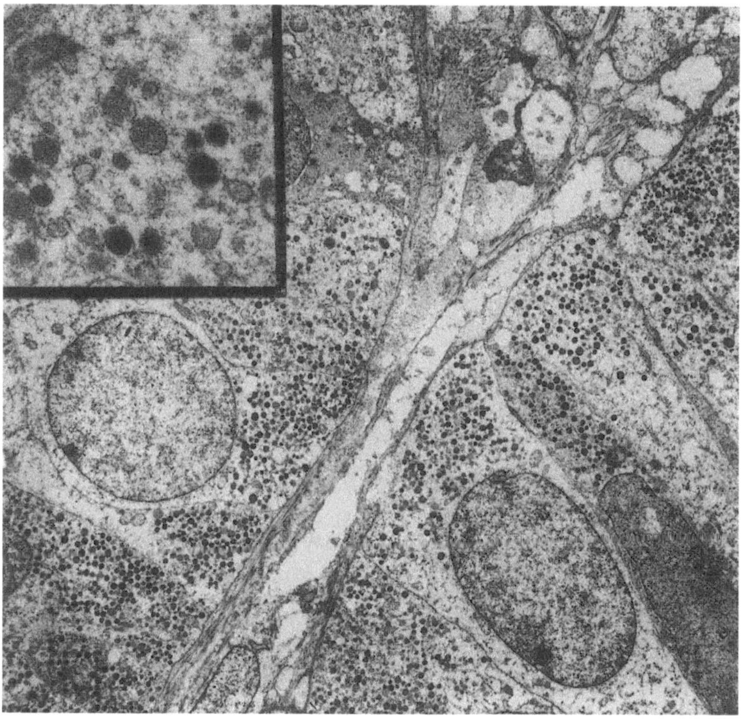

**Fig. 13.** Ultrastructural appearances of trabecular carcinoid tumor showing numerous neurosecretory granules located in the basal part of the cell. × 3200. *Inset*: The granules are uniformly round. × 7900

uniform cuboidal or columnar cells with pale or clear cytoplasm and goblet cells with clear and vacuolated cytoplasm (Fig. 14). The nuclei vary from small and round to large and hyperchromatic. Some cells are distended with mucin and their nuclei are compressed and may be of the signet-ring type. Other cells may be disrupted due to overdistention with mucin (Fig. 14). The cells show argyrophil and argentaffin granules, but there is considerable variation in the frequency and intensity of the staining from tumor to tumor and even within the same tumor.

The glands are surrounded by connective tissue which varies from loose and edematous to dense and fibrous. Some glands may be larger and cystic, containing mucin in their lumen. Small pools of mucin caused by complete disruption of some glands are often present within the connective tissue. Less well-differentiated areas where tumor cells form larger aggregates with numerous signet-ring cells, larger irregular glands lined by atypical cells, and foci of typical Krukenberg tumor are also present (Talerman 1984; Alenghat et al. 1986; Talerman et al., unpublished observations). Although ultrastructural studies showed originally that mucin and neurosecretory granules were present in

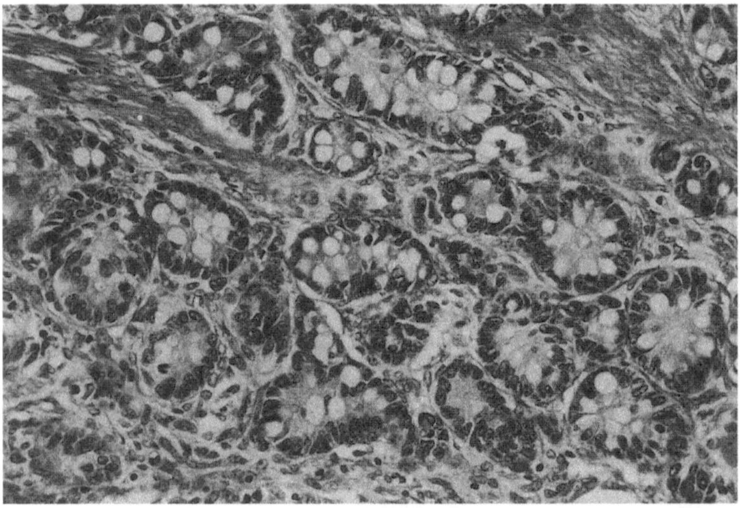

**Fig. 14.** Mucinous carcinoid tumor composed of numerous small glands with prominent goblet cells and surrounded by connective tissue. H&E, ×185

different cells (Talerman 1984), it has been shown subsequently that they may be present in the same cell (Alenghat et al. 1986; Talerman 1987a). The neurosecretory granules are plemorphic and similar to those seen in insular carcinoids (Talerman 1984; Alenghat et al. 1986). Immunocytochemical studies have revealed the presence of cytokeratin, carcinoembryonic antigen, serotonin, gastrin, chromogranin, pancreatic polypeptide, and prolactin (Alenghat et al. 1986; Talerman et al., unpublished observations). Mucinous carcinoid is more malignant than other types of ovarian carcinoid tumors. Except for small tumors associated with mature cystic teratoma, mucinous carcinoid metastasizes widely via small lymphatics and microscopic metastases may be present at the time of diagnosis. In such cases in spite of excision of all the visible tumor deposits, metastases have been noted within 6–12 months and the patients have died of the disease in less than 2 years. Response to chemotherapy has so far been disappointing (Talerman 1984; Alenghat et al. 1986; Talerman et al., unpublished observations).

*10.5.2.4 Metastatic Carcinoid Tumors.* Primary ovarian carcinoids must be distinguished from metastatic carcinoids, most frequently of the insular type (Robboy et al. 1974) but occasionally of the mucinous type (Talerman 1984; Talerman et al., unpublished observations). Metastatic carcinoids invariably involve both ovaries and tumor deposits are diffusely scattered throughout the ovarian tissue. This is detected microscopically, but if the tumor nodules are larger they may be seen on macroscopic examination. The most common sites of origin of metastatic carcinoid tumors to the ovary are small intestinal carcinoids of the insular type and mucinous carcinoids of the vermiform appendix (Robboy et al.

1974; TALERMAN 1984). It is of interest that although the prognosis of mucinous carcinoid tumors of the vermiform appendix is generally favorable, when metastases to the ovaries are present the outcome in invariably fatal (TALERMAN et al., unpublished observations).

## 10.6 Strumal Carcinoid (Struma Ovarii and Carcinoid)

Strumal carcinoid is composed of thyroid tissue intimately admixed with carcinoid tumor which in most cases is of the trabecular type, sometimes of both the trabecular and the insular type, and rarely entirely of the insular type (ROBBOY and SCULLY 1980). Although a controversy has raged over the identity of the thyroid component, its true thyroid nature has been conclusively documented by the demonstration of thyroglobulin within the thyroid follicles (UEDA et al. 1978; ROBBOY and SCULLY 1980; SNYDER and TAVASSOLI 1986). Either component may predominate within the tumor.

Strumal carcinoid is the second most common type of ovarian carcinoid tumor after the insular carcinoid, and more than 60 cases have been reported (ROBBOY and SCULLY 1980; SNYDER and TAVASSOLI 1986). It has the same age

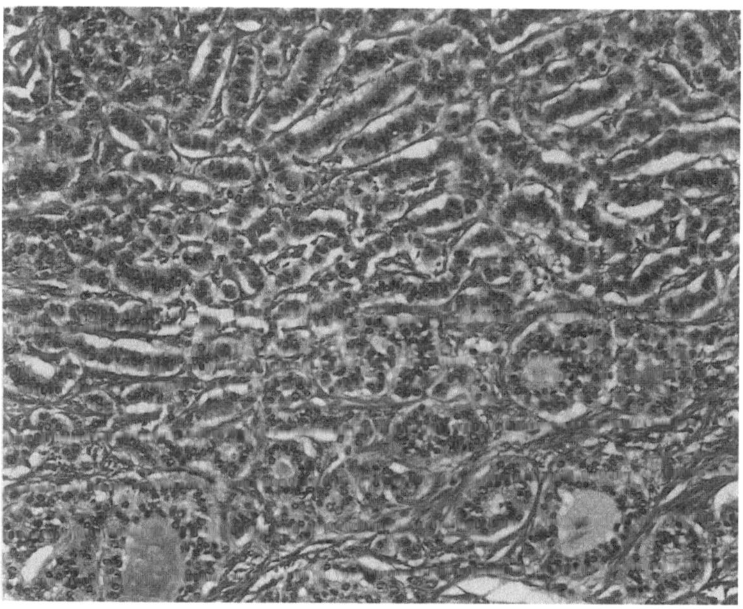

**Fig. 15.** Strumal carcinoid tumor composed of carcinoid tumor showing trabecular pattern (*top*) intimately admixed with thyroid follicles (*bottom*). H&E, × 140

distribution and symptomatology as other ovarian carcinoids. As a rule it is not associated with the carcinoid syndrome and this association has only been documented in a single case (ULBRIGHT et al. 1982). Macroscopically it shows the same features as other ovarian carcinoids, and may constitute a part of a mature cystic teratoma or occur in pure form. The former is more common. Microscopically it is composed of thyroid tissue which is intimately admixed with carcinoid tumor most frequently of the trabecular type (Fig. 15). Argyrophil granules are present not only in the cells forming the carcinoid trabeculae but also in some of the cells lining the thyroid follicles, and 50% of the tumors contain argentaffin granules (ROBBOY and SCULLY 1980). In occasional tumors amyloid is present in the stroma (DAYAL et al. 1979). Ultrastructural examination shows neurosecretory granules not only within the carcinoid component but also in some cells lining the thyroid follicles (SNYDER and TAVASSOLI 1986; STAGNO et al. 1987). Excision of the tumor results in a complete cure. Metastases have only been reported in a single case and even this patient has been cured (ROBBOY and SCULLY 1980).

## 10.7 Other Types of Monodermal Teratoma

In recent years a number of other types of monodermal teratoma have been recognized (AGUIRRE and SCULLY 1982; KLEIMAN et al. 1984; TALERMAN, unpublished observations). It should also be pointed out that between 10% and 20% of mucinous tumors of the ovary show intestinal differentiation and are probably of germ cell origin (SCULLY 1979; TALERMAN 1987a). Five percent of mucinous tumors are associated with dermoid cysts or carcinoids (SCULLY 1979).

### *10.7.1 Monodermal Teratomas with Neuroectodermal Differentiation*

Both malignant (AGUIRRE and SCULLY 1982; KLEIMAN et al. 1984, 1990) and benign (ULIRSCH and GOLDMAN 1982; TILTMAN 1985) tumors of this type have been described during the past decade. The benign tumors consisted of a cyst lined entirely either by mature glial tissue and described as a neurogenic cyst (ULIRSCH and GOLDMAN 1982), or by ependymal tissue (TILTMAN 1985). It is very important to recognize the benign nature of such tumors and to differentiate them from their malignant counterparts.

The malignant tumors in this category consist of malignant neuroectodermal tumor (AGUIRRE and SCULLY 1982) and of ependymoma (KLEIMAN et al. 1984; DEKMEZIAN et al. 1986).

*10.7.1.1 Malignant Neuroectodermal Tumor.* AGUIRRE and SCULLY (1982) described five ovarian tumors occurring in patients in the second decade and showing pure neuroectodermal differentiation characterized by histologic patterns resembling those of glioblastoma, medulloblastoma, and neuroblastoma present alone or in combination. Small foci of more mature glia or ependyma, as well as small foci of mature teratoma, may also be seen in these tumors. The tumors pursue an aggressive course and prognosis is poor (AGUIRRE and SCULLY 1982). Although such tumors may be confused with other ovarian tumors composed of small cells, special stains for neural tissue and immunocytochemical stains for glial fibrillary acidic protein (GFAP) and neurofilaments are helpful in reaching the current diagnosis.

*10.7.1.2 Ependymoma.* Four cases of pure ovarian ependymoma representing one-sided development of a teratoma have been reported (KLEIMAN et al. 1984; DEKMEZIAN et al. 1986). The patients were all in the third and fourth decades and presented with abdominal pain and a palpable abdominal mass. Three patients had intra-abdominal metastases and in one case the tumor was confined to the ovary. The tumors were cystic containing fleshy mural nodules or papillary processes arising from the cyst wall. Microscopically they showed typical features of ependymoma arising in the central nervous system (Fig. 16). Perivascular pseudorosettes consisting of a blood vessel surrounded by tumor cells with long radiating processes and antipodally arranged nuclei characteristic of ependymoma were prominent, and central lumen (Homer Wright) rosettes were also seen (Fig. 16). Mitotic activity varied from one to three per ten high power fields. Special stains for neural tissue and for GFAP are helpful in confirming the diagnosis (KLEIMAN et al. 1984). The prognosis of patients with this tumor is much more favorable than that of those with malignant neuroectodermal tumor, and in spite of the presence of metastases on presentation in three of the four patients, only one of them succumbed to the disease.

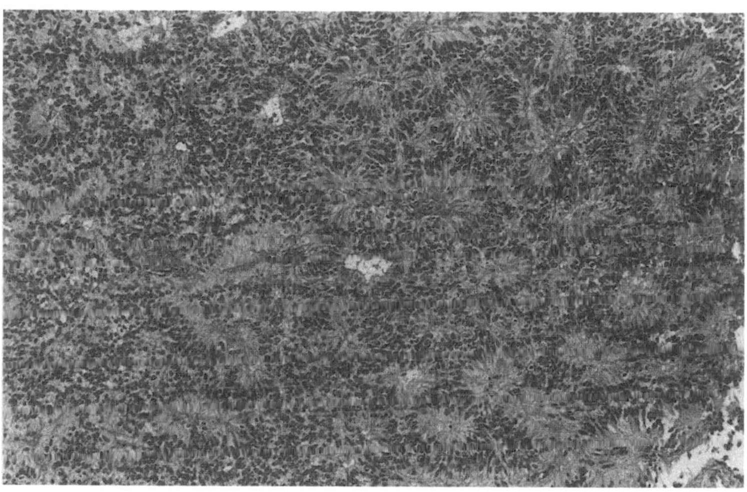

**Fig. 16.** Ependymoma containing typical Homer Wright rosettes and perivascular pseudorosettes. H&E, × 90

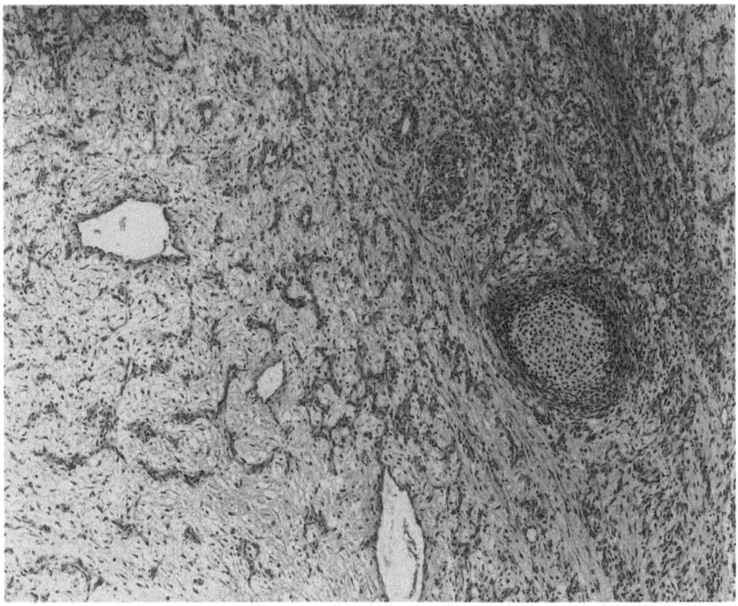

**Fig. 17.** Immature teratoma composed predominantly of vascular tissue. Note the solid cord-like immature vessels mainly devoid of a lumen and surrounded by loose connective tissue. A nest of immature cartilage (*right*) provides a clue to the diagnosis. H&E, × 75

### *10.7.2 Monodermal Teratoma Composed of Vascular Tissue*

Another type of monodermal teratoma is represented by neoplasms composed entirely or predominantly of immature vascular tissue. They occur in children and young adults, and the patients present with symptoms and signs suggestive of an ovarian tumor. The tumors may vary in size, and are smooth, soft, solid, and gray–pink, but may be hemorrhagic. Microscopically they consist of collections of small vascular spaces lined by immature endothelial cells and surrounded by connective tissue, which varies from loose and edematous to dense and fibrous. The lining of the vascular spaces may be multilayered and the endothelial cells may form small projections bulging into the lumen. Small collections of endothelial cells, some forming abortive lumina and some devoid of a lumen, are also seen within the connective tissue and may predominate (Fig. 17). The endothelial cells show a considerable degree of cellular and nuclear pleomorphism, and mitotic activity is usually evident. Occasionally hematopoietic activity may be seen within some of the vascular spaces. When these tumors contain small teratomatous foci (Fig. 17) their nature is more readily apparent, but when they occur in pure form, especially when the endothelial cells form a more solid pattern with fewer obvious vascular spaces (Fig. 17), the nature of the lesion is more difficult to recognize. Occasionally these tumors may be composed of immature pericytes and resemble a hemangiopericytoma. Further sectioning of the tumor, which may reveal a more typical vascular pattern, and immunocytochemical stains for factor VIII and *Ulex Europaeus* may be helpful in reaching the correct diagnosis. This is important because monodermal teratomas composed of immature vascular tissue or with a predominant vascular component behave on the whole in a less aggressive manner compared with high-grade immature teratomas and hemangioendothelial sarcomas of the ovary, with which they tend to be confused. As in most immature teratomas, the grade of the tumor is an important prognostic feature.

## 11 Mixed Germ Cell Tumors

This group comprises all germ cell tumors composed of more than one germ cell element, and because of this all the neoplasms included in this category are malignant. Although in the past mixed or combined germ cell tumors were considered to be rare, recent studies indicate that they are not uncommon (KURMAN and NORRIS 1976b; SCULLY 1979; GERSHENSON et al. 1984; ULBRIGHT et al. 1986; TALERMAN 1987a). More extensive sampling and careful histologic examination are considered to be the main contributory factors to these developments. The importance of recognizing the presence of multiple neoplastic germ cell elements within a germ cell tumor needs little emphasis, as it provides the correct diagnosis and forms a basis for the appropriate therapy. It can also explain the presence or absence of tumor markers like AFP or β-hCG in the serum and may help to explain similarities and differences in tumor content between the primary tumor and its metastases. Therefore extensive and judicious sampling and careful histologic examination of germ cell tumors are strongly recommended. At least one section should be taken per centimeter of the longest dimension of the tumor, and additional sections should be taken from any differing parts (TALERMAN 1987a).

## 12 Tumors Composed of Germ Cells and Sex Cord-Stromal Derivatives

Tumors composed of germ cells intimately admixed with sex cord-stromal derivatives are uncommon, and consist of two distinct types:

1. Gonadoblastoma
2. Mixed germ cell–sex cord-stroma tumor (MGC–SCST)

## 12.1 Gonadoblastoma

Gonadoblastoma occurs predominantly in young phenotypic females (80%) and less frequently in phenotypic male pseudohermaphrodites (20%) (SCULLY 1970). The majority of phenotypic females with gonadoblastoma (60%) show signs of virilization. Nearly all patients (96%) are chromatin-negative and have a Y chromosome. The most common karyotypes observed are 46, XY, 45, X/46, XY, and various other forms of mosaicism (SCULLY 1970; TALERMAN 1987a). Gonadoblastoma has been described occasionally in patients with Turner's syndrome, in true hermaphrodites, and in phenotypic females with normal 46, XX karyotype (TALERMAN 1987a). The gonad of origin is often indeterminate, but when discernible it is usually a testis or a streak gonad. The contralateral gonad is a testis, a streak, or is indeterminate. In more than 50% of cases it also contains a gonadoblastoma (SCULLY 1970; TALERMAN 1987a). In a few cases gonadoblastomas has been observed in ovotestes (Fig. 18) or in normal ovaries (TALERMAN 1987a; NAKASHIMA et al. 1989). Gonadoblastoma is a small lesion, sometimes only microscopic, and shows a very typical and distinct histologic appearance which has been described in detail (SCULLY 1970, 1979; TALERMAN 1980, 1987a). It is frequently admixed with dysgerminoma and this is seen in more than 50% of cases. In another 10% it is admixed with other malignant neoplastic germ cell elements (SCULLY 1970; TALERMAN 1987a). When gonado-

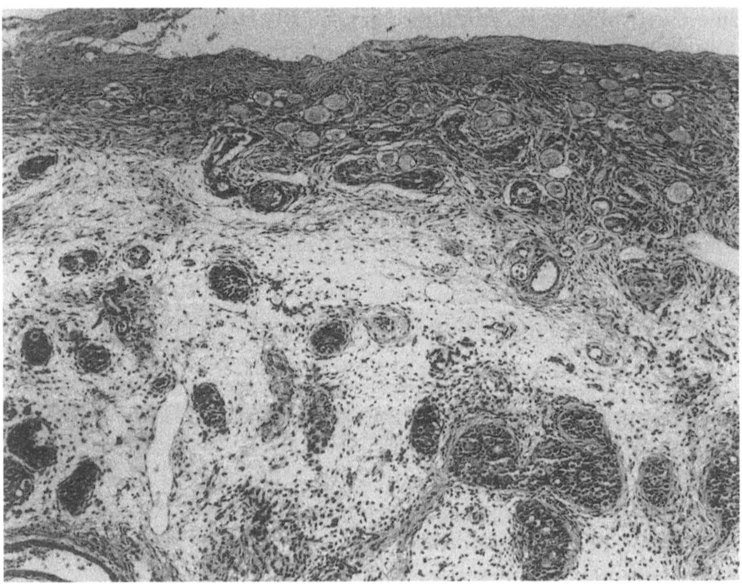

**Fig. 18.** Ovotestis containing gonadoblastoma. Note the primordial follicles (*top*), seminiferous tubules (*left and top*), and gonadoblastoma nests (*right*). H&E, ×40

blastoma is associated with dysgerminoma, the latter tends to metastasize less frequently and later than dysgerminoma arising de novo, and prognosis is very favorable. When gonadoblastoma is admixed with other malignant germ cell elements the treatment is surgical followed by administration of combination chemotherapy used to treat malignant germ cell tumors other than dysgerminoma. Although previously the prognosis of such patients was poor, nowadays it is much more favorable due to the efficacious combination chemotherapy (TALERMAN 1987a).

Bilateral gonadectomy is mandatory in patients with dysgenetic gonads and karyotypes containing the Y chromosome because of its high malignant potential in such subjects and because the gonads are nonfunctional (SCULLY 1970; TALERMAN 1987a). In true hermaphrodites with normal 46, XX female karyotype and unilateral gonadoblastoma, one-sided gonadectomy and biopsy of the contralateral gonad should be performed. If the contralateral gonad is a normal ovary or even an ovotestis it may be left in situ and the patient carefully followed up. A similar course may be followed in occasional phenotypic females with normal, 46, XX karyotype and gonadoblastoma occurring in normal ovary, as normal pregnancies have been reported in such subjects (TALERMAN 1987a; NAKASHIMA et al. 1989). A normal pregnancy has been documented recently in a true hermaphrodite with bilateral ovotestes and bilateral gonadoblastomas (Fig. 18) (TALERMAN et al. 1990).

Although it has been suggested that gonadoblastoma may co-exist with MGC–SCST, the documentation in the only case describing such an association is considered to be highly unsatisfactory and the tumor described and depicted (BHATENA et al. 1985) is in reality a conventional gonadoblastoma.

Gonadoblastoma has never been encountered in extragonadal locations or in metastatic lesions and to date it has only been observed in the gonads.

## 12.2 Mixed Germ Cell–Sex Cord-Stroma Tumor

The MGC–SCST is encountered most frequently in normal ovaries of phenotypic female infants and children with normal 46, XX karyotype. It has also occurred in ovaries of genetically normal young women, some of whom have had normal pregnancies, as well as in descended testes of genetically normal adult males, some of whom are known to have fathered children (TALERMAN 1980, 1987a). MGC–SCST has not been associated with abnormal karyotypes or gonadal dysgenesis. The patients present with an abdominal mass which may be associated with pain. Infants and prepubertal children may present with isosexual precocious pseudopuberty which regresses following the excision of the tumor (TALERMAN 1987a). The tumors are usually large, solid, smooth, and gray-white. Although the tumors are usually unilateral, two patients with bilateral tumors, one an infant and the other a 21-year-old girl, have been encountered in recent years (TALERMAN, unpublished observations). In both cases MGC–SCST was present in pure form and was not associated with other neoplastic germ cell elements. The histologic appearances of MGC–SCST have been described in detail (TALERMAN 1980, 1987a). Although originally MGC–SCST was observed only in pure form and it was considered that, unlike gonadoblastoma, it is not associated with other neoplastic germ cell elements, occasional cases have come to light where MGC–SCST was associated with dysgerminoma (Fig. 19) or other malignant neoplastic germ cell elements (TALERMAN 1980, 1987a). Although the frequency of this complication is far lower than in patients with gonadoblastoma, where it is seen in more than 60% of cases, it should certainly be borne in mind. This complication is rare in infants and children in the first decade, but when the tumor occurs in postpubertal patients it is seen more frequently (TALERMAN 1987a). Dysgerminoma is the most common malignant germ cell element associated with MGC–SCST (Fig. 19), but YST, choriocarcinoma, and mixed germ cell tumors have also been encountered (TALERMAN 1987a). Recently the first case of metastasizing MGC–SCST, occurring in a normal 8-year-old girl, was reported. The metastases were found in the para-aorotic lymph nodes and the peritoneal cavity. The patient was treated by excision of the affected adnexa and intra-abdominal metastatic tumor deposits, followed by combination chemotherapy. She was well without evidence of disease 2 years after surgery (LACSON et al. 1988). Although MGC–SCST is capable of metastatic spread, this is rarely seen and there are

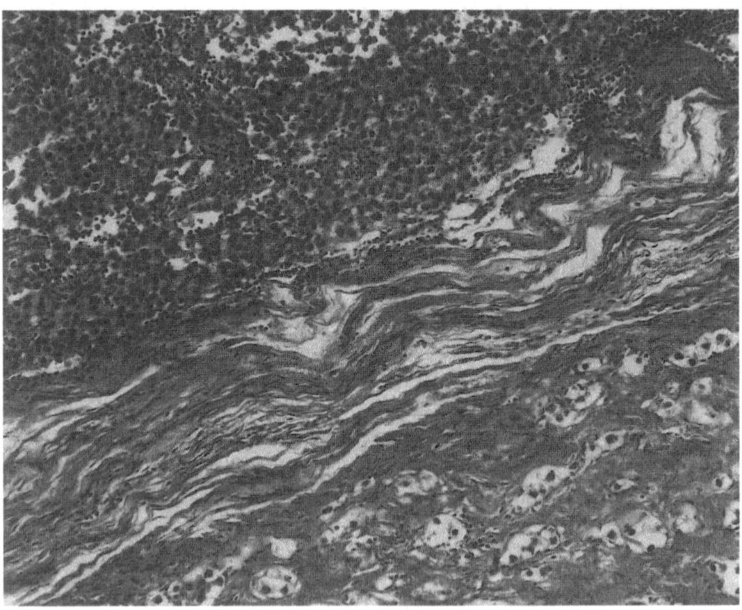

**Fig. 19.** Mixed germ cell–sex cord-stroma tumor (*bottom*) associated with dysgerminoma (*top*). H&E, × 90

cases on record where the tumor was known to be present for a number of years without development of metastatic disease (TALERMAN and VAN DER HARTEN 1977). The recommended treatment for patients with ovarian MGC–SCST is excision of the tumor or unilateral adnexectomy, careful inspection or biopsy of the contralateral ovary, and long-term follow-up of the patient.

The prognosis of patients with MGC–SCST has been very good. Fatal outcome occurred in a few cases when the tumor was associated with malignant neoplastic germ cell elements other than dysgerminoma in the days before combination chemotherapy effective in treating these neoplasms was introduced. Such chemotherapy regimens have proven themselves to be effective in a few known cases of MGC–SCST associated with YST (TALERMAN, unpublished observations) and were successful in the only case of metastasizing MGC–SCST reported to date (LACSON et al. 1988).

It is of interest that to date none of the MGC–SCSTs seen in males have been associated with metastases or with other neoplastic germ cell elements.

## References


Alenghat E, Okagaki T, Talerman A (1986) Primary mucinous carcinoid tumor of the ovary. Cancer 58:777–783

Aguirre P, Scully RE (1982) Malignant neuroectodermal tumor of the ovary, a distinctive form of monodermal teratoma. Report of five cases. Am J Surg Pathol 6:283–292

Asadourian LA, Taylor HB (1969) Dysgerminoma. An analysis of 105 cases. Obstet Gynecol 33:370–379

Atkin NB (1973) High chromosome numbers of seminomata and malignant teratomata of the testis: a review of data on 103 tumors. Br J Cancer 28:275–278

Atkin NB, Baker MC (1983) i (12p): specific chromosomal marker in seminoma and malignant teratoma of the testis? Cancer Genet Cytogenet 10:199–204

Atkin NB, Baker MC (1987) Abnormal chromosomes including small metacentrics in 14 ovarian cancers. Cancer Genet Cytogenet 26:355–361

Awais GM (1983) Dysgerminoma and serum lactic dehydrogense levels. Obstet Gynecol 61:99–101

Battifora H, Sheibani K, Tubbs RR, Kopinski M, Sun T (1984) Antikeratin antibodies in tumor diagnosis. Distinction between seminoma and embryonal carcinoma. Cancer 54:843–848

Beck JS, Fulmer HF, Lee ST (1969) Solid malignant teratoma with "embryoid bodies" and trophoblastic differentiation. J Pathol Bacteriol 99:67–72

Bhatena D, Haning RV Jr, Shapiro S, Hafez GR (1985) Coexistence of a gonadoblastoma and mixed germ cell–sex cord stroma tumor. Pathol Res Pract 180:203–206

Bjorkholm E, Lundell M, Gyftodimos A, Silversward C (1990) Dysgerminoma. The Radiumhemmet series 1927–1984. Cancer 65:38–44

Bradof JE, Hakes TB, Ochoa M, Golbey R (1982) Germ cell malignancies of the ovary. Treatment with vinblastine, actinomycin D, bleomycin, and cisplatin containing chemotherapy combinations. Cancer 50:1070–1075

Clement PB, Young RH, Scully RE (1987) Endometrioid-like variant of ovarian yolk sac tumor. A clinicopathological analysis of eight cases. Am J Surg Pathol 11:767–778

Cohen MB, Mulchahey KM, Molnar JJ (1986) Ovarian endodermal sinus tumor with intestinal differentiation. Cancer 57:1580–1583

Cohen MB, Friend DS, Molnar JJ, Talerman A (1987) Gonadal endodermal sinus (yolk sac) tumor with pure intestinal differentiation; a new histologic type. Pathol Res Pract 182:609–616

Dayal Y, Tashjian AH Jr, Wolfe HJ (1979) Immunocytochemical localization of calcitonin-producing cells in a strumal carcinoid with amyloid stroma. Cancer 43:1331–1338

Dekmezian R, Sneige N, Ordonez NG (1986) Ovarian and omental ependymomas in peritoneal washings: cytologic and immunocytochemical features. Diagn Cytopathol 2:62–68
Fujii S, Konishi I, Suzuki A, Okamura H, Okazaki T, Mori T (1985) Analysis of serum lactic dehydrogenase levels and its isoenzymes in ovarian dysgerminoma. Gynecol Oncol 22:65–72
Gershenson DM, Del Junco G, Herson J, Rutledge FN (1983) Endodermal sinus tumor of the ovary. The MD Anderson experience. Obstet Gynecol 61:194–202
Gershenson DM, Del Junco G, Copeland LJ, Rutledge FN (1984) Mixed germ cell tumors of the ovary. Obstet Gynecol 64:200–206
Gibas Z, Prout FR Jr, Sandberg AA (1984) Malignant teratoma of the testis with an isochromosome No12, i (12p), as the sole structural abnormality. J Urol 131:762–763
Gordon A, Lipton D, Woodruff JD (1981) Dysgerminoma: a review of 158 cases from the Emil Novak Ovarian Tumor Registry. Obstet Gynecol 58:497–504
Jacobs AJ, Newland JR, Green RK (1982) Pure choriocarcinoma of the ovary. Obstet Gynecol Surv 37:603–609
Jacobsen GR, Talerman A (1989) Atlas of germ cell tumors. Munksgaard, Copenhagen
Jenkyn DJ, McCartney AJ (1987) A chromosome study of three ovarian tumors. Cancer Genet Cytogenet 26:327–337
King ME, DiGiovanni LM, Yung JF, Clarke-Pearson DL (1990) Immature teratoma of the ovary grade 3, with karyotype analysis. Int J Gynecol Pathol 9:178–184
King ME, Hubbell MJ, Talerman A (1991) Mixed germ cell tumor of the ovary with prominent polyembryoma component. Int J Gynecol Pathol 10:88–95
Kleiman GM, Young RH, Scully RE (1984) Ependymoma of the ovary: report of three cases. Hum Pathol 15:632–638
Kleiman GM, Young RH, Scully RE (1990) Ovarian neuroectodermal tumors. Mod Pathol 3:52A
Kommoss F, Franklin WA, Talerman A (1989) Estrogen and progesterone receptors in endodermal sinus (yolk sac) tumor. Evaluation of immunocytochemical and biochemical methods. J Reprod Med 34:943–945
Kommoss F, Bibbo M, Talerman A (1990) Nuclear deoxyribonucleic acid content (ploidy) of endodermal sinus (yolk sac) tumor. Lab Invest 62:223–231
Konishi I, Fujii S, Kataoka N, Noda Y, Okamura H, Yamabe H, Mori T (1988) Ovarian mucinous cystadenocarcinoma producing α-fetoprotein Int J Gynecol Pathol 7:182–189
Kurman RJ, Norris HJ (1976a) Endodermal sinus tumor of the ovary. A clinical and pathologic analysis of 71 cases. Cancer 38:2404–2419
Kurman RJ, Norris HJ (1976b) Malignant mixed germ cell tumors of the ovary. A clinical and pathologic analysis of 30 cases. Obstet Gynecol 48:579–589
Kurman RJ, Norris HJ (1976c) Embryonal carcinoma of the ovary. A clinicopathologic entity distinct from endodermal sinus tumor and resembling embryonal carcinoma of the adult testis. Cancer 38:2420–2433
Lacson AG, Gillis DA, Shawwa A (1988) Malignant mixed germ cell–sex cord stromal tumors of the ovary associated with isosexual precocious puberty. Cancer 61:2122–2133
Langley FA, Govan ADT, Anderson MC, Gowing NFC, Woodcock AS, Harilal KR (1981) Yolk sac and allied tumors of the ovary. Histopathology 5:389–401
Linder D, Kaiser-McCaw B, Hecht R (1975) Parthenogenic origin of benign ovarian teratomas. N Engl J Med 292: 63–66
Marin-Padilla M (1965) Origin, nature and significance of the "embryoids" of human teratomas. Virchows Arch [A] 340:105–121
Mazur MT, Talbot WH Jr, Talerman A (1988) Endodermal sinus tumor and mucinous cystadenofibroma of the ovary. Occurrence in an 82-year-old woman. Cancer 62:2011–2015
Miettinen M, Virtanen I, Talerman A (1986) Intermediate filaments in testicular germ cell tumors. In: Talerman A, Roth LM (eds) Pathology of the testis and its adnexa. Churchill Livingstone, New York, pp 181–191
Mostofi FK, Sobin LH (1977) Histological typing of testis tumors. International Histological Classification of Tumors No. 16. World Health Organization, Geneva
Nakashima M, Nagasaka T, Fukata S, Oiwa N, Nara Y, Fukatsu T, Takeuchi J (1989) Ovarian gonadoblastoma with dysgerminoma in a woman with two normal children. Hum Pathol 20:814–816
Nielsen SNJ, Scheithauer BW, Gaffey TA (1985) Gliomatosis peritonei. Cancer 56:2499–2503
Nomura K, Ohama K, Okamoto E, Fujiwara A (1983) Cytogenetic studies of multiple ovarian dermoid cysts in a single host. Acta Obstet Gynecol Jpn 35:1938–1944

Norris HJ, Zirkin HJ, Benson WL (1976) Immature (malignant) teratoma of the ovary. A clinical and pathologic study of 58 cases. Cancer 37:2359–2372

Parrington JM, West LF, Povey S (1984) The origin of ovarian teratomas. J Med Genet 21:4–12

Parrington JM, West LF, Povey S (1986) Chromosome changes in germ cell tumors. In: Jones WG, Milford Ward A, Anderson CK (eds) Germ cell tumors II. Pergamon, Oxford, pp 61–67

Prat J, Bhan AK, Dickersin RG, Robboy SJ, Scully RE (1982) Hepatoid yolk sac tumor of the ovary (endodermal sinus tumor with hapatoid differentiation). A light microscopic, ultrastructural and immunohistochemical study of seven cases. Cancer 50:2355–2368

Robboy SJ, Scully RE (1970) Ovarian teratoma with glial implants on the peritoneum. Hum Pathol 1:643–653

Robboy SJ, Scully RE (1980) Strumal carcinoid of the ovary: an analysis of 50 cases of a distinctive tumor composed of thyroid tissue and carcinoid. Cancer 46:2019–2034

Robboy SJ, Scully RE, Norris HJ (1974) Carcinoid metastatic to the ovary. A clinicopathologic analysis of 35 cases. Cancer 33:798–811

Robboy SJ, Norris HJ, Scully RE (1975) Insular carcinoid primary in the ovary. A clinicopathologic analysis of 48 cases. Cancer 36:404–418

Rutgers JL, Young RH, Scully RE (1987) Ovarian yolk sac tumor arising from endometrioid carcinoma. Hum Pathol 18:1296–1299

Sawada M, Okudaira Y, Matsui Y, Nishiura H, Iwasaki T, Karamatsu H (1985) Cisplatin, vinblastine and bleomycin therapy of yolk sac (endodermal sinus) tumor of the ovary. Gynecol Oncol 20:162–169

Schwartz PE, Morris JM (1988) Serum lactic dehydrogenase. A tumor marker for dysgerminoma. Obstet Gynecol 72:511–515

Scully RE (1970) Gonadoblastoma. A review of 74 cases. Cancer 25:1340–1356

Scully RE (1979) Tumors of the ovary and maldeveloped gonads. Atlas of tumor pathology, second series, fascicle 16. Armed Forces Institute of Pathology, Washington, DC.

Scully RE, Sasano N, Saksela E, Fox H, Russell P, Talerman A, Sobin LH (1990) World Health Organization classification of the tumors of the ovary, fallopian tube and peritoneum. Springer, Heidelberg, Berlin New York (in press)

Serov SF, Scully RE, Sobin LH (1973) Histological typing of ovarian tumours. International histological classification of tumours No. 9. World Health Organization, Geneva

Sessa C, Bonazzi C, Landoni F, Pecorelli S, Sartori E, Mangioni C (1987) Cisplatin, vinblastine and bleomycin combination chemotherapy in endodermal sinus tumor of the ovary. Obstet Gynecol 70:220–224

Simard LC (1957) Polyembryonic embryoma of the ovary of parthenogenetic origin. Cancer 10:215–223

Snyder RR, Tavassoli FA (1986) Ovarian strumal carcinoid: immunohistochemical, ultrastructural, and clinicopathologic observations. Int J Gynecol Pathol 5:187–201

Sporrong B, Falkmer S, Robboy SJ, Alumets J, Hakanson R, Ljungberg O, Sundler F (1982) Neurohormonal peptides in ovarian carcinoids: an immunohistochemical study of 81 primary carcinoids and of intraovarian metastases from six mid-gut carcinoids. Cancer 49:68–74

Stagno PA, Petras RE, Hart WR (1987) Strumal carcinoids of the ovary. An immunohistologic and ultrastructural study. Arch Pathol Lab Med 111:440–446

Stamp GWH, McConnell EM (1983) Malignancy arising in cystic ovarian teratomas. Br J Obstet Gynecol 90:671–675

Takeda A, Ishizuka T, Goto T, Goto S, Ohta M, Tomoda Y, Hoshino M (1982) Polyembryoma of ovary producing α-fetoprotein and HCG: immunoperoxidase and electron microscopic study. Cancer 49:1878–1889

Talerman A (1980) Pathology of gonadal neoplasms composed of germ cells and sex cord stroma derivatives. Pathol Res Pract 170:24–38

Talerman A (1984) Carcinoid tumors of the ovary. J Cancer Res Clin Oncol 107:125–135

Talerman A (1987a) Germ cell tumors of the ovary. In: Kurman RJ (ed) Blaustein's pathology of the female genital tract. Springer, New York Heidelberg Berlin

Talerman A (1987b) Ovarian Sertoli–Leydig cell tumor (androblastoma) with retiform pattern. A clinicopathologic study. Cancer 60:3056–3064

Talerman A, Evans MI (1982) Primary trabecular carcinoid tumor of the ovary. Cancer 50:1403–1407

Talerman A, Okagaki T (1985) Ultrastructural features of primary trabecular carcinoid tumor of the ovary. Int J Gynecol Pathol 4:153–160

Talerman A, van der Hartern JJ (1977) A mixed germ cell–sex cord stroma tumor of the ovary associated with isosexual precocious puberty in a normal girl. Cancer 40:889–894
Talerman A, Huyzinga WT, Kuipers T (1973) Dysgerminoma. Clinicopathologic study of 22 cases. Obstet Gynecol 41:137–147
Talerman A, Haije WG, Baggerman L (1980) Serum α-fetoprotein (AFP) in patients with germ cell tumors of the gonads and extragonadal sites: correlation between endodermal sinus (yolk sac) tumor and raised serum AFP. Cancer 46:380–385
Talerman A, Verp M, Senekjian E, Gilewski T, Vogelzang N (1990) True hermaphrodite with normal female 46, XX karyotype, bilateral gonadoblastomas and dysgerminomas and normal pregnancy. Cancer 66:2668–2672
Taylor MH, DePetrillo AD, Turner AR (1985) Vinblastine bleomycin and cisplatin in malignant germ cell tumors of the ovary. Cancer 56:1341–1349
Teilum G (1965) Classification of endodermal sinus tumor (mesoblastoma vitellinum) and so-called "embryonal carcinoma" of the ovary. Acta Pathol Microbiol Scand 64:407–429
Teilum G (1976) Special tumors of the ovary and testis. Comparative histology and identification, 2nd edn. Munksgaard, Copenhagen
Thomas GM, Dembo AJ, Hacker NE, DePetrillo AD (1987) Current therapy for dysgerminoma of the ovary. Obstet Gynecol 70:268–275
Thurlbeck WM, Scully RE (1960) Solid teratoma of the ovary. Cancer 13:804–811
Tiltman AJ (1985) Ependymal cyst of the ovary. S Afr Med J 68:424–425
Truan LD, Jurco S III, McGavran MH (1982) Gliomatosis peritonei. Report of two cases and review of literature. Am J Surg Pathol 6:443–449
Tsuchida Y, Kaneko M, Yokomori K et al. (1978) α-fetoprotein, prealbumin, albumin, α-1-antitrypsin, and transferrin as diagnostic and therapeutic markers for endodermal sinus tumors. J Pediatr Surg 13:25–29
Ueda G, Sato Y, Yamasaki M et al. (1978) Strumal carcinoid of the ovary. Histological, ultrastructural, and immunohistological studies with antihuman thyroglobulin. Gynecol Oncol 6:411–419
Ulbright TM, Roth LM, Ehrlich CE (1982) Ovarian strumal carcinoid. An immunocytochemical and ultrastructural study of two cases. Am J Clin Pathol 77:662–663
Ulbright TM, Roth LM, Brodhecker CA (1986) Yolk sac differentiation in germ cell tumors. A morphologic study of 50 cases with emphasis on hepatic, enteric, and parietal yolk sac features. Am J Surg Pathol 10:151–164
Ulirsch RC, Goldman RL (1982) An unusual teratoma of the ovary: neurogenic cyst with lactating breast tissue. Obstet Gynecol 60:400–402
Vance RP, Geisinger KR (1985) Pure nongestational choriocarcinoma of the ovary. Report of a case. Cancer 56:2321–2325
Waxman M, Damjanov I, Alpert L, Sardinsky T (1981) Composite mucinous ovarian neoplasms associated with Sertoli–Leydig and carcinoid tumors. Cancer 47:2044–2052
Young RH, Scully RE (1983) Ovarian Sertoli–Leydig cell tumors with a retiform pattern. A problem in histopathologic diagnosis. A report of 25 cases. Am J Surg Pathol 7:755–771
Zaloudek CJ, Tavassoli FA, Norris HJ (1981) Dysgerminoma with syncytiotrophoblastic giant cells. A histologically and clinically distinctive subtype of dysgerminoma. Am J Surg Pathol 5:361–367

# Trophoblastic Disease

Y. TOMODA, T. ISHIZUKA, S. GOTO, and Y. FURUHASHI



## 1 Introduction

Trophoblastic disease originates from the placental villi and possesses the following features:

1. The paternal genes are inherited, and from the standpoint of graft immunity the disease has the characteristics of a homograft tumor.

2. These tumors produce human chorionic gonadotropin (hCG), and the level of hCG is a valuable marker for diagnosis as well as for assessment of therapeutic effect and remission.

3. Chemotherapy is very effective, and even metastatic cases may be cured by chemotherapy alone.

Current Topics in Pathology
Volume 85, Ed. N. Sasano

4. The tumors apparently progress from hydatidiform mole to invasive mole to choriocarcinoma, and therfore by controlling the hydatidiform mole stage it is possible to detect early choriocarcinoma or even prevent its occurrence.

## 2 Classification of Trophoblastic Disease

There is no completely accepted international standard yet for the classification of trophoblastic disease. First the classification of the World Health Organization (WHO) is outlined and then the classification used in Japan is discussed.

### 2.1 The WHO Classification

The WHO classification of 1983 is shown in Table 1.

**Table 1.** Classification of gestational trophoblastic disease (WHO 1983)

| |
|---|
| 1. Hydatidiform mole |
| a) Complete hydatidiform mole |
| b) Partial hydatidiform mole |
| 2. Invasive mole |
| 3. Gestational choriocarcinoma |
| 4. Placental site trophoblastic tumor |

1. *Hydatidiform Mole.* This is a general term that includes two distinct entities, i.e., complete hydatidiform mole and partial hydatidiform mole. The features common to both forms are the edematous state of some or all of the placental villi and trophoblastic hyperplasia.

a) *Complete Hydatidiform Mole.* This is an abnormal conceptus without any embryo or fetus, and with gross edematous swelling of the placental villi. There is also usually pronounced hyperplasia of both layers of the trophoblast. The villous edema leads to the formation of central cisterns and the concomitant compression of maturing connective tissue that has lost its vascularity.

b) *Partial Hydatidiform Mole.* This is an abnormal conceptus with an embryo or fetus that tends to die early. The placenta shows focal villous edema leading to cistern formation, and there is focal trophoblastic hyperplasia usually involving the syncytiotrophoblast only. The unaffected villi appear to be normal and vascularity of the villi decreases following fetal death.

2. *Invasive Mole.* This is a tumor or a tumor-like process invading the myometrium and characterized by trophoblastic hyperplasia and the persistence of placental villous structures. It commonly arises from a complete hydatidiform mole but may do so from a partial mole. This condition does not often

progress to choriocarcinoma. It may metastasize but it does not often exhibit the behavior of a true cancer, and it may even regress spontaneously.

3. *Gestational Choriocarcinoma*. This is a carcinoma arising from the trophoblastic epithelium that shows both cytotrophoblastic and syncytiotrophoblastic elements. It may arise from conceptions that give rise to a live birth, a stillbirth, an abortion at any stage, an ectopic pregnancy, or a hydatidiform mole, or it may possibly arise from invasive mole.

4. *Placental Site Trophoblastic Tumor*. This is a tumor originating from the placental bed trophoblast and is composed mainly of cytotrophoblastic cells. It encompasses lesions with a low to high grade of malignancy.

## 2.2 The Japanese Classification

In Japan, the classification of the Japanese Society of Obstetrics and Gynecology was prepared in 1963 and revised in 1979. Then, in 1980, a Joint Committee of this Society and the Japanese Pathological Society was organized, and the classification, definition, and diagnostic criteria for trophoblastic disease were formulated by the Committee in 1982. The 1982 classification is shown in Table 2. Trophoblastic disease is classified into hydatidiform mole, choriocarcinoma, and persistent trophoblastic disease, with complete mole, partial mole, and invasive mole being collectively categorized as hydatidiform mole to emphasize their mutual relationship.

**Table 2.** Classification of trophoblastic disease (Japan Society of Obstetrics and Gynecology 1982)

1. Hydatidiform mole
   (1) Complete (total) hydatidiform mole
      a) Noninvasive complete (total) mole
      b) Invasive complete (total) mole
   (2) Partial hydatidiform mole
      a) Noninvasive partial mole
      b) Invasive partial mole
2. Choriocarcinoma
   (1) Gestational choriocarcinoma
      a) Uterine choriocarcinoma
      b) Extrauterine choriocarcinoma
      c) Intraplacental choriocarcinoma
   (2) Nongestational choriocarcinoma
      a) Choriocarcinoma of germ cell origin
      b) Choriocarcinoma derived from dedifferentiation of other carcinoma
      c) Unclassified choriocarcinoma
3. Persistent trophoblastic disease
   (1) Postmolar persistent hCG
   (2) Clinical invasive mole
   (3) Clinical choriocarcinoma

Addendum: Placental site trophoblastic tumor

Syncytial endometritis and microscopic mole are not included within the scope of trophoblastic disease. In many patients with trophoblastic disease, focal tissue samples may not be obtained, and even if they are, a firm diagnosis may not always be possible because of histologic changes due to treatment or other causes. In order to distinguish such cases clinically and to obtain information for improving therapy, the category of persistent trophoblastic disease was set up. If the presence of a focus of disease cannot be confirmed, the patient is classified as having postmolar hCG persistence, while when a focus of disease can be identified it is classed as clinical invasive mole or clinical choriocarcinoma according to the choriocarcinoma diagnosis score (Table 3) (ISHIZUKA 1976).

The pathology of placental site trophoblastic tumor has not yet been clarified. Outside Japan it tends to be treated as a single disease unit, and in the 1982 Japanese classification it was included as an addendum to the classification of trophoblastic disease.

The 1982 classification is valuable but rather complicated, and it is usually simplified into complete mole, partial mole, invasive mole, choriocarcinoma, and persistent trophoblastic disease. This simplified form of the Japanese classification is very similar to the WHO classification.

## 3 Hydatidiform Mole

### 3.1 Pathology

Hydatidiform mole is a disease featuring cystic edema of the placental villi and is divided into complete mole and partial mole.

The pathologic features of hydatidiform mole include (a) trophoblastic proliferation, (b) edematous degeneration of the villous stroma, and (c) a paucity of blood vessels.

In complete mole, all the villi are cystic, and neither embryo nor fetus nor umbilical cord are present. Histologically, all villi are edematous and cystic, and interstitial blood vessels are lacking. Proliferation and atypia of villous cells are often noted, but the degree of such changes is not uniform (Fig. 1). In typical cases, the proliferation of syncytial elements accompanied by vacuolation and extension of villi can be observed.

In complete mole, the karyotype is 46,XX in about 96% of cases and 46,XY in the other 4%. There are no maternal chromosomes present, and all such tumors are androgenetic (KAJII and OHAMA 1977; WAKE et al. 1978; JACOBS et al. 1978). As the mechanisms of its occurrence, normal monoploid spermatozoa becoming diploid after fertilization (YAMASHITA et al. 1979; LAWLER et al. 1979) and the simultaneous fertilization of an ovum by two spermatozoa (OHAMA et al. 1981) have been suggested.

**Table 3.** Choriocarcinoma risk score table (ISHIZUKA 1976)

| Score | 0 | 1 | 2 | 3 | 4 | 5 |
|---|---|---|---|---|---|---|
| Probability of choriocarcinoma | ~50% | ~60% | ~70% | ~80% | ~90% | ~100% |
| Antecedent pregnancy[a] | Hydatidiform mole | | | Abortion | | Term delivery |
| Latent period[b] | Under 6 months | | | | 6 months to 3 years | Over 3 years |
| Primary lesion | Corpus uteri, parametrium | | | Ovary, fallopian tube | Cervix | Extrapelvic |
| Metastatic site | None, lung, intrapelvic | | | | | Extrapelvic except lung |
| Pulmonary metastases | | | | | | |
| Diameter | None | | | | | |
| | Under 20 mm | | | 20–30 mm | | Over 30 mm |
| Uniformity (size)[c] | Uniform | | | | Nonuniform | |
| Number | Under 20 | | | | | Over 20 |
| Urinary hCG[d] | Under $10^6$ m IU/ml | $10^6$–$10^7$ m IU/ml | | Over $10^7$ m IU/ml | | |
| Menstrual cycles during latent period (BBT) | Irregular (irregular) | | | | | Regular for at least 2 cycles (diphasic) |

*Indication* : Case of trophoblastic disease in which the lesions were verified by pelvic angiography, plain chest x-ray, computed tomography, ultrasonography, etc

*Scoring method* : The score for each individual item is determined and the total score for each patient is then calculated

*Discrimination* : Total score ≦ 4 points $\frac{1}{m}$ clinical invasive mole

Total score ≧ 5 points $\frac{1}{m}$ clinical choriocarcinoma

[a] The pregnancy preceding development of trophoblastic disease

[b] Time interval from the termination of the antecedent pregnancy to the diagnosis

[c] Over 1 cm difference in the diameter of pulmonary metastases is judged as nonuniform

[d] If the patient's hCG value was negative several times during the latent period, she is scored 5 points for this item

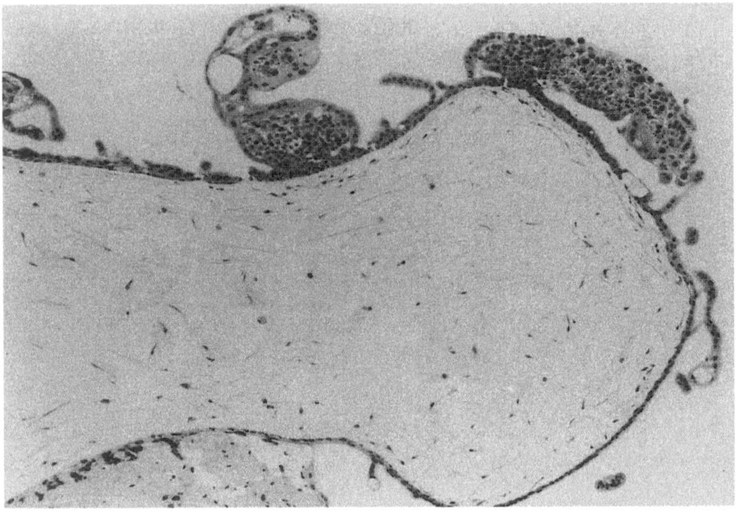

**Fig. 1.** Hydatidiform mole. This villus is swollen, devoid of vessels, and partly covered by proliferating trophoblast. H&E × 100

In Partial mole, the villi are only partly cystic and an embryo, fetus, or umbilical cord is not uncommonly recognized. Most of the cystic villi are lacking in interstitial blood vessels, but generally vascularization of at least part of the villous interstitial area is noted. If an embryo or fetus is present but all the villi are cystic, the lesion is classified as a partial mole. If nucleated erythrocytes are noted within villous blood vessels, this also provides the basis for a diagnosis of partial mole.

The karyotype of partial mole is mostly triploid, but tetraploidy, trisomy, and a normal karyotype are also found.

## 3.2 Incidence

Numerous reports have been published around the world relating to the incidence of hydatidiform mole. Table 4 shows a list of reports from regional registration systems (HARA et al. 1986; Registration Committee for Trophoblastic Disease of the Japan Society of Obstetrics and Gynecology 1987; ACOSTA-SISON 1967, LLEWELLYN-JONES 1965; TEOH et al. 1971; KOLSTAD and HOGNESTAD 1965; RINGERTZ 1970; YEN and MACMAHON 1968; MCCORRISTON 1968; FRANKE et al. 1983; BAGSHAWE et al. 1986). The incidence of hydatidiform mole ranges from 1 case per 340 to 1580 births and the rate varies from nation to nation, but

**Table 4.** Incidence of hydatidiform mole around the world

| Country | Author (year) | Number of hydatidiform moles | Incidence with respect to pregnancy | Incidence with respect to live births | |
|---|---|---|---|---|---|
| Japan | Nagoya University (1986) | 5 803 | | 1:350 | Aichi prefecture |
| Japan | Registration Committee for Trophoblastic Disease (1987) | 16 078 | | 1:342 | 20 prefectures in Japan |
| Philippines | ACOSTA-SISON (1967) | 141 | 1:200 | | Philippine General Hospital |
| Malaysia | LLEWELLYN-JONES (1965) | 188 | 1:600 | | Kuala Lumpur District Hospital |
| Singapore | TEOH et al. (1971) | 206 | | 1:823 | Kandang Kerbau Hospital |
| Norway | KOLSTAD and HOGNESTAD (1965) | 405 | | 1:1300 | Norwegian Cancer Registry |
| Sweden | RINGERTZ (1970) | 631 | 1:1560 | 1:1398 | Swedish Cancer Registry |
| U.S.A. | YEN and MACMAHON (1968) | 122 | 1:1512 | 1:1077 | 12 hospitals in Rhode Island |
| U.S.A. (Hawaii) | MCCORRISTON (1963) | 94 | 1:1326 | | 4 hospitals in Hawaii |
| Netherlands | FRANKE et al (1983) | 308 | 1:2270 | 1:1580 | Trophoblastic Disease Center |
| U.K. | BAGSHAWE et al. (1986) | 970 | | 1:649 | England and Wales |

it is evident that the incidence is higher in Asia than in Europe and the United States, and is especially high in Southeast Asia.

### 3.3 Management

The management after molar delivery centers around the detection of postmolar trophoblastic disease, such as invasive mole, choriocarcinoma, or persistent trophoblastic disease.

The cumulative distribution of patients according to the time from molar evacuation to the diagnosis of postmolar trophoblastic disease is shown in percentages in Fig. 2. In the case of invasive moles, 89.8% of all patients were diagnosed by the end of the 3rd month, and 97.8% by the end of the 6th month after molar evacuation. On the other hand, only 42% of choriocarcinomas were found by the end of the 1st year and 72.3% by the end of 2 years, indicating that the possibility of developing a choriocarcinoma still exists more than 2 years after molar evacuation. It is only 4 years after evacuation that the cumulative percentage for choriocarcinoma diagnosis reaches 94.3%.

A flow chart outlining the management after molar delivery is shown in Fig. 3.

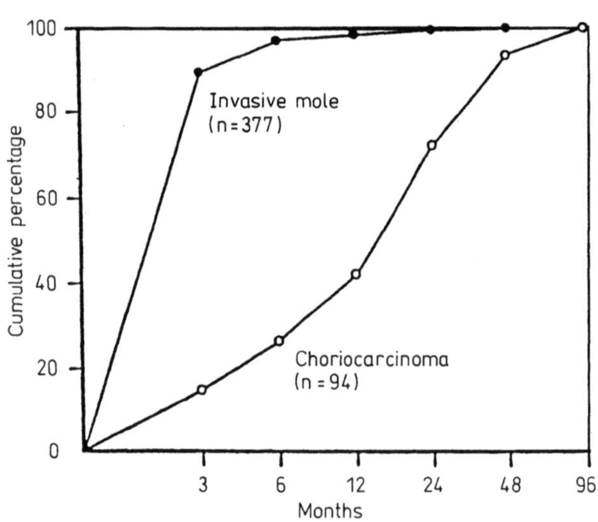


**Fig. 2.** Cumulative distribution of patients according to the time from evacuation of the mole to the diagnosis of postmolar trophoblastic disease

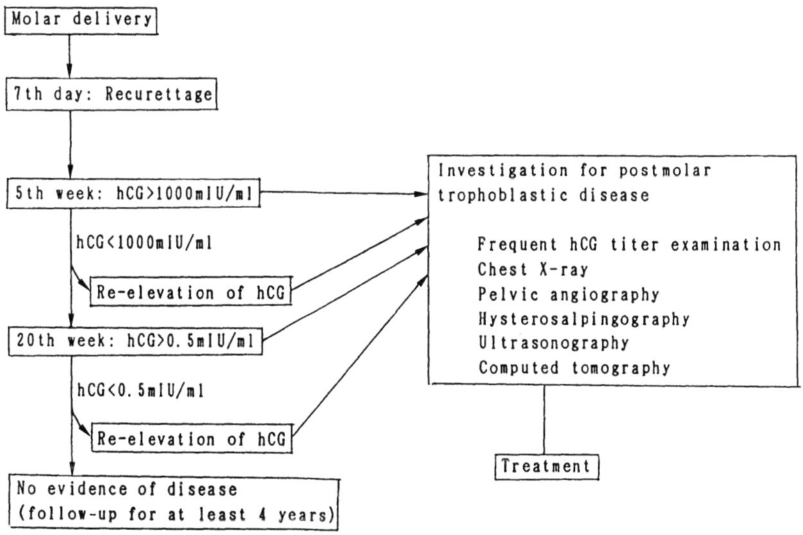


**Fig. 3.** Flow chart of management after molar delivery

### 3.4 Prognosis

Aichi Prefecture is located in the central part of Japan, and its population is about 6.5 million. In Aichi Prefecture, a registration system for trophoblastic disease was established covering the whole prefecture, and has been in operation since August 1962 (Ishizuka 1976). In the first 20 years of operation of the system, 5792 cases of hydatidiform mole were registered. Registered patients were followed up for a minimum of 6 years and 602 cases (10.4%) of postmolar trophoblastic disease were found. There were 106 choriocarcinomas (1.8%), 490 invasive moles (8.5%), and six undetermined cases (0.1%). The incidence of successive invasive moles was 7.8% (227 of 2918 cases) during the first 10 years, and increased to 9.2% (263 of 2874 cases) in the second 10-year period. On the other hand, the incidence of choriocarcinoma declined from 2.4% (69 of 2918 cases) to 1.3% (37 of 2874 cases). This decrease in the incidence of choriocarcinoma was attributed to the effective treatment of invasive moles and to the ongoing supervision of patients following the diagnosis of hydatidiform mole.

Lurain et al. (1983) have reported that chemotherapy was required in 142 (19.2%) of 738 patients after molar evacuation. Such treatment was performed in 602 (10.4%) of the 5792 patients in Aichi Prefecture. Among the patients of Nagoya University Hospital, the percentage receiving chemotherapy was 21.3%. This discrepancy was probably due to differences between the central hospital and regional hospital registration procedures, since the reports of both Nagoya University Hospital and LURAIN et al. included patients with spontaneous remission.

## 4 Invasive Mole

### 4.1 Pathology

Invasion of molar villi into the myometrium is known as invasive mole, and such lesions sometimes penetrate through the uterine wall to spread outside the uterus. Histologically, a villous pattern can be noted in the disease focus in the myometrium (Fig.4), and the invasion and proliferation of villous cells in the uterine muscular tunic is usually observed. Villi may be either invasive or not, and may be either well-formed or only the bare outline of normal villi (Fig. 5). If villous cells are proliferating destructively, cellular atypia is obvious, and there is accompanying hemorrhage and necrosis, the lesion is an invasive mole if the presence of a villous pattern can be recognized. Sometimes invasion is not noted macroscopically and the villous pattern may be detected only by histologic examination. Since abnormal tissue may be present in only a

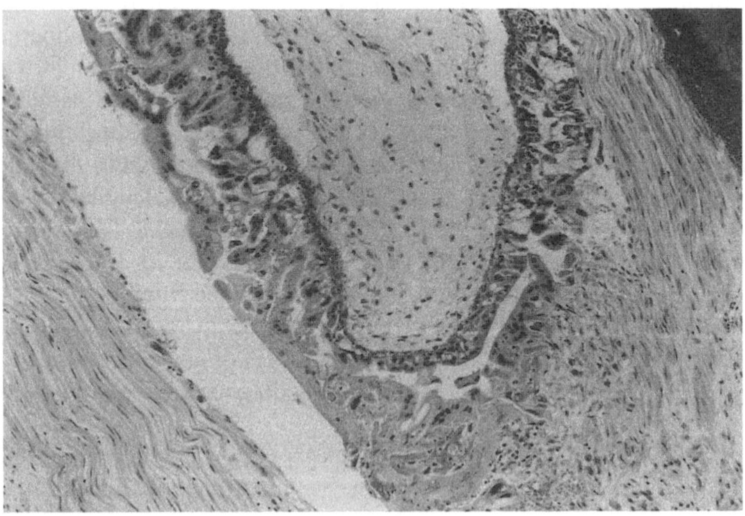

**Fig. 4.** Invasive mole. The molar villus is associated with considerable trophoblast proliferation. It lies within the myometrium. H&E × 400

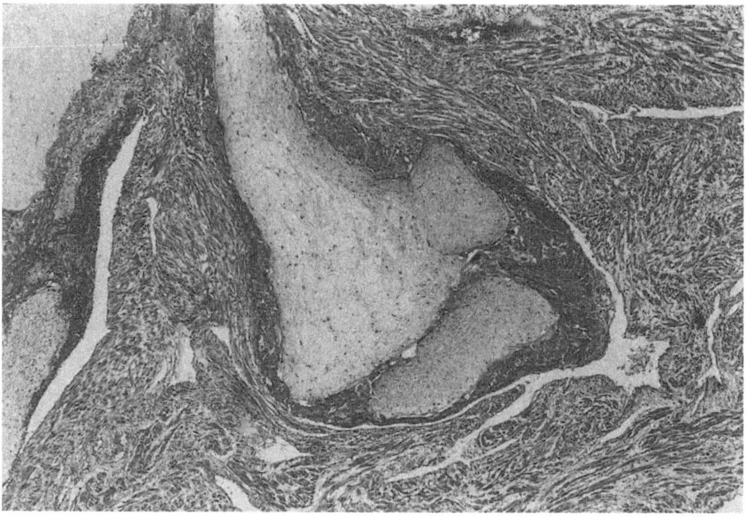

Fig. 5. Invasive mole. The shadow of thee villus can be recognized. H&E × 100

very small region, it is necessary to examine as many tissue segments as possible.

An invasive mole is sometimes metastatic. It is considered to metastasize by vascular emboli, and commonly involves the lungs or the vagina. Direct invasion of the parametrium is also observed. Among the 260 cases of invasive mole treated at Nagoya University Hospital, metastasis was noted in 103 cases (39.6%). Metastasis to the lungs was noted in 85 cases (32.7%), metastasis to the vagina in 12 cases (4.6%), and invasion of the parametrium in 14 cases (5.4%).

## 4.2 Treatment

In women not wishing to become pregnant again, hysterectomy is performed if the tumor is found to be limited to the uterus and is determined to be removable surgically. In this case, since the confirmation of ovulation by measurement of the basal body temperature is an important method of post operative follow-up, it is necessary to leave at least one ovary in situ, except in elderly patients. After operation, chemotherapy should be started as soon as possible (usually 7–10 days after surgery).

Since invasive mole often occurs in patients in their twenties, the use of hysterectomy poses problems. If the patient wishes to preserve her reproductive capacity, the uterus is not removed and primary chemotherapy is attempted. Hertz et al. (1963) first proposed the use of primary chemotherapy for trophoblastic disease, and this idea was then adopted by HAMMOND et al.(1973), GOLDSTEIN (1972), and others. Such therapy is now established as the treatment of choice for trophoblastic disease. In Japan, this treatment was introduced by Ishizuka and his colleagues, and a report on the use of primary chemotherapy in 123 cases was presented in 1974 by KASEKI. At present, more than 38% of patients with invasive mole are treated by primary chemotherapy in Japan (Registration Committee for Trophoblastic Disease of the Japan Society of Obstetrics and Gynecology 1987). The rate of onset of choriocarcinoma after treatment of invasive mole shows almost no difference between the surgically treated group and the primary chemotherapy group (Report on the study financially assisted by the Cancer Research Fund of the Ministry of Health and Welfare for the fiscal year 1980).

When primary chemotherapy fails to achieve its objectives, it then becomes necessary to perform a hysterectomy. Whether chemotherapy is used after operation or the primary treatment, it is vital to continue it until the criteria for remission are fulfilled.

### 4.3 Prognosis

Regarding the mortality of invasive mole, PARK has reported that 17 out of 47 cases were fatal in 1950. As a result of progress in therapy, BAGSHAWE (1969) could report no fatalities in a personal series. In the latest nationwide report for Japan (Registration Committee for Trophoblastic Disease of the Japanese Society of Obstetrics and Gynecology 1987), the 5-year survival rate of patients with histologically diagnosed invasive mole was 97.6%, and that of patients with clinically diagnosed invasive mole, 98.5%. There were only two deaths from invasive mole before 1968 in the authors' series, both of which were due to sepsis. Since 1969, no such fatalities have been experienced.

Invasive mole patients are considered to be a highrisk group for the development of choriocarcinoma, and although the prognosis of invasive mole itself is good, its treatment and follow-up should be performed very carefully. It is suggested that the progression to choriocarcinoma may be prevented by the effective treatment of invasive mole.

The authors have investigated the rate of recurrence of invasive mole (HIROKAWA et al. 1986). Seventeen out of 320 patients (5.3%) were found to have recurrent diseases, comprising 7 to the 135 patients (5.1%) with histologically confirmed invasive mole and 10 of the 185 (5.4%) with clinically diagnosed invasive mole.

Six of the 17 patients (35.3%) in whom choriocarcinoma developed following the initial treatment of invasive mole eventually died.

A uterine choriocarcinoma is shown in Fig. 6 which developed following the surgical removal of a histologically confirmed invasive mole (Fig. 7).

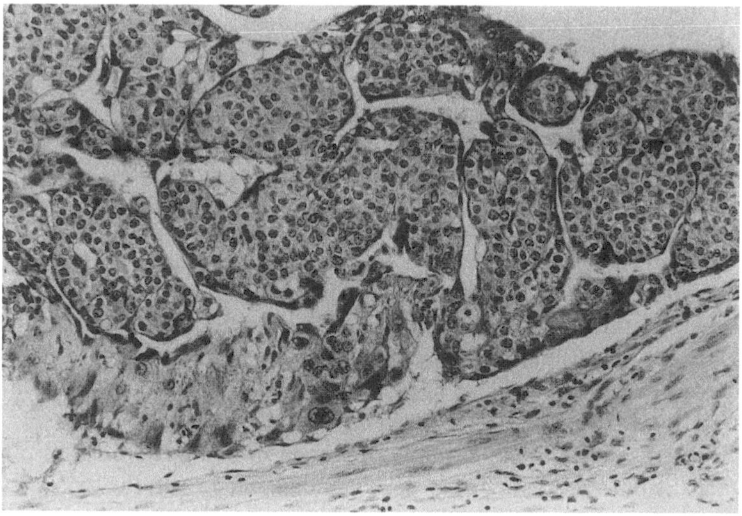

**Fig. 6.** Microscopic view of choriocarcinoma in the resected uterus after recurrence. H&E $\times$ 400

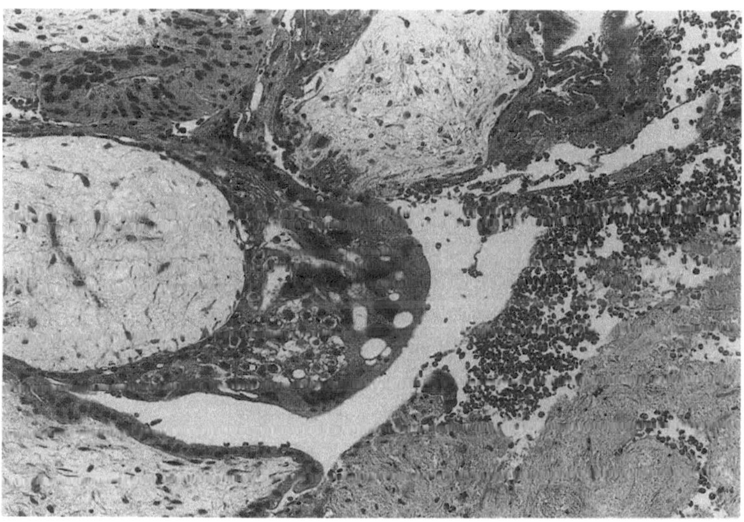

**Fig. 7.** Microscopic view of invasive mole in the resected tumor from uterus during the first treatment. H&E $\times$ 400

# 5 Choriocarcinoma

## 5.1 Pathology

### *5.1.1 Macroscopic and Histologic Appearances*

Choriocarcinoma is a malignant tumor consisting of trophoblastic cells; histologically it is composed of proliferative and destructive foci of tumor cells which can be recognized as syncytiotrophoblast and Langhans' cells without any demonstrable villous pattern (Fig. 8). In uterine choriocarcinoma, macroscopic infiltration of the tumor into the myometrium is noted, and usually hemorrhage and necrosis are evident. Occasionally, choriocarcinoma is composed only of cells that closely resembles Langhans' cells.

The diagnosis of choriocarcinoma must be made on the basis of multiple tissue specimens from a tumor focus; a diagnosis made on the basis of examination of the uterine contents alone should not be regarded as reliable. NISHIKAWA et al. (1985) investigated some of the histopathologic features of choriocarcinoma and studied their relationship to prognosis by selecting 13 different parameters concerning the degree of differentiation and the form of the trophoblast, the manner of trophoblastic invasion, and the host response. Seventy patients with uterine lesions (survivors: 49; deceased: 21) were investigated and four parameters were shown to have significance by the chi-square

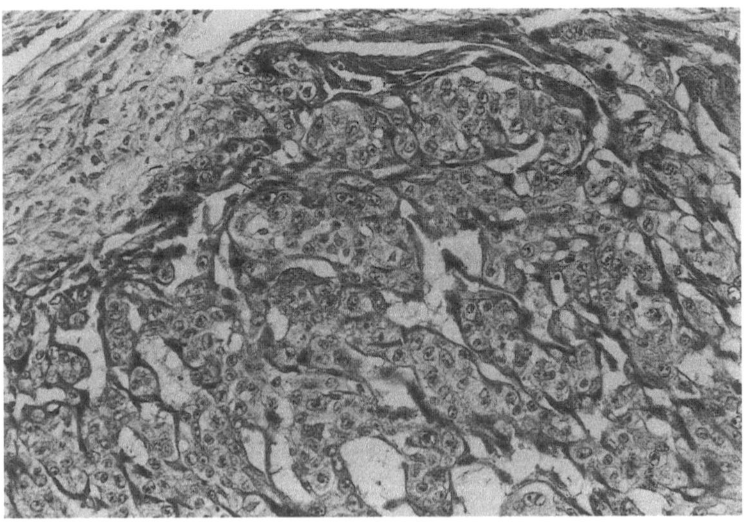

**Fig. 8.** Choriocarcinoma. Syncytiotrophoblasts and cytotrophoblasts proliferate in a close arrangement. H&E × 400

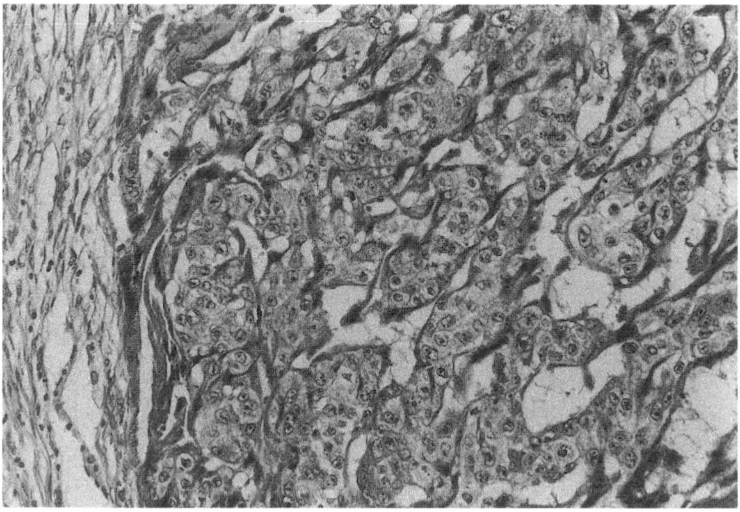

**Fig. 9.** Island formation. Each mass of trophoblasts is surrounded by an attenuated layer of syncytiotrophoblasts. H&E × 400

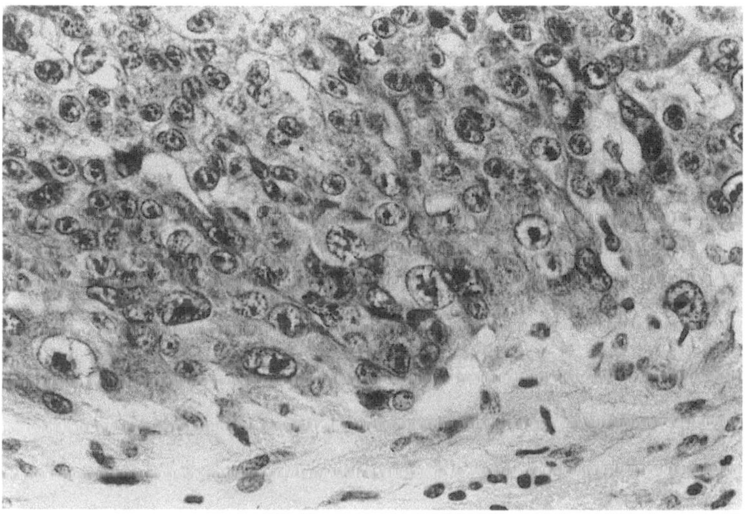

**Fig. 10.** Massive proliferation of intermediate-type trophoblasts. The intermediate-type trophoblasts proliferate close to each other, forming a nest. H&E × 400

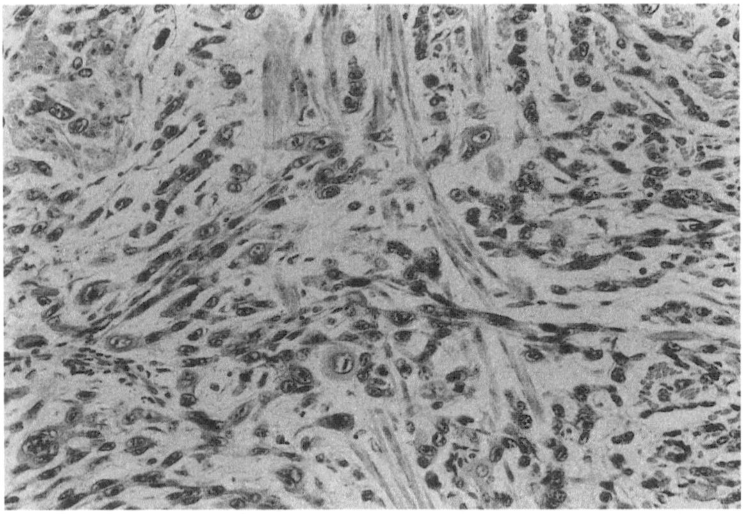

**Fig. 11.** Right-angled infiltration of intermediate-type trophoblasts surrounding muscle fibers. Intermediate-type trophoblast proliferates from the *left* to the *right* in the photomicrograph and infiltrates the muscle fibers at *right* angles. H&E × 400

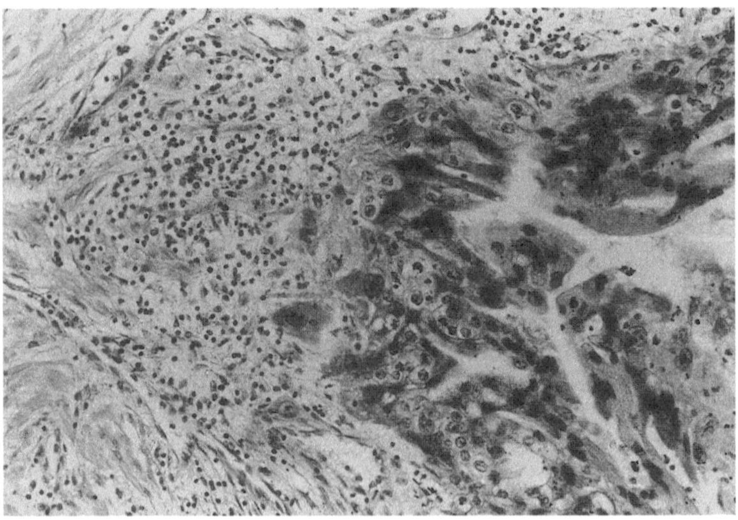

**Fig. 12.** Atypia of trophoblasts at the tumor margins. Trophoblasts at the trip of tumor invasion show marked cellular atypia and partly infiltrate muscle fibers. H&E × 400

test. The following were selected as criteria: (a) island formation (Fig. 9), (b) massive proliferation of intermediate-type trophoblastic cells (Fig. 10), (c) infiltration of trophoblastic cells at right angles into the surrounding myometrium (Fig. 11), and (d) atypia of trophoblastic cells at the tumor margins (Fig. 12). It was found that island formation was seen in patients with choriocarcinoma which had a good prognosis, while extensive proliferation of intermediate-type trophoblastic cells and atypia of trophoblastic cells at the tumor margins were indicators of a poor prognosis. Infiltration of trophoblastic cells into the surrounding myometrium was also found at a high incidence in the patients with a worse prognosis.

### *5.1.2 Hormone Production*

In order to investigate hormone production by trophoblastic cells in choriocarcinoma, KURMAN et al. (1984) studied the immunocytochemical localization of hCG and human placental lactogen (hPL) in placental site trophoblastic tumor, hydatidiform mole, and choriocarcinoma. It was found that the syncytiotrophoblast could produce hCG and hPL in large amounts, whereas intermediate trophoblast cells expressed predominantly hPL and focal areas of hCG. Cytotrophoblast cells were devoid of hCG and hPL, except in choriocarcinoma, which showed focal weak staining for hCG. In choriocarcinoma, the syncytiotrophoblast characteristically contained abundant amounts of hCG and occasionally also hPL, but invariably in smaller amounts.

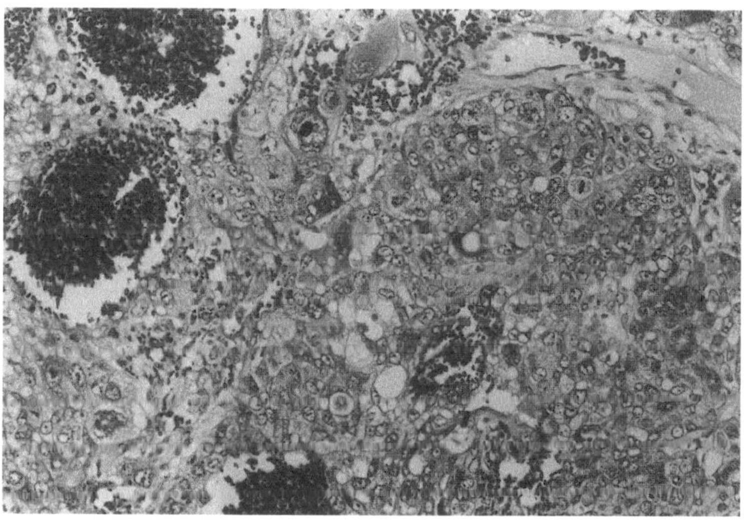

**Fig. 13.** Pulmonary metastasis. The mass of trophoblasts can be recognized adjacent to hematoma at the left. H&E × 400

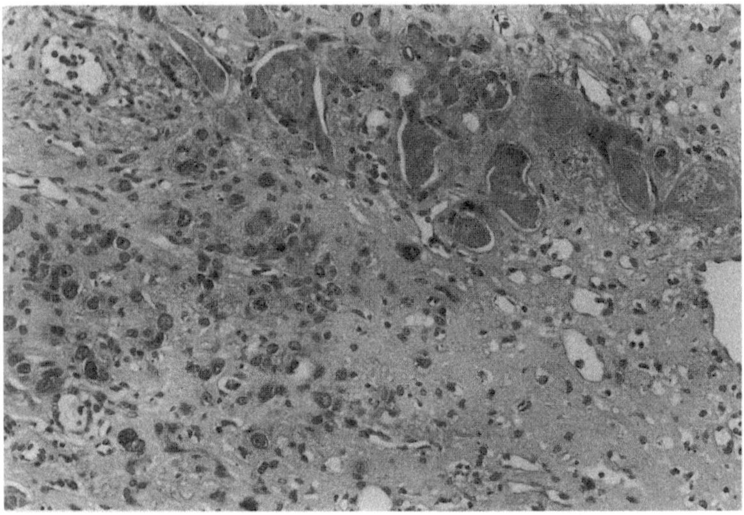

**Fig. 14.** Pulmonary metastasis. Partly degenerated trophoblasts lie at the *left*. H&E × 400

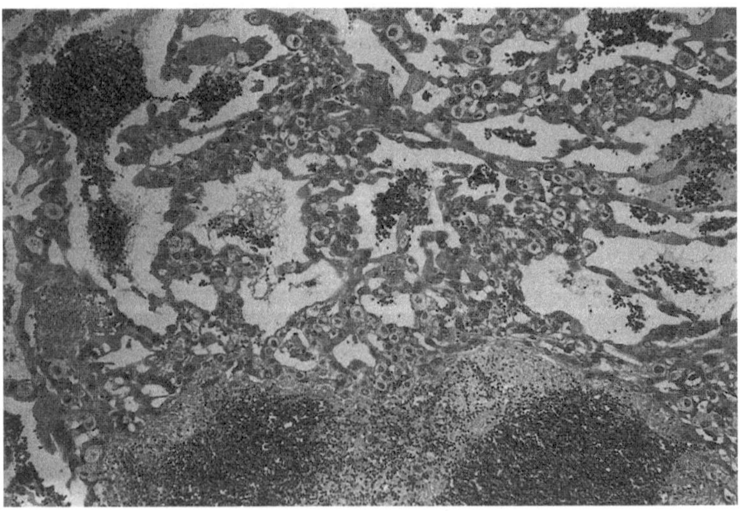

**Fig. 15.** Intracranial metastasis. The mass of trophoblasts lie within the hematoma. H&E × 100

Investigations using cultured cell strains of choriocarcinoma showed that progesterone and estrogen were produced in a culture medium containing 10% fetal calf serum although there was a quantitative difference between strains of choriocarcinoma cells (BAHN et al. 1981; SUGIURA et al. 1988)

Choriocarcinoma is likely to metastasize to the lung and brain, and it is often accompanied by hemorrhage at the metastatic site. In pulmonary metastatic foci, trophoblastic cells are often present around the hematoma (Fig.13). In patients undergoing pulmonary surgery, when hCG levels fall very low after chemotherapy, only trophoblastic cells are sporadically observed around the hematoma in occasional cases (Fig. 14). In brain metastatic foci, trophoblastic cells are often diffusely present in the hematoma (Fig. 15).

### 5.1.3 *Metastasis*

At Nagoya University Hospital, metastasis was noted at the time of admission in 133 out of 186 cases (71.5%). Pulmonary metastases were found in 125 cases (67.2%), intracranial metastases in 9 cases (4.8%), intrapelvic metastases in 26 cases (14.0%), and vaginal metastases in 22 cases (11.8%). Hepatic, small intestinal, and renal metastases were present in one case each (0.5%). Autopsy was conducted in 43 patients who died of choriocarcinoma. Pulmonary metastases were found in 42 cases (97.7%), intracranial metastases in 30 cases (69.8%), hepatic metastases in 16 cases (37.2%), renal metastases in 14 cases (32.6%), and intestinal metastases in 17 cases (39.5%). A total of 47 metastatic foci were found in the brain in 30 patients who underwent autopsy. The intracranial metastatic foci were distributed as follows: The most frequent site was the parietal lobe (36.2%), followed by the occipital lobe (29.7%), the frontal lobe (10.6%), the temporal lobe (8.5%), the cerebellum (8.5%), and the brain stem (6.3%). These intracranial metastatic foci were divided into four categories: superficial, intermediate, deep, and cerebellar metastases. Deep metastases inaccessible to surgical removal, including those located in the basal ganglia, the internal capsule, and the brain stem, accounted only 10% of cases. Of the 30 cases in which autopsy was performed, 18 (60%) had a single lesion, while in 12 (40%) the metastatic foci were multiple. The initial neurologic symptoms caused by brain metastases include headache, followed by focal weakness, disturbance of consciousness, convulsions, and dizziness. CT images of intracranial metastases are shown in Fig. 16.

Concerning the metastasis of choriocarcinoma, BAGSHAWE (1969) compiled the results of 100 patients (including 16 fatal and 14 autopsy cases). He reported pulmonary metastases in 66 cases, intracranial metastases in 14 cases, vaginal metastases in 18 cases, intrapelvic metastases in 19 cases, hepatic metastases in 4 cases, renal metastases in 3 cases, and intestinal metastases in 6 cases. The frequency of metastasis was intermediate between the admission and autopsy data from our studies.

The typical pulmonary metastasis of a choriocarcinoma is a large round lesion that often resembles a snowball or cannonball on x-ray. Multiple coin

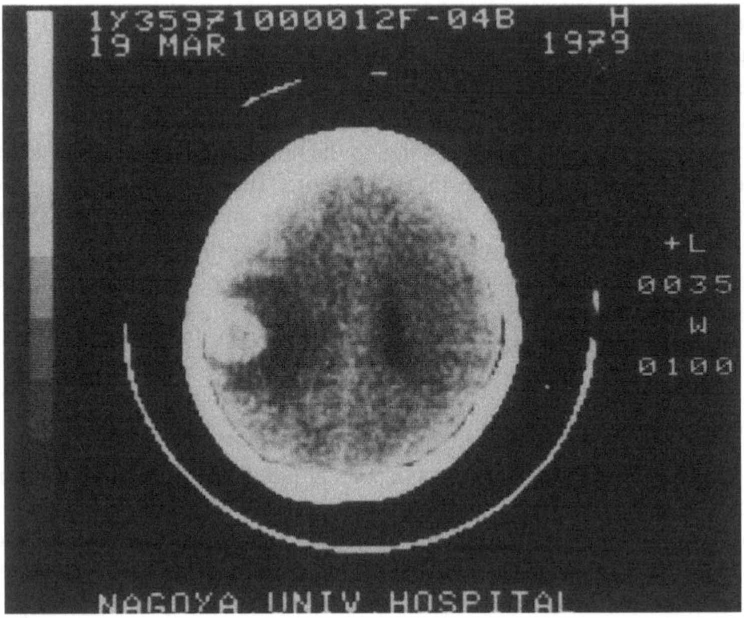


**Fig. 16.** Intracranial metastasis on CT

lesions are also found, while a miliary pattern is rarely seen. The common pulmonary metastatic sites of trophoblastic disease are the outer regions of the middle and lower lung fields.

The signs of pulmonary metastasis include chest pain, hemoptysis, and cough.

Pulmonary metastases were classified into four types according to their size and the clarity of their margins. Metastases were defined as small when their maximum diameter was under 2 cm, as patchy when they ranged from 2 to 5 cm in diameter with poorly defined margins, as nodular when they ranged from 2 to 5 cm in diameter with well-defined margins, and as massive when they were larger than 5 cm. All subjects entered after 1965 were analyzed using this classification. Small metastases were found in 43 cases (40.6%), patchy metastases in 14 cases (13.2%), nodular metastases in 34 cases (32.1%), and massive metastases in 15 cases (14.2%).

The pulmonary metastases were single in 31 cases, two or three lesions were seen in 42 cases, and four or more lesions were seen in 33 cases.

The changes in the x-ray appearance of pulmonary metastases with treatment were also assessed. Lesions initially showed both high and low density areas within a circular pale shadow, and this appearance was thought to represent a freshly bleeding focus. As time passed, such lesions became darker and more diffuse. When chemotherapy was effective, the pulmonary lesions faded away gradually, becoming progressively smaller if the initial lesion was large and clearing rapidly if it was small. Fibrosis was noted to develop subsequently, and the margins of the lesions became irregular while producing traction on the surrounding tissues. Finally, the lesions became minute regions of fibrosis, showing as faint scars.

SUNG et al. (1982) analyzed the chest x-ray appearance of trophoblastic disease in a large series of patients, and classified the early appearance of choriocarcinoma into patchy and nodular types, while the late appearance was classified into cotton ball and tumefied types. They reported that, in cases not responding to chemotherapy, the patchy or nodular appearance changed to a cotton ball or tumefied appearance. In contrast, in patients responding to chemotherapy, cotton ball or tumefied lesions first became patchy or nodular and then eventually disappeared.

Pulmonary metastases can be diagnosed by plain chest x-ray or the use of tomograms, and CT may sometimes show a metastatic focus which cannot be diagnosed by these methods. Chest CT is particularly effective in detecting lesions concealed by the cardiac and mediastinal shadows, or lesions located near the diaphragm or pleura.

Typical pulmonary metastatic lesions are shown in Fig. 17.

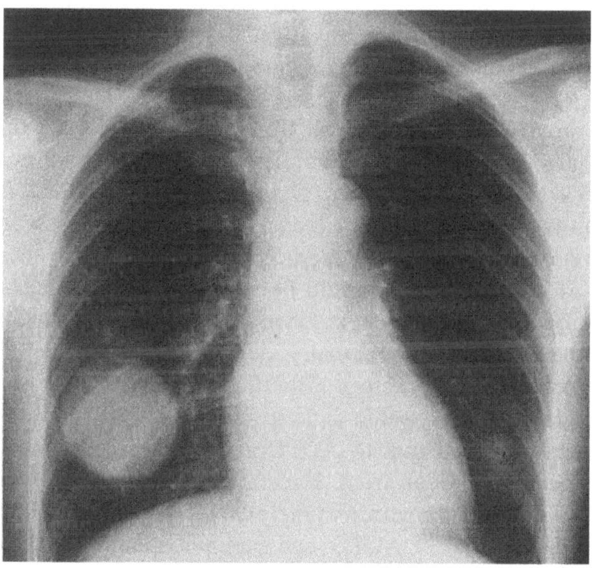

**Fig. 17.** Typical x-ray of pulmonary metastases

## 5.2 Treatment

### 5.2.1 Chemotherapy

The methods of treatment employed so far for choriocarcinoma include surgery, chemotherapy, irradiation, and immunotherapy, with surgery and chemotherapy playing the pivotal roles today. In the treatment of malignant tumors, the therapeutic results for choriocarcinoma have always been superior to those for other cancers. The better results seen in the treatment of choriocarcinoma are due mainly to the sensitivity of this tumor to chemotherapy and to monitoring of disease progression using hCG, which is a reliable tumor marker.

Improvements in the treatment of choriocarcinoma owe much to the development of anticancer agents. Li et al. (1956) reported good results for the administration of methotrexate (MTX), which is an antagonist of folic acid metabolism, to two patients with choriocarcinoma and one with invasive mole. Subsequently, Hertz et al. (1958) reported that a complete remission was attained with MTX in 3 out of 19 cases of choriocarcinoma and one out of three cases of invasive mole. Ross et al. (1962) administered actinomycin D (ACTD) to 13 patients with trophoblastic disease that was resistant to MTX or vinblastine, and obtained a complete remission in six cases. Hertz (1967) reviewed the therapeutic results in trophoblastic disease over an 8-year period, and reported that the advent of ACTD had contributed to a dramatic improvement in the remission rates for choriocarcinoma and invasive mole. The efficacy of ACTD was subsequently recognized throughout the world, and the foundation of today's chemotherapy for trophoblastic disease was thus set in place.

To treat tumors resistant to single agents or advanced disease, multiple drug regimens have been administered and many types of combination chemotherapy have been devised.

Our present chemotherapy regimen for choriocarcinoma is as follows. Initially, MTX and ACTD are simultaneously administered for 4-days. Since MTX occasionally induces hepatic injury, ACTD is administered alone if worsening of liver function is observed. For an advanced case with widespread metastases, cyclophosphamide is sometimes added to MTX and ACTD. The interval between courses of chemotherapy should be as short as possible. In general, after an interval of 10 days, the next course is started. However, excessive shortening of the interval may actually delay the next cycle of treatment because of side-effects. The factors affecting the duration of the interval between cycles are mainly leukopenia and thrombocytopenia.

Treatment of choriocarcinoma resistant to ACTD and MTX is extremely difficult, and various regimens have been tried. Bagshawe (1977) added four agents (hydroxyurea, vincristine, Adriamycin, and melphalan) in cases showing resistance to MTX and ACTD, or to MTX, ACTD, and cyclophosphamide. They administered these drugs cyclically for 10 days, and reported that this regimen (Chamoma) was effective.

With the steady introduction of new drugs, various combination chemotherapy regimens have been reported. NEWLANDS and BAGSHAWE (1979) reported a regimen comprising vinblastine, MTX, and cis-diamminedichloroplatinum (CDDP). Use of etoposide for choriocarcinoma was started from 1976, and it was found to be an effective first-line agent for choriocarcinoma (NEWLANDS and BAGSHAWE 1980). Application of etoposide in cases of drug-resistant choriocarcinoma has also been tried (NEWLANDS 1982). We have tested some of these agents and also attempted new combinations, but could not obtain the same good results shown in the other reports. Etoposide is useful both as a single agent for the treatment of new cases and in combination with other drugs for the treatment of resistant cases. It is a drug that seems worth using more in the future. Recently, studies have been reported on the pharmacokinetics of etoposide (BRINDLEY et al. 1985), and combination regimens utilizing etoposide have been introduced, like the EMA/CO therapy of BAGSHAWE (1987).

### *5.2.2 Surgical Treatment of Metastasis*

We perform surgical treatment in selected patients with metastatic disease. Among the sites of metastasis of choriocarcinoma, pulmonary and intracranial metastases are particularly important.

At Nagoya University Hospital, pulmonary metastases were noted in 125 of the cases treated from 1957 to 1984. Chemotherapy was the first-line treatment overall, and surgery was simultaneously performed on 32 patients.

In the patients achieving remission with chemotherapy alone, the urinary hCG level dropped below the detectable limit within 10 weeks after it fell below 1000 IU/liter. On the other hand, in eventually fatal cases not achieving remission with chemotherapy alone, the hCG level tended to rise before 10 weeks after going below 1000 IU/liter or else did not drop below the detectable limit after this time. It was therefore concluded that surgery is required if the hCG level does not drop below the detectable limit within 10 weeks of declining below 1000 IU/liter. THOMFORD et al. (1965) proposed four indications for the surgical treatment of pulmonary metastatic tumors: (a) the patient must be a good risk for surgical intervention, (b) the primary malignancy must be controlled, (c) there must be no evidence of metastatic disease elsewhere, and (d) radiologic evidence of pulmonary metastasis should be limited to one lung. On the basis of these indications, the authors established their own set of indications for surgery in pulmonary metastatic choriocarcinoma, as shown in Table 5 (TOMODA et al. 1986). In 32 patients having pulmonary surgery, treatment results were compared between the patients satisfying the four criteria and those who did not. Among 20 cases satisfying the four conditions, the remission rate was 100%, but for the other patients the remission rate was only 33%.

Regarding surgical intervention for pulmonary metastases, SHIRLEY et al. (1972) operated on four cases and reported remission in three of them. However, they did not recommend surgery because chemotherapy is extremely effective, and there is always the possibility of lesions elsewhere that cannot be detected

**Table 5.** Conditions for achieving good results by thoracotomy in pulmonary metastasis of choriocarcinoma

1. Patients whose urinary hCG value is below 1000 mIU/ml for over 10 weeks and still detectable.
2. The patient must be a good risk for surgical intervention.
3. There is no evidence of primary and metastatic foci elsewhere in the body.
4. The metastases are resectable in one operation.

by investigations. HAMMOND et al. (1980) performed pulmonary surgery in 11 cases, and obtained remission in four of them. XU et al. (1985) reported that from 1962 to 1982 pulmonary metastatic choriocarcinoma was found to be resistant to chemotherapy in 43 of their patients who subsequently underwent surgery. There were no early postoperative deaths, and the 5-year survival rate was 50% (16/32).

As the principal mode of treatment of pulmonary metastases from choriocarcinoma, multiple agent chemotherapy is performed initially. After the hCG level has fallen below 1000 IU/liter, surgery can be performed in cases satisfying the above-mentioned criteria, and then further chemotherapy is given until remission is achieved. The timing of surgery is very important, and it must be emphasized that satisfactory results will not be achieved if it is performed too early or too late.

Conventionally, intracranial metastasis of choriocarcinoma was regarded as fatal, and once cerebral metastases developed the outcome was almost always an early death. However, with progress in neurosurgery as well as advances in chemotherapy, cures have come to be reported occasionally.

At Nagoya University Hospital (ISHIZUKA et al. 1983), intracranial metastases were observed in 42 of 186 patients (22.6%), and an autopsy study revealed that most intracranial metastatic foci were surgically respectable.

WEED and HAMMOND (1980) reported remission in 7 out of 14 cases with brain metastasis treated with chemotherapy alone, and stated that four out of the five cases also undergoing surgery achieved remission. ATHANASSIOU et al. (1983) reported remission in 17 out of 69 cases with intracranial metastasis, and in five out of seven cases that underwent surgery.

Our therapeutic policy regarding intracranial metastases is as follows. In cases with increased intracranial pressure, craniotomy or decompressive surgery is performed to relieve the immediate danger. Soon after surgery, 30–40 Gy of cranial irradiation is administered together with chemotherapy. In cases without increased intracranial pressure, remission can be obtained by the use of chemotherapy and radiotherapy alone, so it remains debatable whether immediate surgery is indicated. When metastases occur in patients who show resistance to chemotherapy, surgical intervention should be considered, but this subject requires further investigation.

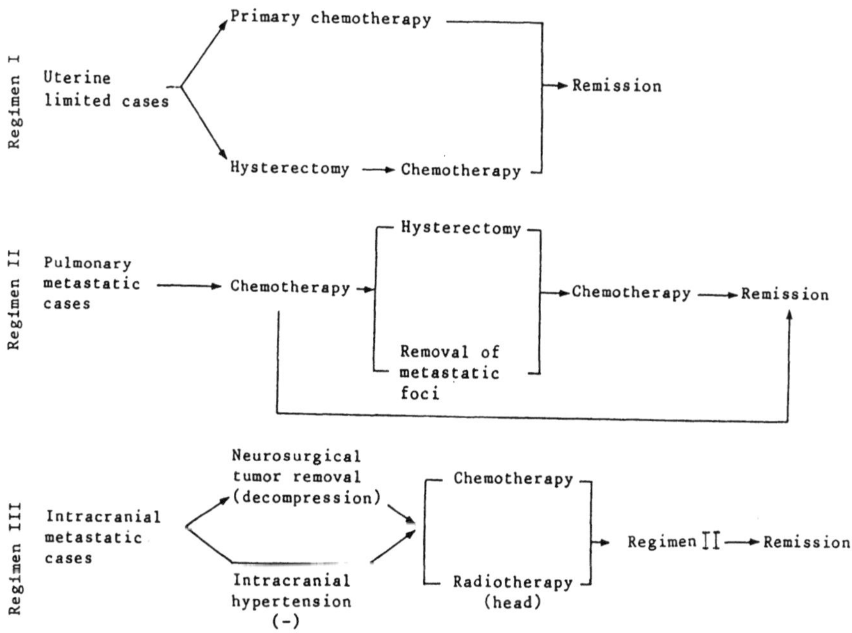


**Fig. 18.** Flow chart of therapeutic regimens for choriocarcinoma

### *5.2.3 Systemic Treatment*

An outline of our current therapeutic methods is shown in Fig. 18, with regimens I–III being selected depending on the degree of progression of the disease.

In patients with disease limited to the uterus, when primary chemotherapy is chosen because of the patient's wish to keep her reproductive capability, the response to chemotherapy must be accurately evaluated and surgery must be used if required.

In patients with pulmonary metastases, it is important to perform chemotherapy appropriately and to keep firmly in mind the criteria for surgery mentioned above.

When metastasis to the brain with raised intracranial pressure occurs, the first priority is surgery to save the patient's life, and radiotherapy is also worth considering.

It is extremely important to start treatment according to the correct principles from the beginning, and to determine the timing of treatment adequately.

## 5.3 Prognosis

The outcome in patients with trophoblastic disease treated at Nagoya University Hospital is shown in Table 6 by dividing patients into an invasive mole group

**Table 6.** Results of treatment for trophoblastic disease

| | Choriocarcinoma | | Invasive mole | |
|---|---|---|---|---|
| | Survivors | Nonsurvivors | Survivors | Nonsurvivors |
| 1957–1964 | 5 (21.7%) | 18 (78.3%) | 35 (97.2%) | 1 (2.8%) |
| 1965–1971 | 40 (59.7%) | 27 (40.3%) | 135 (99.3%) | 1 (0.7%) |
| 1972–1975 | 28 (63.6%) | 16 (36.4%) | 88 (100%) | 0 (0.0%) |
| 1976–1984 | 43 (82.7%) | 9 (17.3%) | 120 (100%) | 0 (0.0%) |
| Subtotal | 116 | 70 | 378 | 2 |
| Total | 186 | | 380 | |

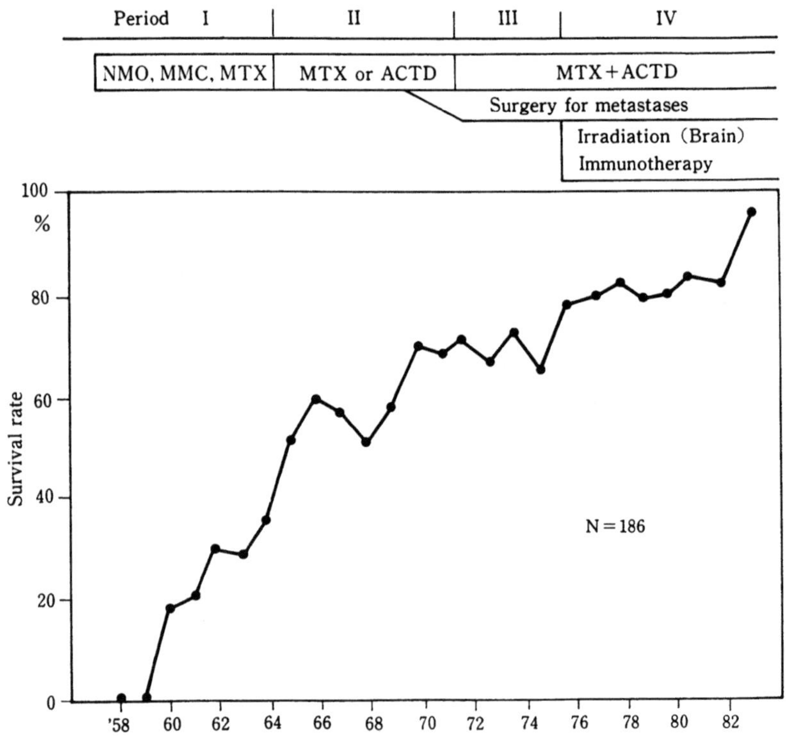


**Fig. 19.** Improvement of survival rate in choriocarcinoma accompanying the progress in treatment. *NMO*, nitrogen mustard; *MMC*, mitomycin *C*; *MTX*, methotrexate; *ACTD*, actinomycin D

and a choriocarcinoma group. A total of 219 cases of clinical invasive mole and 43 cases of clinical choriocarcinoma were judged by the choriocarcinoma risk score table. The years from 1957 to 1984 can be divided into four periods according to the progress in the therapeutic techniques. In the first period, nitrogen mustard, mitomycin C, and MTX were mainly used, while in the second period ACTD was introduced. In the third period, the concomitant use of ACTD and MTX began, and surgical treatment was applied to metastatic sites, while in the fourth period multidisciplinary treatment was adopted by combining surgery with irradiation, chemotherapy, and/or immunotherapy.

For invasive mole, nearly 100% of patients survived even in the first period, and a mortality of 0% has been achieved since 1972. By contrast, for choriocarcinoma, the mortality was 80% in the first period. It dropped to 40% in the second period when the use of ACTD began, and then fell to under 20% in the fourth period. There is thus still a marked difference evident between survival in patients with invasive mole and patients with choriocarcinoma.

By following the latest regimen, more than 90% of choriocarcinoma patients can be cured (Fig. 19). This level is a useful reference for comparison with the results of treatment of other cancers, and the authors believe that the efforts by the researchers in this field can provide a model for those in other fields.

## References


Acosta-Sison H (1967) Trophoblastic or chorionic tumors as observed in the Philippines. In: Holland JF, Hreshchyshyn MM (eds) Choriocarcinoma. Springer, Heidelberg Berlin New York, (UICC Monograph Series, vol 3, pp 33–36)

Athanassiou A, Begent RHG, Newlands Es, Parker D, Rustin GJS, Bagshawe KD (1983) Central nervous system metastases of choriocarcinoma—23 years' experience at Charing Cross Hospital. Cancer 52:1728–1735

Bagshawe KD (1969) Metastatic Choriocarcinoma. In: Choriocarcinoma. Edward Arnold, London, pp 93–103

Bagshawe KD (1977) Treatment of trophoblastic tumors. Recent Results Cancer Res 62:192–199

Bagshawe KD (1987) Chemotherapy and general treatment—current and future developments. In: Takagi S, Freidberg V, Haller U, Knapstein PG, Sevin BV (eds) Gynecologic oncology, surgery and urology. Central Foreign Books, Tokyo, pp 243–249

Bagshawe KD, Dent J, Webb J (1986) Hydatidiform mole in England and Wales 1973–1983. Lancet II:673–677

Bahn RS, Worsham A, Speeg KV, Ascoli M, Rabin D (1981) Characterization of steroid production in cultured human choriocarcinoma cells. J Clin Endocrinol Metab 52:447–450

Brindley CJ, Antoniw P, Newlands ES, Bagshawe KD (1985) Pharmacokinetics and toxicity of the epipodophyllotoxin derivative etoposide in patients with gestational choriocarcinoma and malignant teratoma. Cancer Chemother Pharmacol 15:66–71

Franke HR, Risse EKJ, Kenemans P, Vooijs GR, Stolk JG (1983) Epidemiologic features of hydatidiform mole in the Netherlands. Obsestet Gynecol 62:613–616

Goldstein DP (1972) The chemotherapy of gestational trophoblastic disease. JAMA 220:209–213

Hammond CB, Borchert LG, Tyrey L, Creasman WT, Parker RT (1973) Treatment of metastatic trophoblastic disease: good and poor progonosis. Am J Obstet Gynecol 115:451–457

Hammond CB, Weed JC, Currie JL (1980) The role of operation in the current therapy of gestational trophoblastic disease. Am J Obstet Gynecol 136:844–858

Hara T, Kaseki S, Tomoda Y, Nishikawa Y, Ishizuka T, Ishizuka N (1986) Determinants of risk for developing invasive mole and choriocarcinoma following hydatidiform mole. Asia Oceania J Obstet Gynecol 12:241–250

Hertz R (1967) Eight years experience with the chemotherapy of choriocarcinoma and related trophoblastic tumors in women. In: Holland JF, Hreshchyshyn MM (eds) Choriocarcinoma. Springer, Heidelberg Berlin New York (UICC Monograph Series, vol 3, pp 66–71)

Hertz R, Bergenstal DM, Lipsett MB, Price EB, Hilbish TF (1958) Chemotherapy of choriocarcinoma and related trophoblastic tumors in women. JAMA 168:845–854

Hertz R, Ross GT, Lipsett MB (1963) Primary chemotherapy of nonmetastatic trophoblastic disease in women. Am J Obstet Gynecol 86:808–814

Hirokawa K, Tomoda Y, Kaseki S, Ishizuka T, Nishikawa Y, Goto S (1986) Recurrence of invasive moles and choriocarcinomas. Asia Oceania J Obstet Gynecol 12:11–20

Ishizuka N (1976) Studies on trophoblastic neoplasia. In: Hirayama T (ed) Cancer in Asia. University of Tokyo Press, Tokyo (Gann Monograph on Cancer Research No 18, pp 203–216)

Izhizuka T, Tomoda Y, Kaseki S, Goto S, Hara T, Kobayashi T (1983) Intracranial metastasis of choriocarcinoma—a clinicopathologic study. Cancer 52:1896–1903

Jacobs PA, Hassold TJ, Matsuyama AM, Newland IM (1978) Chromosome constitutions of gestational trophoblastic disease. Lancet II:49

Kajii T, Ohama K (1977) Androgenetic origin of hydatidiform moles. Nature 286:633–634

Kaseki S (1974) Primary chemotherapy of trophoblastic disease—experience with 123 cases. Acta Obstet Gynecol Jpn 26:1069–1076

Kolstad P, Hognestad J (1965) Trophoblastic tumors in Norway. Acta Obstet Gynecol Scand 44:80–88

Kurman RJ, Young RH, Norris HJ, Main CS, Lawrence WD, Scully R (1984) Immunocytochemical localization of placental lactogen and chorionic gonadotropin in the normal placenta and trophoblastic tumors, with emphasis on intermediate trophoblast and the placental site trophoblastic tumor. Int J Gynecol Pathol 3:101–121

Lawler SD, Pickthall VJ, Fisher RA, Povey S, Evans MW, Szulman AE (1979) Genetic studies of complete and partial hydatidiform moles. Lancet II:580

Li MC, Hertz R, Spencer DB (1956) Effect of methotrexate therapy upon choriocarcinoma and chorioadenoma. Proc Soc Exp Biol Med 93:361–366

Llewellyn-Jones D (1965) Trophoblastic tumors—geographical variations in incidence and possible aetiological factors. J Obstet Gynecol Br Commonw 72:242–248

Lurain JR, Brewer JI, Trok EE, Halpern B (1983) Natural history of hydatidiform mole after primary evacuation. Am J Obstet Gynecol 145:591–595

McCorriston CC (1968) Racial incidence of hydatidiform mole. Am J Obstet Gynecol 101:377–382

Newlands ES (1982) New chemotherapeutic agents in the management of gestational choriocarcinoma. Semin Oncol 9:239–243

Newlands ES, Bagshawe KD (1979) Activity of high-dose cisplatinum in combination with vincristine and methotrexate in drug-resistant gestational choriocarcinoma. A report of 17 cases. Br J Cancer 40:943–945

Newlands ES, Bagshawe KD (1980) Anti-tumor activity of the epipodophyllin derivative VP16-213 in gestational choriocarcinoma. Eur J Cancer 16:401–405

Nishikawa Y, Kaseki S, Tomoda Y, Ishizuka T, Asai Y, Suzuki T, Ushijima H (1985) Histopathologic classification of uterine choriocarcinoma. Cancer 55:1044–1051

Ohama K, Kajii T, Okamoto E et al. (1981) Dispermic origin of XY moles. Nature 292:551–552

Park WW, Lees JC: Choriocarcinoma. A general review, with an analysis of 516 cases. Arch Path 49:73–104, 205–241 (1950)

Registration Committee for Trophoblastic Disease of the Japan Society of Obstetrics and Gynecology (1982) Report of the Registration Committee for Trophoblastic Disease. Acta Obstet Gynecol Jpn 34:1805–1812

Registration Committee for Trophoblastic Disease of the Japan Society of Obstetrics and Gynecology (1987) Report of the Registration Committee for Trophoblastic Disease. Acta Obstet Gynecol Jpn 39:871–880

Report of a WHO scientific group (1983) Gestational trophoblastic disease. WHO technical report series 692, Geneva, pp 11–12

Report on the study financially assisted by the Cancer Research Fund of the Ministry of Health and Welfare for the fiscal year 1980

Ringertz N (1970) Hydatidiform mole, invasive mole and choriocarcinoma in Sweden. Acta Obstet Gynecol Scand 49:195–203

Ross GT, Stolbach LL, Hertz R (1962) Actinomycin D in the treatment of methotrexate-resistant trophoblastic disease in women. Cancer Res 22:1015–1017
Shirley RL, Goldstein DP, Collins JJ (1972) The role of thoracotomy in the management of patients with chest metastases from gestational metastatic disease. J Thorac Cardiovasc Surg 63:545–550
Sugiura M, Goto S, Saito M, Kato S, Hattori S, Tomoda Y (1988) Establishment and characterization of three new human gestational choriocarcinoma cell lines. Acta Obstet Gynecol Jpn 40:1447–1454
Sung HC, Wu PC, Hu MH, Su HT (1982) Roentgenologic manifestations of pulmonary metastases in choriocarcinoma and invasive mole. Am J Obstet Gynecol 142:89–92
Teoh ES, Dawood MY, Ratnam SS (1971) Epidemiology of hydatidiform mole in Singapore. Am J Obstet Gynecol :415–420
Thomford NR, Woolner LB, Clagett OT (1965) The surgical treatment of metastatic tumors in the lungs. J Thorac Cardiovasc Surg 49:357–363
Tomoda Y, Kaseki S, Goto S, Ishizuka T, Furuhashi Y, Kato S (1986) Approach for attaining complete cure of trophoblastic disease. In: Ichinoe K (ed) Trophoblastic disease. Igaku-Shoin, Tokyo, pp 111–120
Wake N, Takagi N, Sasaki M (1978) Androgenesis as a cause of hydatidiform mole. JNCI 60:51–57
Weed JC, Hammond CB (1980) Cerebral metastatic choriocarcinoma: intensive therapy and prognosis. Obstet Gynecol 55:89–94
Xu LT, Sun CF, Wang YE, Song HZ (1985) Resection of pulmonary metastatic choriocarcinoma in 43 drug-resistant patients. Ann Thorac Surg 39:257–259
Yamashita K, Wake N, Araki T, Ichinoe K, Kuroda M (1979) Human lymphocyte antigen expression in hydatidiform mole: androgenesis following fertilization by a haploid sperm. Am J Obstet Gynecol 135:597–600
Yen S, MacMahon B (1968) Epidemiologic features of trophoblastic disease. Am J Obstet Gynecol 101:126–132

# Cytology in Gynecological Disorders

M.K. SIDAWY



## 1 Cervical Cytology—an Update on Selected Topics

### 1.1 Introduction

This chapter is by no means an exhaustive, comprehensive review of cervical cytology. Instead, it is limited to the discussion of the recent advances in respect

Current Topics in Pathology
Volume 85, Ed. N. Sasano

of some selected topics, such as the introduction of the "Bethesda System" for reporting the cytologic findings in cervicovaginal smears, and the recognition of adenocarcinoma in situ of the cervix and its diagnostic pitfalls. The subject of human papillomavirus infection is discussed in detail in the chapter by T. OKAGAKI; therefore in the relevant section in this chapter the emphasis is upon the cytologic features that are associated with the infection, and the application of molecular biology techniques to detect and identify the type of human papillomavirus in cytologic samples.

The first attempt to describe and define morphologic criteria in exfoliated squamous epithelial cells from the genital tract dates back to 1847. In that year POUCHET reported changes in the vaginal cell pattern during different phases of the menstrual cycle. PAPANICOLAOU and TRAUT (1943) reported cycle-dependent epithelial changes in the vagina. Currently, exfoliative cytology in gynecological practice has an established place for the early detection of cervical carcinoma and its precursors, and is an efficient and highly successful large-scale screening technique which has contributed to the decline in the incidence of invasive squamous carcinoma in the last two decades. The reliability of cervical cytology, however, for the detection of premalignant and malignant disease depends strongly upon the skill and experience of the sample taker, the site of the lesion, the technique used for collecting material, the quality of the smear, and the efficiency of the cytology laboratory.

## 1.2 Collection of Material

The cervical smear should be obtained preferably 2 weeks after the first day of the last menstrual period and definitely not during menstruation. Vaginal medications, contraceptives, or douches should not be used 48 h prior to the appointment. Intercourse is not recommended the night before the examination. Lubricant should not be introduced into the vagina; instead water may be used to lubricate and warm the speculum. Treatment with acetic acid or iodine as an aid to colposcopy must be deferred until the specimen has been obtained. It is important to obtain a smear that is not obscured by blood, mucus, or inflammatory exudate. It is necessary to obtain a specimen from both the ectocervix and the endocervix. Because most intraepithelial squamous lesions arise at or near the squamocolumnar junction (transformation zone), an optimal cervical smear should sample that area.

## 1.3 Smearing, Fixation, and Staining

The ectocervical and endocervical specimens should be spread on a glass slide uniformly and as thinly as possible without undue force. The material must then be fixed immediately to prevent air drying. Air drying causes artifacts and cellular distortion and prevents accurate assessment of the specimen. 95%

ethanol is accepted as an ideal cellular fixative. Spray fixatives are also widely accepted. For the best results the nozzle of the spraying apparatus should be held approximately 12 in. from the slide. The use of commercially available hair spray is discouraged because of the variability in the ingnedients. These cosmetic aerosols may result in very poor specimen preservation. The preparation is stained by the Papanicolaou technique.

## 1.4 Specimen Adequacy

There is no universally accepted definition of an unsatisfactory gynecological smear for cytologic evaluation. Considerable disagreement exists regarding the presence of endocervical or metaplastic cells as a criterion for a satisfactory sample. The importance of the presence of endocervical columnar cells for smear adequacy has been discussed since 1972 (Gondos et al. 1972). Some investigators have suggested that cervical smears without endocervical columnar cells are not always inadequate (Kivlahan and Ingram 1986). Other studies (Killough et al. 1988) show that although an abnormal cytologic diagnosis may be made in the absence of endocervical or metaplastic cells in a sample, the overall diagnostic yield from these cases is lower than the diagnostic yield from smears that include these cells. The end result of using samples lacking such cells is an increased number of false-negative diagnoses due primarily to sampling error. Consequently the question arises as to what should a physician do when faced with screening cervical smear that contains no endocervical cells? The financial and pragmatic burden of recalling those patients is significant. The ethical and potential medicolegal implications of not recalling them are profound.

The recently proposed Bethesda classification for reporting cervical/vaginal cytology (1988) includes a statement on the adequacy of the specimen and recommends that the cytologist requests a repeat smear when reporting an unsatisfactory specimen. A sample is considered unsatisfactory less than optimal when "No endocervical component" is present in a premenopausal woman who has a uterine cervix. This indicates that none of the following elements is present: (a) endocervical cells, (b) endocervical mucus, or (c) squamous metaplastic cells.

There are three major factors affecting the yield of endocervical columnar cells:

- The hormonal influence:
  pregnant and menopausal women often have smears without endocervical cells (Allingham and King 1985).
- The sample taker: well-trained sample takers obtain higher rates of smears containing endocervical cells than do general practitioners (Kirk and Boon 1981).
- The method and/or instrument used for taking the sample.

A variety of devices are available to obtain cervical samples. The two devices most commonly employed to obtain a sample from the ectocervix are the wooden and plastic spatulas. Currently, a variety of devices are available to obtain a sample from the endocervical canal: a saline-moistened cotton-tipped applicator, the Cytobrush, the Cytopick, the Cervex brush, and a plastic or glass pipette attached to a suction bulb. Both the Cytobrush and the Cytopick are constructed as screw conveyors; when rotated in the endocervical canal, the moving bristles of the Cytobrush and the corkscrew sharp edges of the Cytopick effectively dislodge cells from the epithelial lining. The Cervex brush offers the advantage of sampling both the ectocervix and 0.5 cm of the endocervix simultaneously with one device; a disadvantage of this device is that, due to the thickness of the bristles, it is absolutely mandatory to remove the mucus from the external os to avoid thick smears that are difficult to screen.

### 1.5 Comparison of Methods of Endocervical Sampling

A number of studies have shown that the yield of endocervical cells and/or metaplastic cells can be increased by using a Cytobrush for the endocervical sampling (KRISTENSEN et al. 1989). Compared with cervical samples obtained by conventional methods, the Cytobrush smears contain significantly more endocervical cells and have less drying artifacts. The rate of suboptimal smears (those without endocervical cells) falls from 12.0% to 1.7% when the endocervical brush is used instead of the endocervical swab (TAYLOR et al. 1987). BOON et al. 1989) analyzed five sampling methods for the preparation of cervical smears and concluded that the methods using Cytobrush and Cytopick give superior results in the detection of CIN III; the study also showed a correlation between CIN III detection and the presence of endocervical cells in the smear. The Cytobrush is also more effective than the bulb aspirator technique in obtaining endocervical cells, particularly in pregnant and postmenopausal patients, and in predicting the histologic severity of the cervical lesions (SELVAGGI et al. 1989). The results of other studies, however, question whether improved sampling of the squamocolumnar junction results in any increased detection of cervical disease (LAI-GOLDMAN et al. 1988). It is important to note that while the presence of endocervical columnar cells on a cervical smear increases the sensitivity for the detection of epithelial abnormality, their presence is not an absolute assurance of adequate sampling (DETWEILER et al. 1989).

### 1.6 Reporting and Interpretation of Cytologic Findings

In the final assessment of a smear the cytologist should consider the smear background, the arrangement of the cells, their numbers, and their pattern of distribution. The diagnosis should not be based upon the appearance of an individual cell because there is no single hallmark characteristic of every cell from a given lesion. The cytologic diagnosis must be based on the sum total of the cytologic criteria. Cellular atypia is based upon changes in the nucleus and cytoplasm. Nuclear characteristics of atypia are nuclear enlargement and hyperchromasia. It should be remembered that the impression of hyperchromasia depends on two factors, namely nuclear volume and chromatin content, and is to some extent determined by degenerative changes. Increased nuclear–cytoplasmic ratio, nuclear polymorphism or anisokaryosis, and abnormal chromatin pattern and distribution are other criteria of atypia.

Papanicolaou divided his classification into groups I–V for purposes of cytologic reporting; however, his classification is no longer an adequate way of reporting cervicovaginal smear findings. It does not communicate a diagnosis, and there is no agreement as to exactly what the different classes mean, with cytopathologists and clinicians attaching a galaxy of interpretations and numerous subheadings to Papanicolaou classes II and III. Nowadays, most cytologic findings are interpreted by arranging the results into defined groups based on the system of histologic reporting.

The Bethesda System for reporting the laboratory evaluation of cervicovaginal smears was developed at the December 1988 National Cancer Institute Workshop for cervical/vaginal cytology. Driving the new system are the recognized inadequacies of the Papanicolaou classification, as well as the need to standardize the terminology of the cytology reports to allow more efficient communication between the laboratory and clinicians.

The format of the report proposed by the Bethesda System is as follows:

*STATEMENT ON SPECIMEN ADEQUACY*
- **Satisfactory for interpretation**
- **Less than optimal**
- **Unsatisfactory**

**Explanation for "Less Than Optimal/Unsatisfactory Samples":**
- Scant cellularity
- Poor fixation or preservation
- Presence of foreign material (e.g., lubricant)
- Partially or completely obscuring inflammation
- Partially or completely obscuring blood
- Excessive cytolysis or autolysis
- No endocervical component in a premenopausal woman who has a cervix
- Not representative of the anatomic site
- Other:____________________

*GENERAL CATEGORIZATION*
- **Within normal limits**
- **Other:____________________**
    - See descriptive diagnosis
    - Further action recommended

*DESCRIPTIVE DIAGNOSES*

- *INFECTION*
- **Fungal**
  - Fungal organisms morphologically consistent with *Candida sp.*
  - Other:______________________________
- **Bacterial**
  - Microorganisms morphologically consistent with *Gardnerella sp.*
  - Microorganisms morphologically consistent with *Actinomyces sp.*
  - Cellular changes suggestive of *Chlamydia sp.* infection, subject to confirmatory studies
  - Other:______________________________
- **Protozoan**
  - *Trichomonas vaginalis*
  - Other:
- **Viral**
  - Cellular changes associated with cytomegalovirus
  - Cellular changes associated with herpes simplex virus
  - Other:______________________________

  [Note: For human papillomavirus (HPV), refer to Epithelial Cell Abnormalities, Squamous Cell]
- **Other:**______________________________
- ***REACTIVE AND REPARATIVE CHANGES***
- **Inflammation**
  - Associated cellular changes
  - Follicular cervicitis
- **Miscellaneous (as related to patient history)**
  - Effects of therapy
  - Ionizing radiation
  - Chemotherapy
  - Effects of mechanical devices (e.g., intrauterine contraceptive device)
  - Effects of nonsteroidal estrogen exposure (e.g., diethylstilbestrol)
  - Other:______________________________
- ***EPITHELIAL CELL ABNORMALITIES***
- ***Squamous cell***
- **Atypical squamous cells of undetermined significance.**
  (recommended follow-up and/or type of further investigation):______________________
- **Squamous intraepithelial lesion (SIL)**
  [comment on presence of cellular changes associated with HPV if applicable]
- **Low-grade squamous intraepithelial lesion, encompassing:**
  (1) Cellular changes associated with HPV

(2) Mild (slight) dysplasia/cervical intraepithelial neoplasia grade 1 (CIN 1)

- **High-grade squamous intraepithelial lesion, encompassing:**
  (1) Moderate dysplasia/CIN 2
  (2) Servere dysplasia/CIN 3
  (3) Carcinoma in situ/CIN 3
- **Squamous cell carcinoma**

*Glandular cells*

- **Presence of endometrial cells in one of the following circumstances:**
  - Out-of-phase in a menstruating woman
  - In a postmenopausal woman
  - No menstrual history available
- **Atypical glandular cells of undetermined significance**
  (recommended follow-up and/or type of further investigation:____________________
  - Endometrial
  - Endocervical
  - Not otherwise specified
- **Adenocarcinoma**
  - Specify probable site of origin: endocervical, endometrial, extrauterine
  - Not otherwise specified
- **Other epithelial malignant neoplasm:**____________________
- ***NONEPITHELIAL MALIGNANT NEOPLASM***
  (SPECIFY:)____________________

**HORMONAL EVALUATION (APPLIES TO VAGINAL SMEARS ONLY)**

- Hormonal pattern compatible with age and history
- Hormonal pattern incompatible with age and history
  Specify:____________________
- Hormonal evaluation not possible
  - Cervical specimen
  - Inflammation
  - Insufficient patient history
- ***OTHER:***____________________

The Bethesda System uses descriptive diagnostic terminology oriented toward patient management. The system introduced the term *squamous intraepithelial lesion* in order to break away from the mold of other used terminologies and to accommodate several groups in cytology. On one side there are those who advocate the term *cervical intraepithelial neoplasia* (CIN) graded I, II, or III, who emphasize that cervical epithelial changes up to and including carcinoma in situ form a continuous spectrum. Others feel that it is inappropriate to call a low-grade lesion "neoplasia" since such lesions may regress spontaneously, and they use the term *dysplasia* graded as mild, moderate, severe, and carcinoma in situ.

The terminology defines two groups of squamous intraepithelial lesions—low-grade and high-grade. The low-grade squamous intraepithelial lesion incorporates mild dysplasia and CIN I; it also incorporates the diagnosis of human papillomavirus infection. High-grade squamous intraepithelial lesion encompasses moderate and severe dysplasia, carcinoma in situ, as well as CIN II and III. Reducing the number of gradations to two levels may increase the reproducibility of diagnoses.

The Bethesda System limits use of the term *atypia* to those cases where other diagnoses cannot be rendered. *Atypia* is not applied to defined inflammatory changes or neoplasia or its precursor states. The term *atypical squamous cells of undetermined significance* is reserved for cases in which abnormal findings cannot be defined clearly. Follow-up and/or further investigation is recommended to determine the significance of the atypical cells.

## 1.7 Sources of False-Positive Interpretation in Cervical Smears

Cellular changes associated with inflammation, regeneration, and squamous metaplasia are often misinterpreted as atypical (dysplasia, CIN, or HPV-associated changes). Therefore, it is important to recognize these changes cytologically in order to avoid overcalling them.

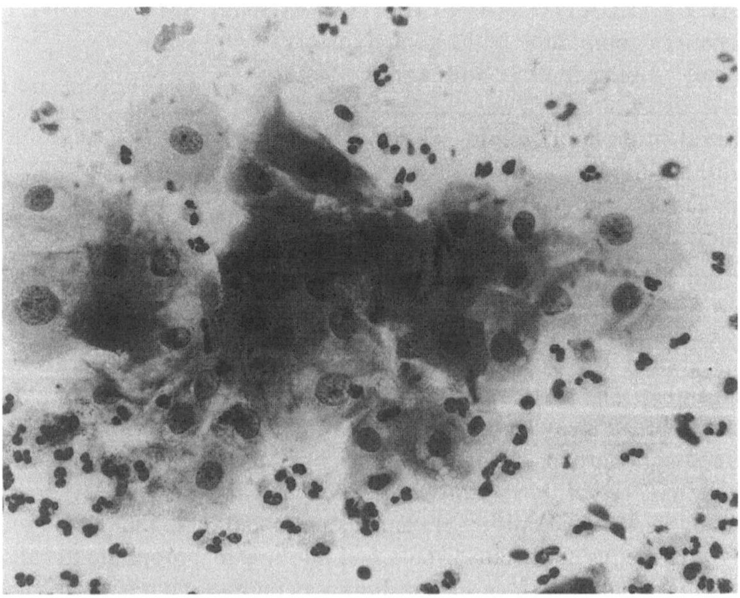

**Fig. 1.** Reactive cellular changes associated with inflammation. The intermediate squamous cells reveal enlarged nuclei. *Trichomonas vaginalis* is present elsewhere in the smear. × 40

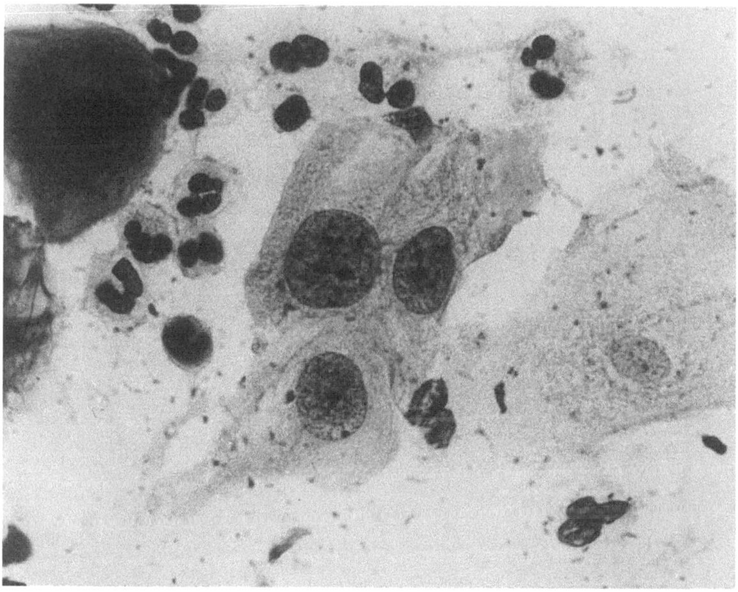

**Fig. 2.** Reactive cellular changes associated with inflammation. Note the enlarged nuclei, the open network chromatin pattern, and small nucleoli. × 100

### *1.7.1 Cellular Changes Associated with Inflammation*

Inflammatory reactions affecting the vagina and the cervix are characterized by changes in the epithelial cells which are reflected in the staining of the cytoplasm and in alterations in nuclear and cytoplasmic structures. These changes include cytoplasmic basophilia due to the activity of the ribosomes, an open network chromatin pattern, and the presence of nucleoli which reflect the activity of the nucleus (Figs. 1, 2). These changes are reversible; however, if the cell is exposed to further stress, regressive and degenerative changes follow. Such changes are characterized by vacuole formation in the cytoplasm and by intense cytoplasmic eosinophilia, and eventually the cytoplasm liquifies and disappears. The nuclei show karyolysis, karyorrhexis, and pyknosis. The presence of multinucleated epithelial cells is also a sign of chronic inflammation. They point to the disordered mitotic activity. They are also common in dysplasia, after irradiation, and as a result of folic acid deficiency.

### *1.7.2 Cellular Changes Associated with Regeneration*

Cells from regenerating epithelium are characterized by relatively large, active nuclei with one or several nucleoli and finely granular chromatin. They often occur in sheets and clusters (Fig. 3).

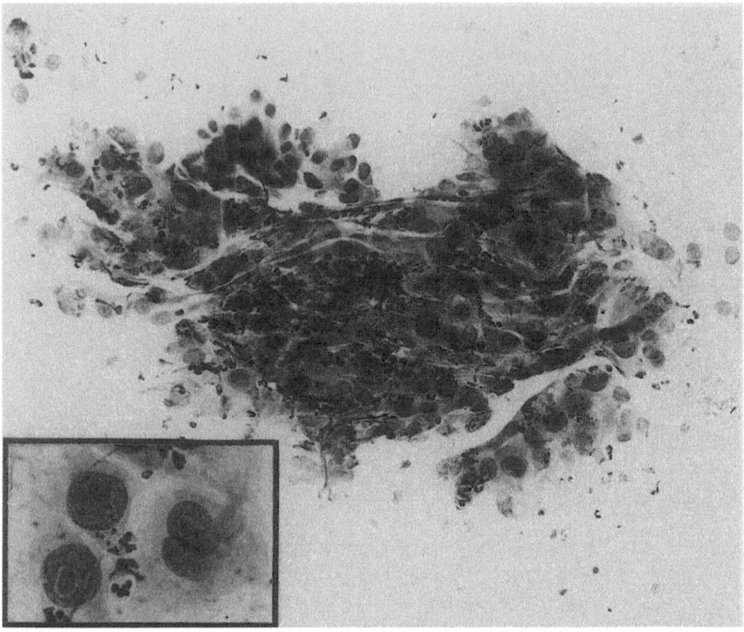

**Fig. 3.** Cellular changes associated with repair. Sheet of squamous metaplastic cells exhibiting significantly enlarged nuclei. Acute inflammatory cells are present. × 20 *Inset*: High power showing the characteristic prominent nucleoli. × 40

### *1.7.3 Squamous Metaplasia*

The cytoplasm of metaplastic cells stains intensely cyanophilic with pronounced accentuation at the cell margin. An inner zone of paler endoplasm is also distinguished from an outer zone of dark ectoplasm, a feature commonly misinterpreted as koilocytosis. The nucleus is central, round, and finely granular; it may show occasional chromocenters, but nucleoli are not present. Metaplastic cells tend to lie in loose groups. The shape of the cells is dependent on its degree of maturation. Immature cells are usually round or oval. As the metaplastic cells mature, the chief criterion which distinguishes them from normal squamous cells at the same stage of maturation is the fact that the cytoplasm is denser.

### *1.7.4 Chlamydial Cervicitis*

*Chlamydia trachomatis* is a recognized pathogen in the female genital tract and is a major cause of involuntary sterility. The organism requires special handling and grows in special cell cultures. Chlamydia-infected cells reveal enlarged hyperchromatic nuclei with uniformly distributed chromatin and are often

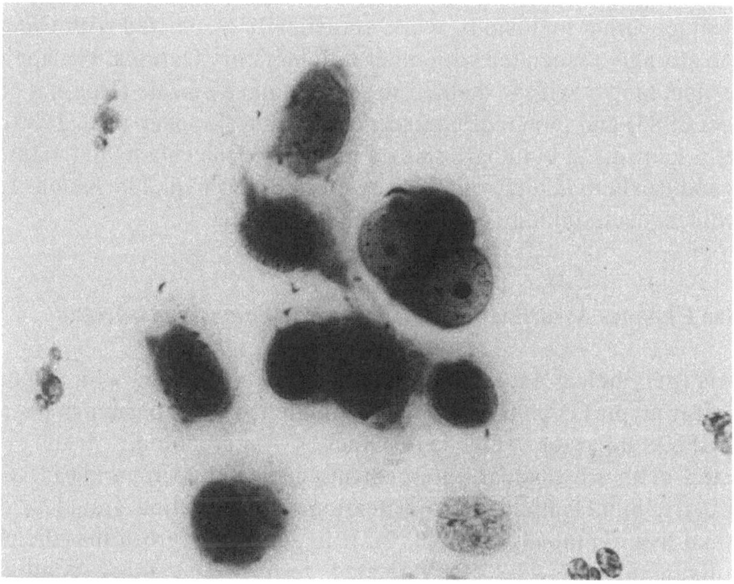

**Fig. 4.** Metaplastic squamous cells showing intracytoplasmic inclusions suggestive of *chlamydia sp.* infection (subject to confirmatory studies). × 100

classified as atypical. Efforts have been made to define the cytologic criteria for the recognition of *Chlamydia trachomatis* on Papanicolaou-stained cervical smears (GUPTA et al. 1979; NAIB 1970). However, the reported morphologic criteria are not generally accepted, and it is quite difficult to distinguish true chlamydial inclusions in cells in gynecological smears from other types of intracytoplasmic inclusions with similar morphologic features. Therefore, considerable controversy exists as to the feasibility of using diagnostic cytology for the detection of chlamydial infection. It is important to recognize that even in cases in which cell cultures or serologic tests are positive, all inclusion bodies seen cytologically cannot be identified as produced by chlamydia. Chlamydial inclusions are most frequently seen in metaplastic squamous cells (Fig. 4). They are occasionally seen in parabasal squamous cells, columnar cells, and intermediate squamous cells. Various types of intracytoplasmic inclusions are reported as indicative of chlamydial infection: coccoid bodies, vacuoles with a central target formation, vacuoles with granular inclusions, and nebular inclusions that are composed of a mixture of fine and large granular particles, which represent elementary and initial bodies in the infection cycle. In general, chlamydial inclusion borders are thin or absent, and thin-walled or membrane-lined vacuoles are not necessarily evident by light microscopy. When the border of a vacuole is thick, the inclusion more like contains mucin. Recent studies (SHIINA 1985; HENRY et al. 1989) indicate that the nebular-type inclusions may represent actual chlamydial organisms recognizable in routine cervical smears and that the cytologic diagnosis of chlamydial infection is possible by the detection of these inclusions. Other inclusions, while statistically associated with *Chlamydia*, are also strongly associated with other inflammatory features. The application of the immunoperoxidase method to the destained smears (DORMAN et al. 1985; SHIINA 1985) and immunofluorescence staining (LINDNER et al. 1985) for chlamydial organisms to cytologic smears may prove the chlamydial nature of inclusions and can help in differentiating suspected chlamydial inclusions from mucin vacuoles, bacterial masses, and degenerated cells.

## 1.8 Cellular Changes Associated with Human Papillomavirus Infection

Koilocytosis (perinuclear and cytoplasmic clearing, associated with some degree of nuclear atypia) is considered the cytologic evidence of human papillomavirus (HPV) infection (Fig. 5). Other cytomorphologic features of HPV-infected cells are nuclear enlargement, nuclear hyperchromasia, giant squamous cells, binucleation, multinucleation, keratohyaline granules, dyskeratosis, and hyperkeratosis (Figs. 6, 7). It is generally agreed that the morphologic distinction between HPV-related lesions and other conditions masquerading as such can be difficult, even to the most experienced observer. Studies correlating the results of the cytomorphologic features with the HPV

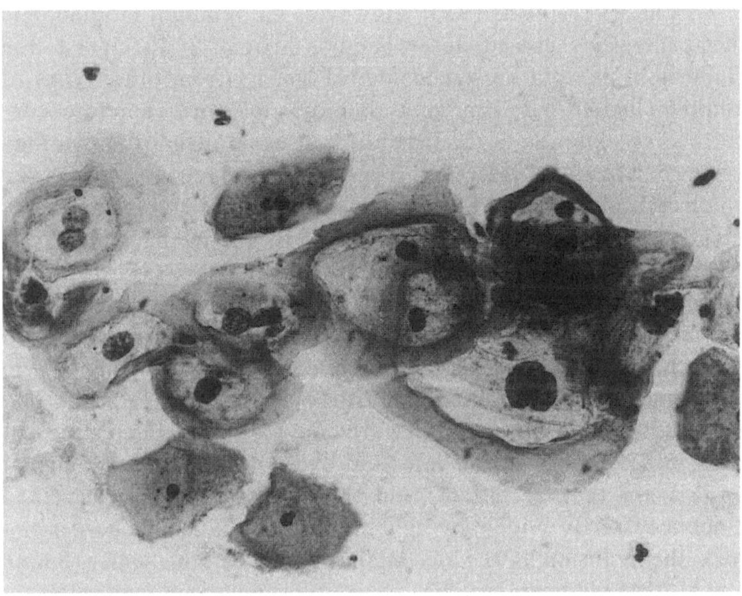

**Fig. 5.** Koilocytosis: perinuclear and cytoplasmic clearing, with nuclear atypia. × 40

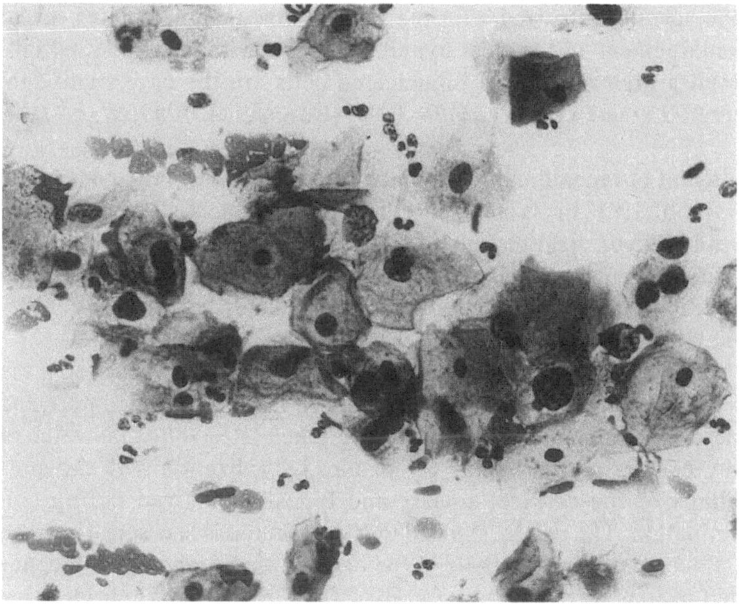

**Fig. 6.** Cellular changes associated with HPV infection. Nuclear enlargement, nuclear hyperchromasia, and binucleation. × 40

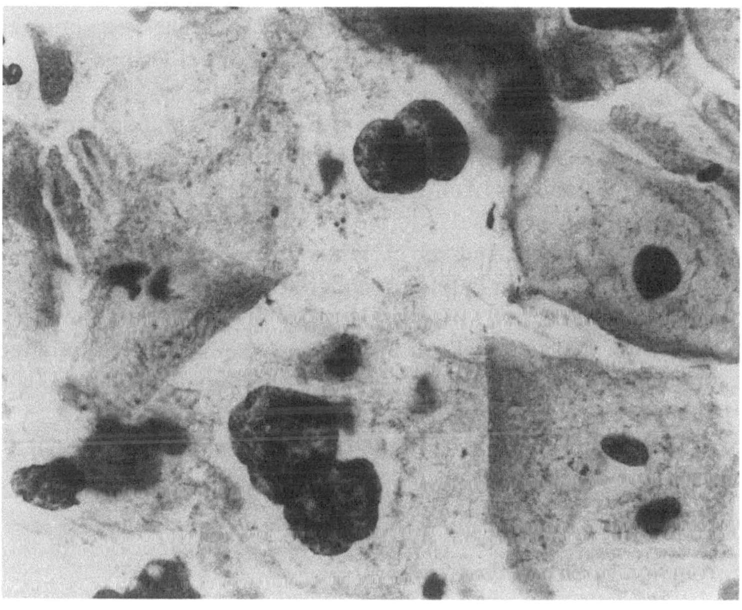

**Fig. 7.** Cellular changes associated with HPV infection. The nuclei are enlarged, hyperchromatic, and reveal an irregular nuclear membrane. × 100

DNA hybridization using Southern blot, reverse blot, and dot blot assays on cervical scrape specimens paired with the Papanicolaou-stained slides reveal that nuclear enlargement and nuclear hyperchromasia (with or without perinuclear halos) and a high number of binucleated cells are the only significant independent predictors of a positive HPV DNA (BOSCH et al. 1989; WARD et al. 1989).

With the advent of recombinant DNA technology, it is currently possible to identify the type of HPV in tissues and cytologic specimens. Several studies using Southern blot hybridization, in situ hybridization, slot blot hybridization, reverse blot, and polymerase chain reaction have been applied to cytologic material. The results corroborate the already well-established association between specific HPV types and particular cervical neoplastic lesions.

Dot blot hybridization performed on cervical smears and swabs, using the ViraPap and the Viratype (Life Technology, Inc.), is a relatively simple and inexpensive test. Recent studies have been undertaken to establish the value of this method by comparing the results of dot blot hybridization with the morphologic findings of the cervical smears and biopsies obtained during colposcopic examination. The results showed that the method is less sensitive than morphology, since approximately half of the cases with morphologic evidence of HPV-related lesions were negative for HPV DNA by dot blot hybridization in cervical swabs (MESONERO et al. 1991). DUGGAN et al.(1988) also concluded that the recovery of HPV DNA using the dot blot hybridization method is low in a group with a high frequency of CIN. Therefore, cervical swab DNA hybridization may be a useful adjunct to morphologic and colposcopic evaluation; however, at the present time, cytology continues to be the best screening method for the detection of HPV-related squamous epithelial lesions.

Polymerase chain reaction allows in vitro amplification of specific DNA synthesis and is currently the most sensitive molecular technique for HPV detection (KATZ et al. 1989). However, the technique is not available in most laboratories because it requires well-trained personel and it is difficult to integrate it into traditional settings due to the problem of contamination.

The application of new technology certainly increases the sensitivity of detecting HPV-related lesions in cytologic material, since cytologic examination alone for HPV has a sensitivity of 74% (JENSON 1989). However, these tests are expensive and time consuming. Their utility for screening large populations and as a treatment-prioritizing procedure for HPV infection is debated (CRUM et al. 1989). Currently, HPV detection and typing are recommended as an adjunct to cytology when there is an equivocal cervical smear and not for general screening.

### 1.9 Adenocarcinoma In Situ of the Cervix

Invasive adenocarcinoma of the cervix is preceded by a precancerous phase during which successful treatment is possible. The concept of adenocarcinoma in situ (AIS) of the cervix was first introduced by FRIEDELL and MC KAY (1953). The precursors of AIS, however, are poorly defined, and diagnostic criteria have not yet been established. AIS has no clinical or colposcopic features, and hence cytology plays an important role in the diagnosis of this lesion. The correct means for investigating for AIS and related lesions predicted on the basis of cytologic findings is a diagnostic cone biopsy.

The cytologic features of AIS were initially described in very general terms by BARTER and WATERS (1970). The first paper devoted to the cytologic criteria necessary for the prospective cytologic diagnosis of AIS of the uterine cervix was published by KRUMINS et al. (1977). AYER et al. (1987) refined further the diagnostic criteria and described two distinct patterns of AIS, based on the architectural and nuclear features: well-differentiated AIS and poorly differentiated AIS.

Well-differentiated AIS is characterized architecturally by (a) tightly crowded sheets with marked cellular pseudostratification, (b) isolated strips with palisading and pseudostratified nuclei, and (c) rosette formation. The nuclei are enlarged, oval, and hyperchromatic. The chromatin is evenly distributed, and the chromatin pattern varies from finely to coarsely granular. Nucleoli may be present (Figs. 8, 9). Poorly differentiated AIS is characterized by enlarged, pleomorphic, hyperchromatic nuclei and prominent nucleoli. In general, the architectural features are not helpful in distinguishing between well-differentiated and poorly differentiated AIS, except that the exfoliated sheets

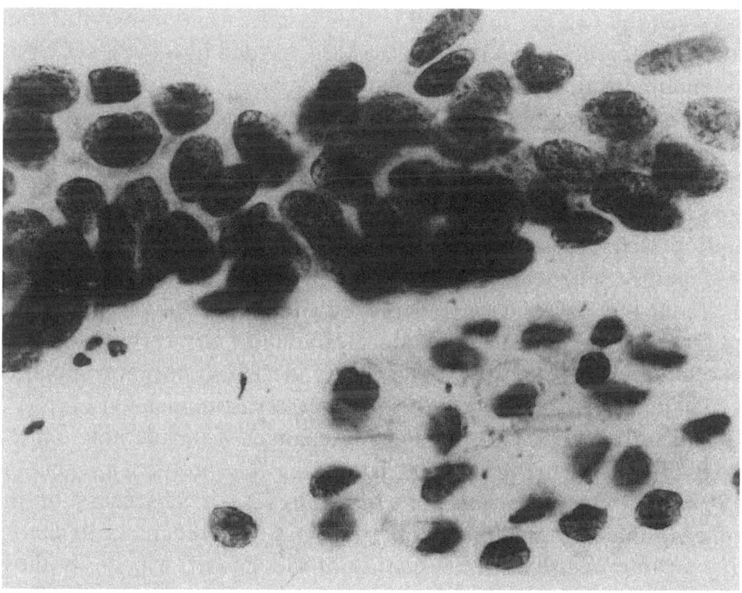

**Fig. 8.** AIS of the cervix. Tightly crowded sheet of epithelial cells with stratified, enlarged, and hyperchromatic nuclei. Compare to the nuclei of normal endocervical cells (*bottom right*). × 100

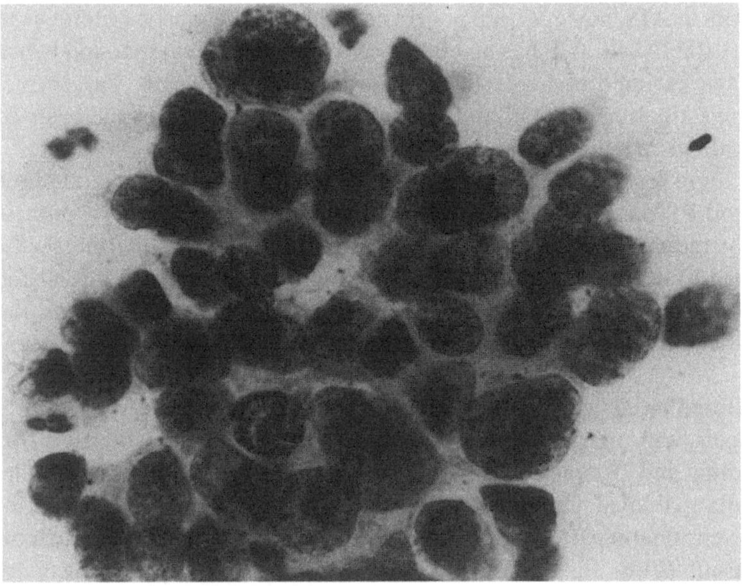

**Fig. 9.** AIS of the cervix. Stratified cells with high nuclear–cytoplasmic ratio, coarsely granular chromatin, and rosette formation. × 100

tend to be more loosely crowded in the latter. The nuclear features enable the distinction between the two entities. Within the classification of well-differentiated and poorly differentiated AIS, the cases are divided into three subtypes: endocervical, endometrial, and intestinal.

Several authors cast considerable doubt upon the cytologic identification of AIS. Underdiagnosis of this type of lesion has been reported. BOON et al. (1981) found the underdiagnosis of glandular abnormalities to be common both by cytologists and by histopathologists. In recent years, however, improved endocervical sampling techniques have greatly increased the yield of endocervical smears. Consequently, endocervical glandular atypias are being recognized with greater frequency. It must be recognized that potential pitfalls in the cytologic diagnosis of precursors to adenocarcinoma of the cervix exist. An improvement of diagnostic sensitivity in respect of these lesions is accompanied by a decrease in specificity, and it may be difficult to distinguish between AIS of the cervix and inflammatory or metaplastic changes. Considerable experience in cytology is required to avoid errors in this area. The problem has become more acute in recent years because of (a) an increased awareness of the possibility of encountering glandular cells that may be precursors to malignancy, and (b) an improvement in the quality of the smears, especially those obtained with the newly marketed endocervical brushes (LEE 1988). Pitfalls in the diagnosis of AIS include cervical endometriosis, various types of metaplasia (Figs. 10, 11), changes due to a previous biopsy (PACEY et al. 1988), and

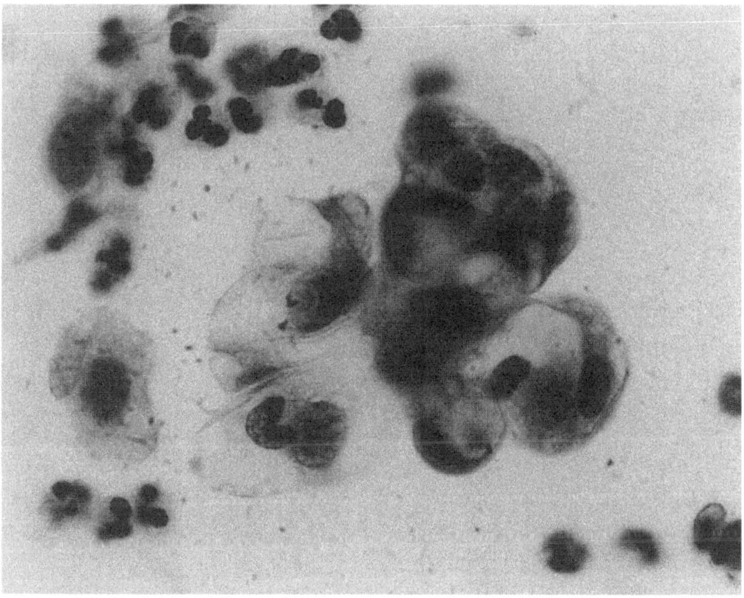

**Fig. 10.** Endometrial cells showing syncytial metaplasia are noted in the cervical smear of an 80-year-old woman. The smear was originally reported as "suspicious for malignancy." × 100

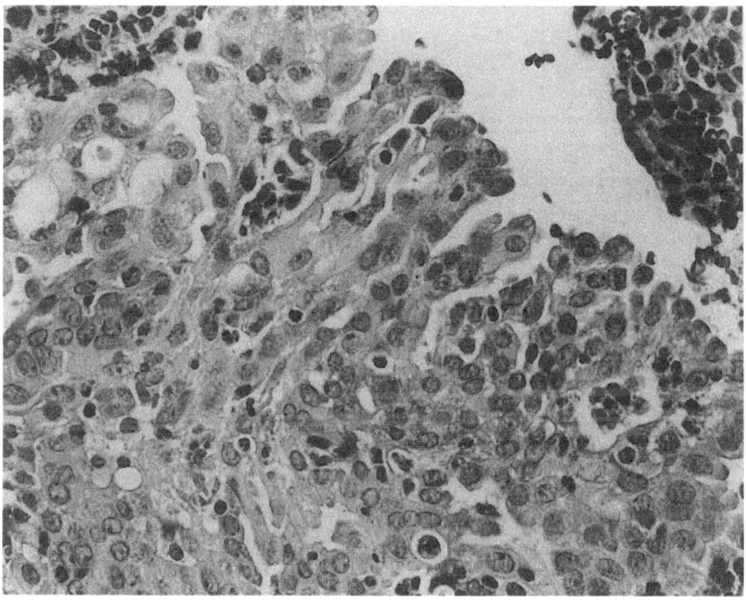

**Fig. 11.** Endometrial curettings from the same patient whose smear is illustrated in Fig. 10. The endometrium shows syncytial surface (papillary) metaplasia. The cells are identical to those noted in the cervical smear. There was no evidence of carcinoma. H&E, × 40

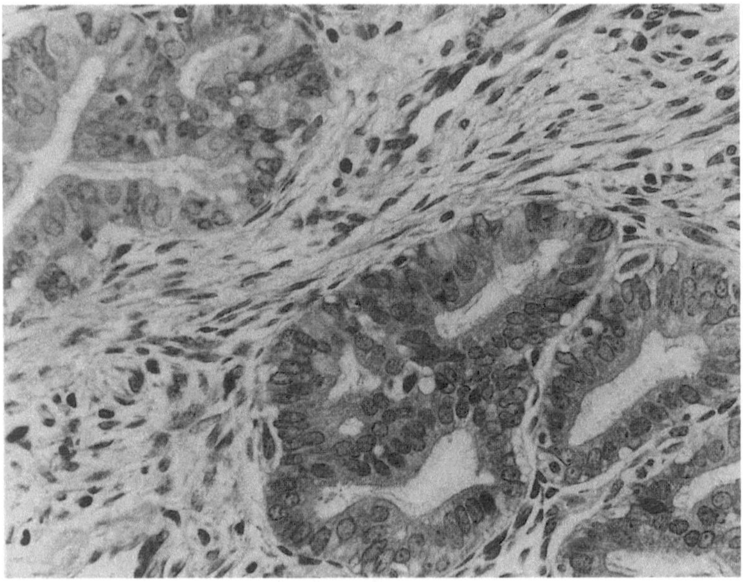

**Fig. 12.** Section of tubal metaplasia of the cervix. The cervical smear of this patient was reported in an outside laboratory as AIS of endocervix. The illustrated cone biopsy of the cervix reveals extensive tubal metaplasia and no evidence of malignancy. H&E, × 40

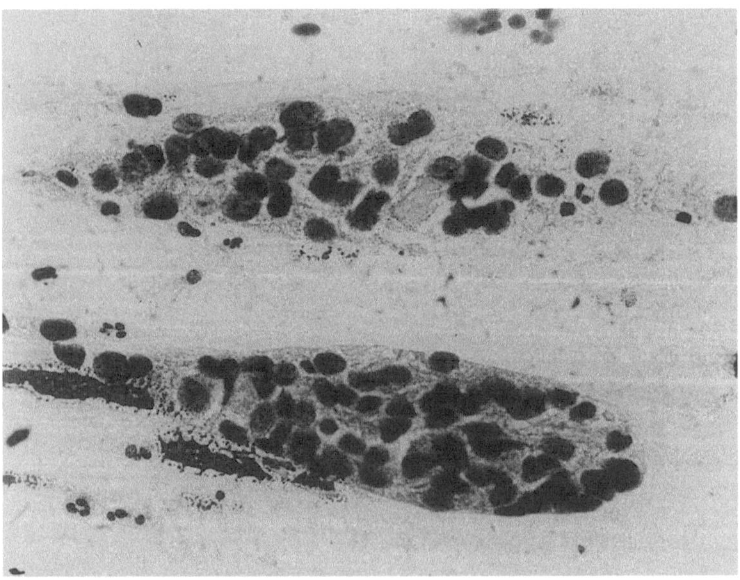

**Fig. 13.** Microglandular endocervical hyperplasia. Atypical glandular cells with enlarged nuclei and vacuolated cytoplasm. × 40

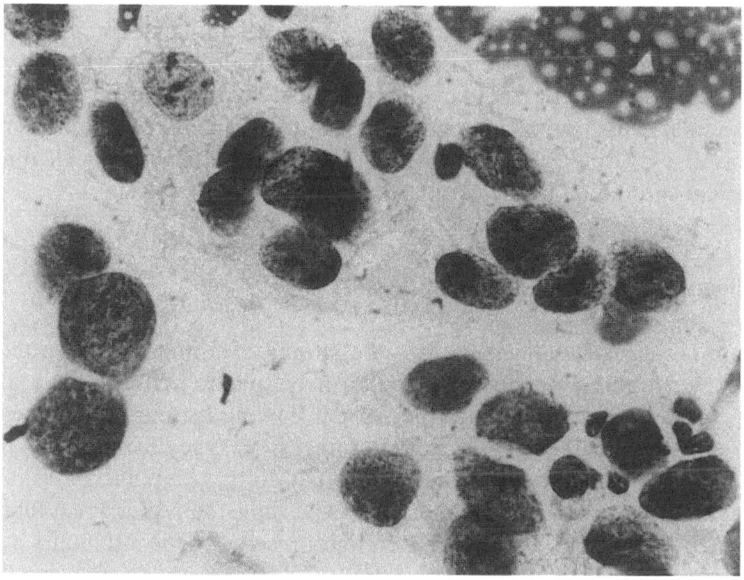

**Fig. 14.** Invasive adenocarcinoma of the cervix. Glandular cells with enlarged hyperchromatic nuclei and vacuolated cytoplasm. × 100

microglandular endocervical hyperplasia (RIZZO et al. 1989). Endometriosis of the cervix desquamates as clusters and large sheets of crowded glandular cells showing nuclear enlargement, mild hyperchromasia, and prominent nucleoli. The cells are present in smears irrespective of the time of the menstrual cycle and, unlike endometrial cells derived from the endometrium, they appear in a well-preserved state. Tubal metaplasia presents cytologically as enlarged endocervical cells arranged in sheets, strips, and rosettes. The nuclei are hyperchromatic, crowded, and pseudostratified. These features can easily lead to an erroneous diagnosis of AIS. The presence of ciliated epithelium, however, must alert to the possibility of tubal metaplasia (Fig. 12). A past history of cone biopsy should demand caution when interpreting follow-up smears. The endocervical canal may be shortened by such a procedure, so that endometrial tissue is more exposed to the direct action of the spatula. The cytologic features of high endocervical cells are not well known, and the features of endometrial cells obtained by direct scrape vary from those shed spontaneously. Review of the cone biopsy histology may help avoiding pitfalls whenever interpreting difficult smears taken after a cone biopsy. Microglandular endocervical hyperplasia is a benign proliferation of endocervical glands, commonly associated with oral contraceptive use and pregnancy. The literature cites several cases false-positive histologic diagnoses due to microglandular endocervical hyperplasia. This lesion should be included in the differential diagnosis of glandular atypia seen in cervical smears, although some authors believe that microglandular endocervical hyperplasia does not produce false-positive cytologic findings (PACEY et al. 1988). On smears microglandular endocervical hyperplasia appears as atypical glandular cells with enlarged nuclei and vacuolated cytoplasm (Fig. 13). It is also difficult always to distinguish AIS from invasive well-differentiated adenocarcinoma of the cervix (Fig. 14) (LEE et al. 1989).

### 1.10 Microinvasive Adenocarcinoma of the Cervix

Microinvasion is defined as invasion into the stroma of 5 mm or less in the absence of demonstrable evidence of vascular or lymphatic permeation or of confluent microinvasion over a broad front. The following features, when seen in conjunction with AIS, are suggestive of microinvasion: syncytia of glandular cells, small cells in very crowded sheets, and papillary groupings of cells. However, based on these features it is not always possible to predict or exclude microinvasion. The predictive accuracy for microinvasive adenocarcinoma by applying these criteria is about 50% (AYER et al. 1988).

## 2 Peritoneal Washing Cytology

### 2.1 Introduction

Peritoneal washing cytology has been used since the early 1950s for the management of gynecological cancer. In 1975 the International Federation of Gynecologists and Obstetricians incorporated the results of peritoneal washing cytology in the staging classification for ovarian carcinoma. It is now an accepted procedure in the staging of female genital tract neoplasms at the time of initial surgery. It is also a part of the second-look laparotomy in patients treated for gynecological malignancies (ZISELMAN et al. 1984). CREASMAN and RUTLEDGE (1971) stated that peritoneal cytologic findings correlate well with prognosis in corporeal, ovarian, and cervical malignant lesions.

The main purpose of cytologic investigation is to determine the presence of absence of tumor; however, the diagnosis of other conditions may be accomplished. In the absence of disease the peritoneal fluid is limited to an insignificant lubricating layer that cannot be aspirated. The role of specimen collection and preparation in the accurate interpretation of these samples cannot be overemphasized. Acellular specimens relate to the washing procedure itself, which requires thoroughness and consistency on the part of the surgeon. The cytopathologist can aid in the care of the ovarian cancer patient by including in the report on the peritoneal fluid cytologic specimen not only whether malignant cells are present but also whether mesothelial cells are present. Their presence is the evidence that a peritoneal fluid cytologic specimen was obtained at operation. The presence or absence of mesothelial cells in a peritoneal fluid specimen will convey to the operating physicians more meaningful clinical information and should help to make them more aware of the need to use appropriate techniques for obtaining a representative peritoneal fluid cytologic specimen (McGowan 1989). Ineffective cytopreparation, particularly of bloody specimens, obscures cellullar details and may hamper interpretation. Cytopreparation must be designed to minimize the effects of blood contamination.

While endorsing the concept of peritoneal washing cytology, various authors have reported problems in interpreting these specimens. Reasons for false-negative diagnoses include paucity of malignant cells, difficulty in distinguishing tumor cells from reactive mesothelial cells, or unsatisfactory specimens (problems in cytopreparation and/or insufficient cellularity). The problem of false-positive peritoneal washing cytologies is well recognized, with a rate of 4.5% reported by Creasman and Rutledge (1971); it is associated with reactive mesothelial cells, presence of psammoma bodies, endometriosis, endosalpingiosis, benign epithelial tumors, epithelium spilled from a ruptured cyst or benign tumor, pelvic inflammatory disease with adhesion formation, ectopic pregnancy, adnexal infarction due to torsion, and recent laparotomy (Ravinsky 1986; Zuna et al. 1989b).

Since a positive peritoneal washing may alter the treatment, diagnostic accuracy is essential. A diagnosis of "suspicious" is not helpful and should be avoided. The diagnostic accuracy can be enhanced by the correlation of the cytology with the available cytologic and histologic studies (Zuna et al. 1989b). A clinical history of recent laparotomy or ruptured viscus may also be helpful in correctly interpreting some problem patterns.

## 2.2 Cytology of Negative Peritoneal Washings

Peritoneal washings contain predominantly lymphocytes, histiocytes (macrophages), and mesothelial cells. Fresh and hemolyzed red cells may represent only a traumatic tap. Fibrin is seen as eosinophilic granules or tangled threads and may trap cells, giving a false impression of clumping. Protein forms a hazy matrix in the background.

### *2.2.1 Mesothelial Cells*

Single mesothelial cells are round to oval; they show a clear zone surrounding the cell membrane, probably corresponding to a poorly preserved brush border. The nucleus occupies about half of the cell diameter and is usually centrally located with the cell. The nuclear membrane is prominent; the chromatin net is very fine, with a few small chromocenters and occasionally one or two small nucleoli. When mesothelial cells are scraped from the abdominal cavity, they appear as a tightly cohensive flat sheet composed of one layer of polygonal cells

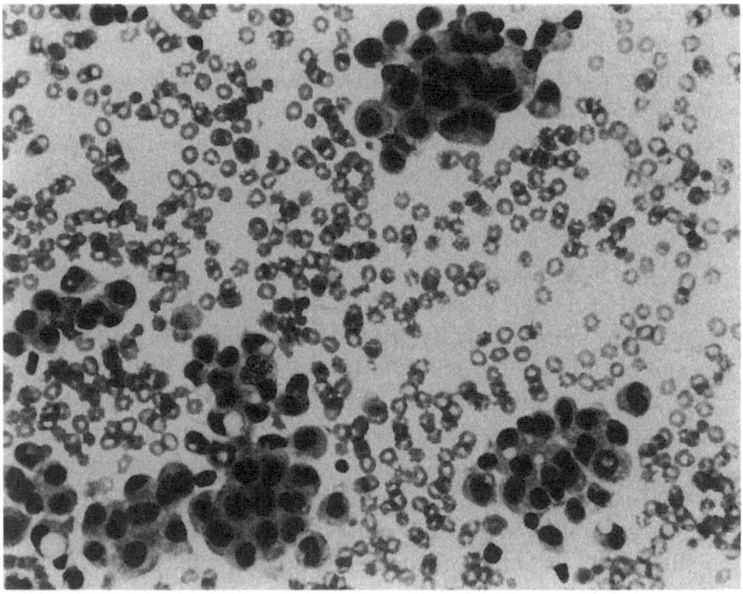

**Fig. 15.** Peritoneal washing. Aggregates of reactive mesothelial cells. Diff-Quick, × 40

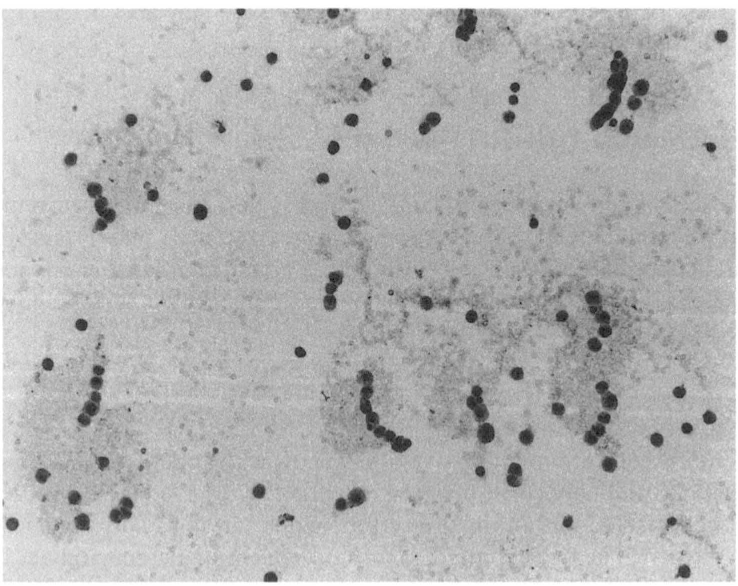

**Fig. 16.** Mesothelial cells arranged in rows. They resemble the "Indian file" arrangement seen in metastatic breast carcinoma. × 20

with delicate, yet sharply demarcated, cytoplasm. Degenerative changes, such as cytoplasmic vacuolation, karyopyknosis, and karyorrhexis can be seen. Some investigators believe that mesothelial cells are capable of multiplying while free-floating in effusions (Koss 1979b) and mitotic figures of normal configuration may be observed. Others (McGrew and Nanos 1983) believe that they are almost never seen in mitosis and 90% of the mitotic figures seen in fluid specimens are in histiocytes. Mesothelial cells show a spectrum of reactivity from small histiocytic looking cells to large cells with enlarged nuclei, coarse chromatin, and prominent nucleoli. Reactive mesothelial cells may have two or three round or oval nuclei of approximately equal size. They may form papillary or rosette-like arrangements that may mimic adenocarcinoma. They may also partially encircle one another and form groups of two to eight cells that can be mistaken for epithelial "pearls" or the "swirling around" groups of adenocarcinoma cells. In smaller clusters, the mesothelial cells often display a molding of cell surfaces. Mesothelial aggregates are usually few in number and are composed of groups of 3–12 cells (Fig. 15). They are rarely made up of a large number of cells. In addition, mesothelial cells may become fastened together in fluids, resulting in the flattening of their opposing surfaces. Since they characteristically occur in rows or "stacks" there is a resemblance to the "Indian file" arrangement of some adenocarcinoma cells (Fig. 16).

Reactive proliferation of mesothelial cells may be so marked that it could cause diagnostic problems. The nuclei, however, lack features of malignancy. The identification of such clusters as mesothelial in origin is based primarily on the uniformity of nuclear size and lack of significant variation in nuclear structure. Reactive mesothelial cells are also recognized cytologically by a peripheral band of cytoplasm that is paler or slightly different in staining quality from the main body of cytoplasm. The cytoplasm is dense and homogeneous. Groups of mesothelial cells have a scalloped border. In addition, careful examination will show a clear zone or cleft in areas where the cells touch one another that is referred to as a "window." The nature of this clear space may represent surface structures (blebs, microvilli) observed on mesothelial cells by scanning electron microscopy. Malignant aggregates are three-dimensional, i.e., made up of several superimposed cell layers which cannot be brought into a single focus (Fig. 17). Round aggregates corresponding to papillary projections or aggregates forming gland-like structures with a central lumen are particularly helpful in identifying malignant tumors.

The effect of chemotherapy and radiotherapy upon the mesothelial cells is characterized by atypical mesothelial cells with bizarre nuclei and a great variety of shapes. In many instances, the cellular atypism is so strong that it greatly reduces the morphologic differences between benign mesothelial cells and metastatic malignant cells. Radiation-induced atypia in mesothelial cells is characterized by cytoplasmic and nuclear enlargement, nuclear atypia, multinucleation, and cytoplasmic and nuclear vacuolation (Fentanes de Torres and Guevara 1981). Changes suggestive of chemotherapy effects in mesothelial cells include cellular enlargement, cytoplasmic vacuolation, nuclear pyknosis

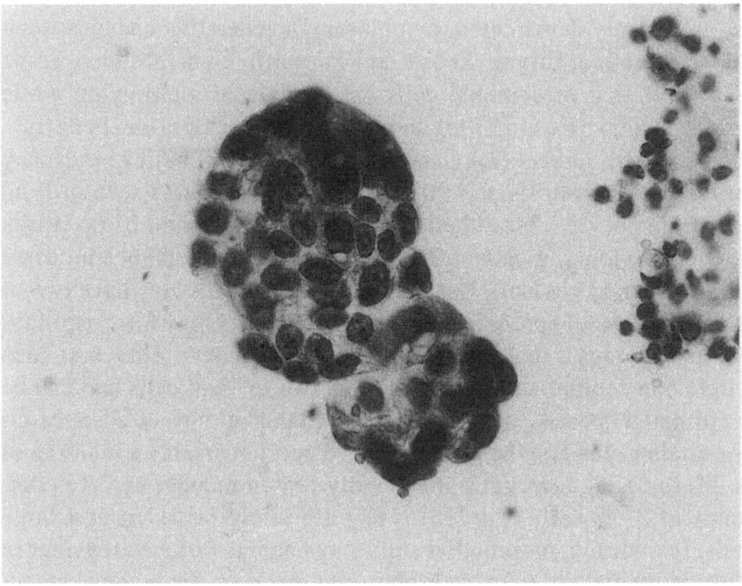

**Fig. 17.** Adenocarcinoma in peritoneal washing specimen. A three-dimensional aggregate composed of superimposed cell layers which cannot be brought into a single focus. × 40

with dense chromatin, nuclear karyorrhexis, and bizarre nuclei with clumped chromatin, and a shrunken membrane. The principal differences between radiation changes and chemotherapy changes are often of such fine degree that no sharp lines can be drawn between them, except perhaps that the nuclei suffer more evidence of cell injury during radiation therapy than during chemotherapy, which primarily affects the cytoplasm (VON HAAM 1990).

### *2.2.2 Histiocytes*

The differentiation between histiocytes and mesothelial cells cannot always be accomplished by light microscopy. The histiocytes usually occur singly or in loosely arranged clusters; they do not have a distinct cytoplasmic membrane and do not show cytoplasmic molding. The nuclei are usually peripheral and may be kidney shaped. The cell may have two to ten nuclei. The cytoplasm stains variously, depending on its phagocytic activity. It is often foamy and contains small, multiple vacuoles. It may also contain a large vacuole and produce a "signet-ring" cell. Hemosiderin-laden histiocytes, when present, indicate intra-abdominal bleeding.

### 2.2.3 *Detached Ciliary Tufts*

Detached ciliary tufts are small fragments of anucleated cytoplasm with a variable number of attached cilia (Fig. 18). They were first reported in nasal secretions of patients with the common cold (HILDING 1930). In 1956, PAPANICOLAOU described the presence of small ciliated tufts in sputum specimens as a manifestation of an overall degenerative process of ciliated respiratory epithelium. He designated this phenomenon "ciliocytophthoria," from the Greek "*phthora,*" meaning destruction. The term "ciliocytophthoria" refers indiscriminately to both ciliated anucleated fragments of cytoplasm and nonciliated fragments containing degenerating nuclei. There are several reported cases of detached ciliary tufts in female peritoneal fluids (pouch of Douglas and peritoneal dialysis fluids). Detached ciliary tufts differ from the respiratory tract "ciliocytophthoria" phenomenon, which occurs generally in response to viral infection, in that they are not accompanied by degenerating nuclear fragments and never show cytoplasmic inclusions (HOLLANDER and GUPTA 1979). In wet preparations, detached ciliary tufts are motile, demonstrate rhythmic, pulsating movement, and may be mistaken for parasites. Several authors (GAUDEFROY and COLICHE 1971; JABAMONI et al. 1977; ROXBY et al. 1986) made this error and described a nonexistent "ciliated parasite." Detached ciliary tufts occur frequently in peritoneal washings from women in the reproductive age group. They most likely represent a physiologic process of cyclic shedding of cilia from the

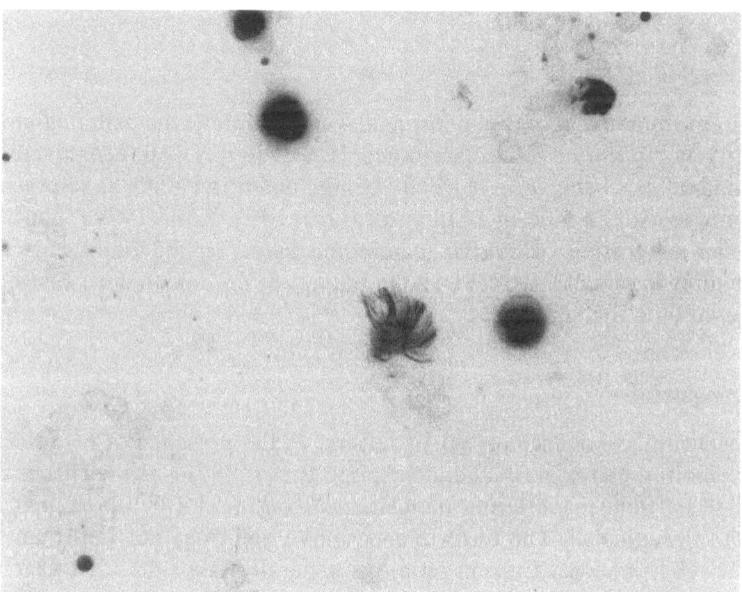

**Fig. 18.** Detached ciliary tuft in peritoneal washing specimen. × 100

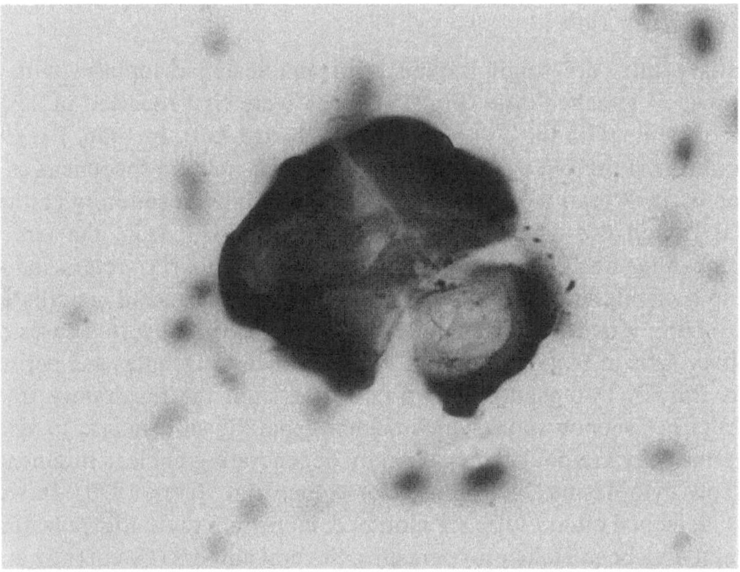

**Fig. 19.** Psammoma body in the peritoneal washing of a patient with endosalpingiosis of the ovaries. × 100

cells of the fallopian tubes during the luteal phase of the menstrual cycle (SIDAWY et al. 1987).

### *2.2.4 Psammoma Bodies*

The presence of psammoma bodies in peritoneal washings alerts the pathologist to the possibility of papillary ovarian carcinoma. However, it is well recognized that psammoma bodies can occur in perfectly benign conditions such as salpingitis, endosalpingiosis, and tubo-ovarian abscess (Fig. 19). Koss (1979b) cautions against the suggestion of ovarian carcinoma based on the findings of pasammoma bodies in material aspirated from the cul-de-sac, since most cases are not associated with malignancy.

### *2.2.5 Endosalpingiosis*

Endosalpingiosis (müllerian inclusions) is defined as the presence of ectopic epithelium resembling that of normal endosalpinx. RIES (1987) was the first to recognize pelvic peritoneal müllerian inclusions. SAMPSON (1930) introduced the term "endosalpingiosis." The term is descriptive and does not imply an origin from the tubal mucosa. Current opinions generally favor the view that endosalpingiosis derives from metaplastic proliferation of mesothelial cells or coelomic epithelium (BURMEISTER et al. 1969; TUTSCHKA and LAUCHLAN 1980).

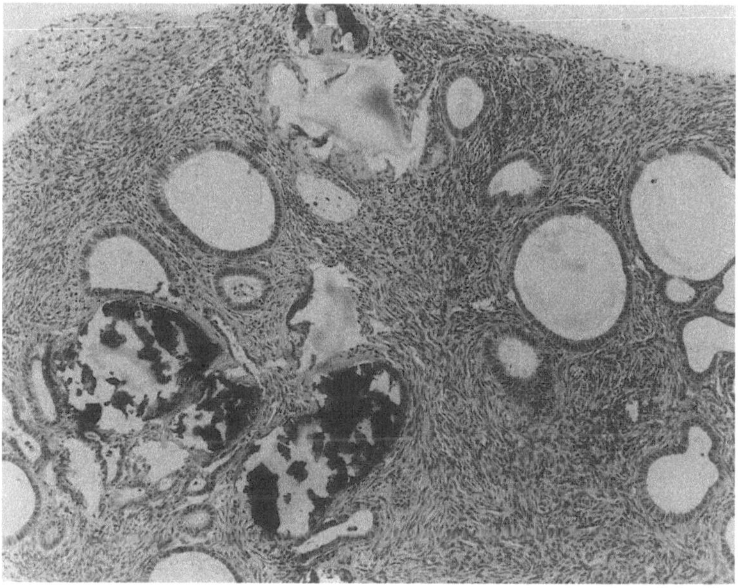

**Fig. 20.** Section of ovary showing endosalpingiosis. Multiple psammoma bodies are present. H&E, × 10

Endosalpingiosis is commonly seen on the ovaries, uterine serosa, omentum, and pelvic lymph nodes (Fig. 20). It is often an incidental finding observed in association with inflammatory tubal disease and ovarian tumors. ZINSSER and WHEELER (1982) reported a 12.5% incidence of endosalpingiosis in surgically removed omenta from female patients. Endosalpingiosis was present in 42.1% of patients with tubal disease and in only 6.4% of patients with ovarian carcinoma. Unlike endometriosis, endoslapingiosis is usually asymptomatic because it does not undergo monthly disintegration. Its significance lies in its confusion with metastatic carcinoma, especially when it presents as extensive ovarian and omental lesions. Although this entity is well described histologically, the cytologic counterpart is not as readily recognized and it represents a source of false-positive diagnoses in peritoneal washings, especially in patients with known ovarian carcinoma. KERN (1969) was the first to report the presence of papillary structures and psammoma bodies in culdocentesis fluid from a patient with psammoma body-associated papillary proliferation of the ovary. More recently, SNEIGE et al. (1986) and SIDAWY and SILVERBERG (1987) described the cytologic appearance of endosalpingiosis identified in peritoneal washings. In several of their cases, these inclusions were initially mistaken for adenocarcinoma.

Cytologically, the peritoneal washings reveal several epithelial clusters and papillary fragments, often with central psammoma bodies (Fig. 21). In addition, psammoma bodies without any association with epithelial or mesothelial cells

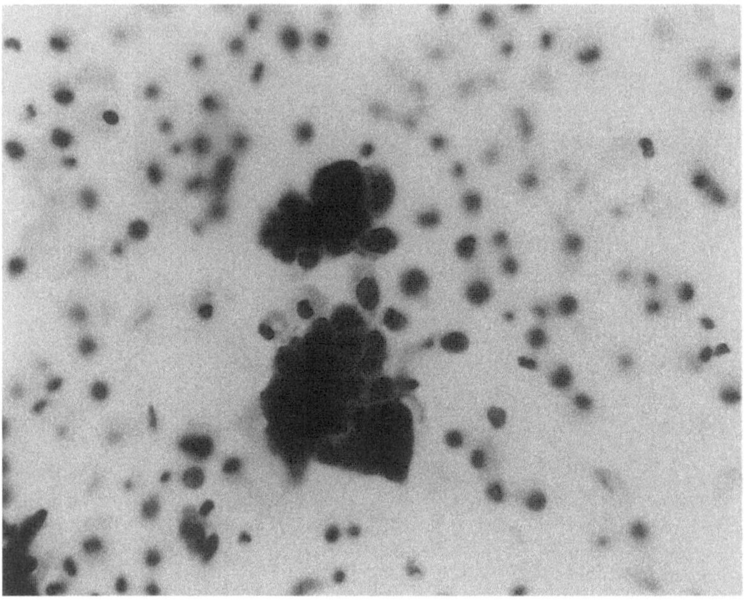

**Fig. 21.** Endosalpingiosis in peritoneal washing. Clusters of epithelial cells with central psammoma bodies. × 40

are also seen. The epithelial cells are arranged in tight clusters composed of one or a few layes. The nuclei are slightly pleomorphic and they display fine, evenly distributed chromatin. Nucleoli, when present, are small. The cytoplasm of the epithelial cells is less abundant than that of the surrounding mesothelial cells. When the epithelial clusters are sparse, they can conceivably go unnoticed and be misinterpreted as groups of mesothelial cells; however, when conspicuous they can be misinterpreted as suspicious or diagnostic of carcinoma, especially ovarian serous tumor of low malignant potential. Endosalpingiosis may be distinguished from low-grade ovarian carcinoma by the tight clustering of the epithelial cells, the absence of single neoplastic cells, and the lack of or minimal cellular plemorphism. In ovarian carcinoma, including tumors of borderline malignancy, the cytoplasm of the neoplastic cells is vacuolated and the nuclei are irregular and exhibit coarse chromatin and prominent nucleoli. Therefore, the presence of papillary fragments with psammoma bodies should not be regarded as diagnostic evidence of disseminated carcinoma, even in a patient with ovarian carcinoma. A diagnosis of malignancy can be based only on accepted cytologic criteria of malignancy of the individual cells.

## 2.3 Cytology of Positive Peritoneal Washings

The rate of positive peritoneal washing cytology increases with increasing stage of disease. The ovary is the primary site most likely to have positive peritoneal cytology, followed by endometrial and cervical carcinoma. The sensitivity of peritoneal washing cytology in ovarian malignancy diminishes in second-look procedures. Positive peritoneal cytology is a poor prognostic indicator for patients with common epithelial tumors, with the exception of serous tumors of low malignant potential (VICIANA et al. 1989). Long-term follow-up has shown the excellent prognosis with ovarian tumors of low malignant potential and the indolent behavior of those with extraovarian spread (HART 1977).

Recurring problems in interpreting peritoneal washings include the differential diagnosis of the spectrum encompassed by reactive mesothelium, endosalpingiosis, serous tumor of low malignant potential, and well-differentiated serous cystadenocarcinoma. The cytologic diagnosis must be based on a combination of the quantity of material, architecture of the cell groups, nuclear atypia, and tissue correlation.

### 2.3.1 *Ovarian Tumors of Low Malignant Potential*

Tumors of low malignant potential are those that have some morphologic features of malignancy but do not show invasion of the adjacent stroma. Numerous peritoneal implants may occur on the peritoneum and on the serosal surfaces of the pelvic organs. These implants are classified as noninvasive and invasive (GERSHENSON and SILVA 1990). In histologic sections, these tumors demonstrate various degrees of architectural complexity, stratification of

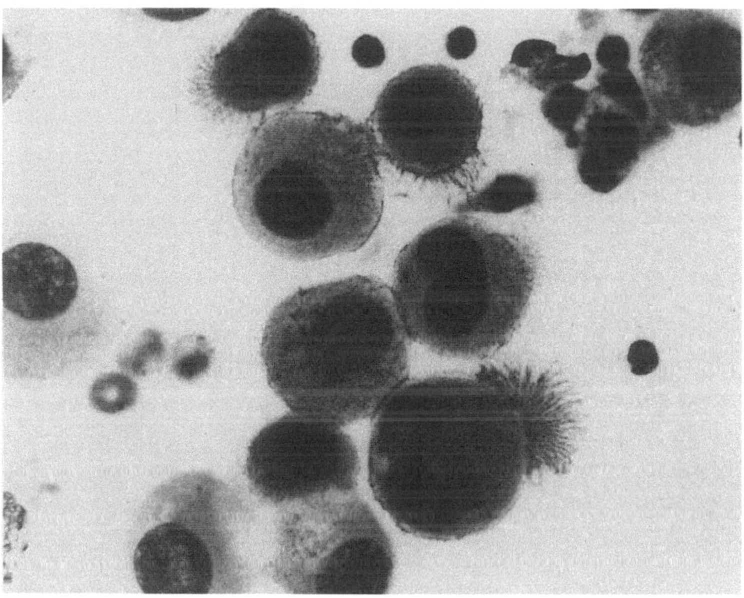

**Fig. 22.** Papillary serous tumor of low malignant potential in peritoneal washing specimen. Ciliated epithelial cells with variation in nuclear size. Diff-Quik, × 100

epithelial cells, mitotic activity, and nuclear atypia. These features are reflected in the washing cytology as clusters showing papillary groupings, branching, and cellular molding. Psammoma bodies are also found. The cytoplasm of the cells is scant and basophilic, and cell borders are usually distinct. The nuclei are usually monomorphic but may show atypia with variation in size and prominent nucleoli (Fig. 22). A cell block may be helpful in identifying papillary fragments, i.e., stromal cores outlined by stratified and occasionally ciliated serous epithelium (COVELL et al. 1985). The clusters of endosalpingiosis (müllerian inclusions), in comparison, lack the cellularity and complex arrangements of serous tumor of low malignant potential.

### *2.3.2 Papillary Serous Cystadenocarcinoma*

In washing cytology, these tumors usually show some cells with obvious malignant features allowing a definite diagnosis. The cell groups are papillary or syncytial and the cell borders are indistinct (Fig. 23). The nuclei are pleomorphic, variable in size and shape, and show crowding and overlapping. The cytoplasm often contains large empty vacuoles. Prominent and often bizarre nucleoli are a very characteristic parameter of all grades of ovarian carcinoma in fluids (Fig. 24). Psammoma bodies may be identified. Although

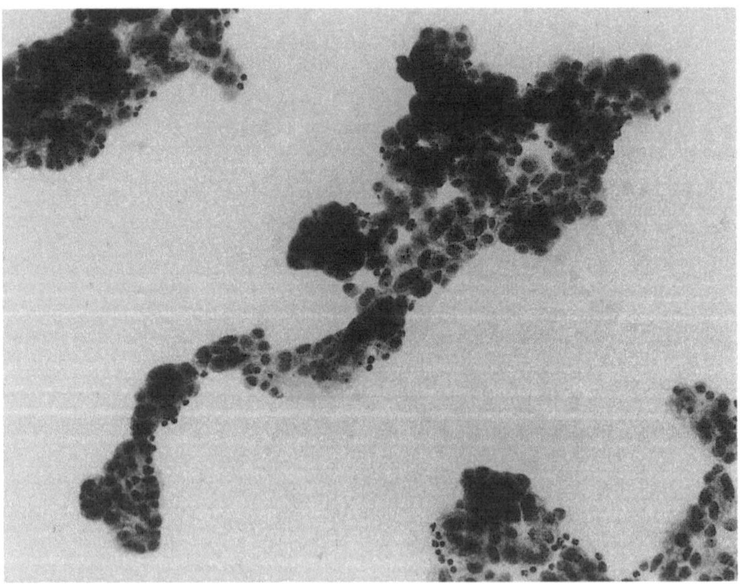

**Fig. 23.** Papillary serous cyst-adenocarcinoma in peritoneal washing specimen. Papillary groups of epithelial cells showing overlapping nuclei. × 20

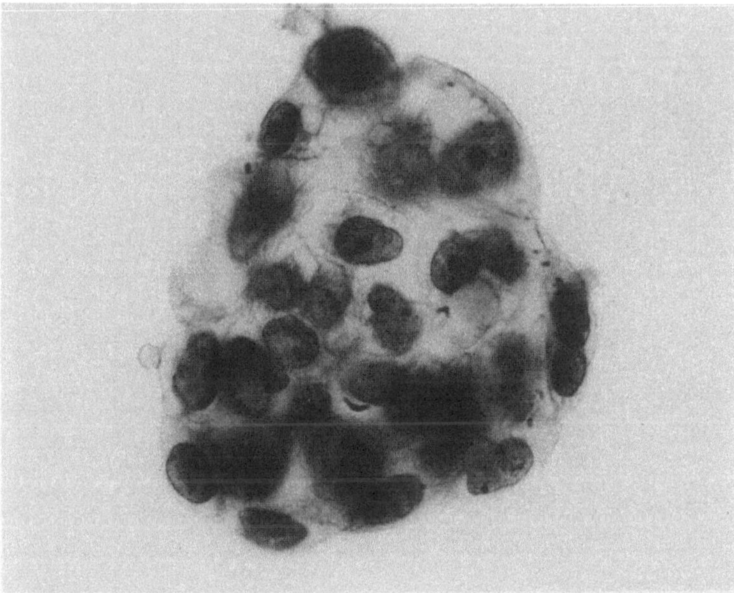

**Fig. 24.** Ovarian adenocarcinoma in peritoneal washing. A three-dimensional group of epithelial cells showing vacuolated cytoplasm and the characteristic prominent nucleoli. × 100

their presence supports the ovary as the primary tumor site, other primaries such as endometrium, breast, and intestine may be associated by psammoma bodies.

Based on cytology alone it is difficult to separate well-differentiated serous carcinomas from serous tumors of low malignant potential. Some authors (Covell et al. 1985) recommend reporting these lesions as papillary serous tumor with a comment that histologic sections are required to establish a diagnosis of frank carcinoma. If the ovarian lesion is malignant, identical cells in the washings are interpreted as malignant. If histologic sections reveal tumor of low malignant potential, matching cellular findings in the washings are reported as being consistent with a borderline tumor. Comparing and correlating the histologic with the cytologic findings is important, since the lesions in the peritoneum may differ fro those seen in the ovary, and either lesion and even more than one entity may shed cells into the cytologic sample.

### 2.3.3 *Pseudomyxoma Peritonei*

Pseudomyxoma peritonei refers to the diffuse accumulation of mucus within the peritoneal cavity secondary to benign or malignant mucinous tumors. The site of origin of the mucinous tumor is commonly the ovary or the appendix.

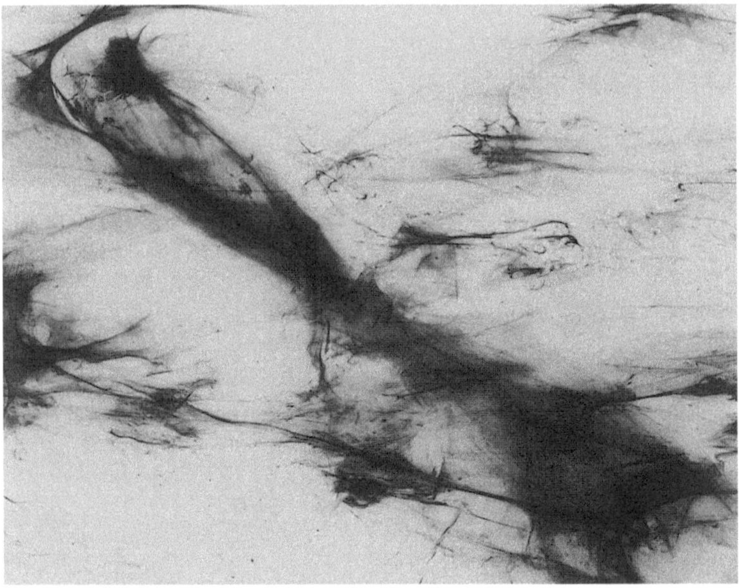

**Fig. 25.** Pseudomyxoma peritonei. Dense strands of mucin. No epithelial cells are present. Diff-Quik, × 4

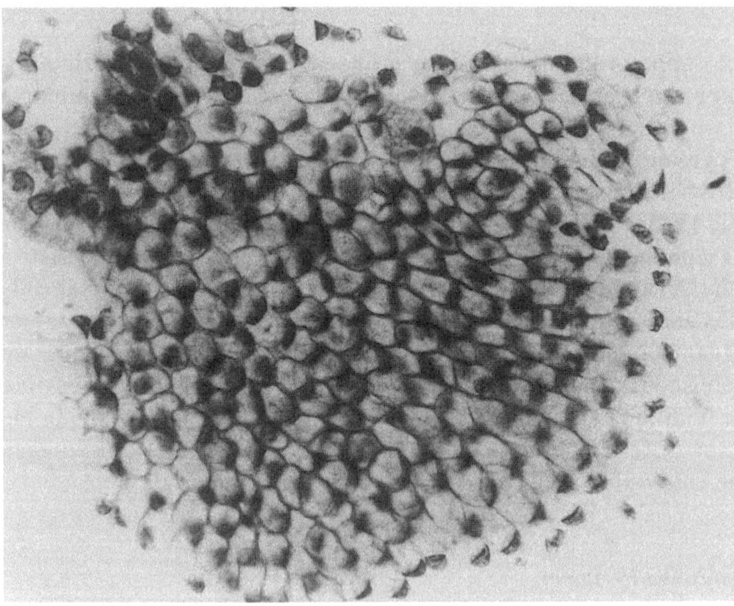

**Fig. 26.** Pseudomyxoma peritonei secondary to a ruptured mucinous cystadenoma of the ovary. A benign group of mucinous epithelial cells is arranged in a honeycomb pattern. The nuclei are small, basally located, and lack atypia. × 100

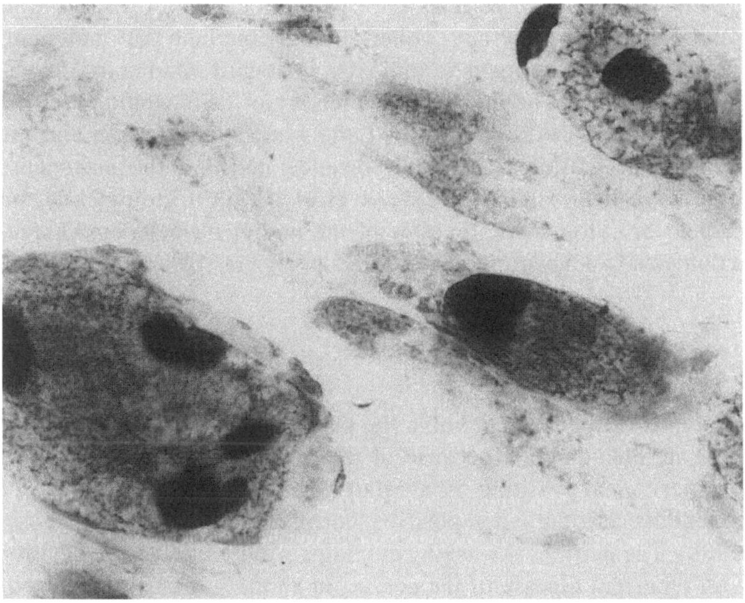

**Fig. 27.** Pseudomyxoma peritonei secondary to a mucinous adenocarcinoma. Signet-ring cells arranged singly and in clusters with vacuolated cytoplasm and hyperchromatic nuclei. × 100

Mucinous tumors arising concomitantly in both ovaries and appendix may also occur. Cytologically, pseudomyxoma peritonei is manifested by the presence of abundant mucin forming dense strands in the background of the smears (Fig. 25). Epithelial cells may or may not be present (Figs. 26, 27).

### *2.3.4 Mucinous Cystadenocarcinoma*

In peritoneal washing cytology, mucinous carcinoma of the ovary is characterized by cellular clusters showing large, clear, cytoplasmic vacuoles and irregular arrangement of nuclei. The nuclei are variable in size and shape and show prominent nucleoli.

### *2.3.5 Endometrial Carcinoma*

Endometrial carcinoma patients with malignant cells in the peritoneal cytologic specimens are at risk of increased recurrence rates and have significantly lower survival rates. However, studies often include patients with all stages of endometrial cancer (Creasman and Rutledge 1971). The prognostic significance of positive peritoneal cytology in stage I endometrial carcinoma patients is unclear. Szpak et al. (1981) suggest that the concentration of malignant cells in the peritoneal washing can be used to determine the risk of recurrence in any given patient, and that the presence of abundant malignant cells has prognostic importance in identifying those patients with pathologic stage I disease who may require more aggressive therapy. Other authors conclude that malignant peritoneal cytology is not a prognostic indicator in stage I endometrial carcinoma (YAZIGI et al. 1983). The manner in which tumor cells would enter the peritoneal cavity in these cases is unclear. Early lymphatic invasion and the concept of transtubal migration of endometrial cancer cells into the peritoneum in early disease have been suggested (SZPAK et al. 1981). Cytologically, no distinctive nuclear or cytoplasmic features of the malignant cells are characteristic for endometrial adenocarcinoma in fluid specimens (SPIELER and GLOOR 1985).

#### 2.3.6 *Cervial Carcinoma*

Cervical carcinomas infrequently involve the peritoneal cavity. Peritoneal involvement is a late phenomenon because of the retroperitoneal nature of the disease. Thus, peritoneal washing is a relatively insensitive technique for detecting cervical disease, but when positive, correlates with a poor prognosis (ZUNA et al. 1988). The peritoneal washing cytology is more likely to be positive in patients with recurrent disease of the cervix. In addition, cases with adenocarcinoma have been reported as being four times more likely to have malignant peritoneal washing cytology than those with squamous carcinoma (ABU-GHAZALEH et al. 1984; IMACHI et al. 1987)

### 2.4 Adjunct Studies

The sensitivity of the cytologic diagnosis of malignancy in serous fluid does not exceed 75% even upon repeated sampling. Adjunct studies may help in the further characterization of atypical cells in effusions. They may be helpful in distinguishing between "reactive" mesothelial cells and malignant cells, and may also highlight occult carcinoma cells in cases in which standard cytologic criteria for malignancy are not present. Cytochemical methods, such as the mucin staining of adenocarcinoma, are only helpful when positive. Cell block preparation in addition to conventional smears may be used to distinguish benign from malignant cells. Such material is processed in a fashion similar to conventional histologic specimens, and can be used for cytochemical and immunologic evaluation.

#### 2.4.1 *Immunocytochemistry*

Recent immunologic methods, employing monoclonal antibodies raised against tumors or cell constituents, have proven to be useful; however, such markers are not always specific and sensitive. Many attempts have been made to establish reliable and reproducible markers; however, no studies have shown universally consistent results.

B72.3 is a monoclonal antibody (MAB) generated against a membrane-enriched fraction of breast carcinoma. This antibody reacts with a high-molecular-weight, glycoprotein, tumor-associated antigen, designated TAG-72, in formalin-fixed, paraffin-embedded tissue sections of adenocarcinomas of the ovary, lung, colon, and breast. Studies have shown that MAb B72.3 demonstrates no reactivity to mesothelial cells or to other cell types in benign, leukemic, or lymphomatous effusions. MAb B72.3 may be useful as an immunocytochemical adjunct for the diagnosis of carcinoma (Masood 1989) in cytologic preparations of human serous effusions, because of its selective reactivity for tumor cells (particularly adenocarcinoma of the breast, lung, and ovary) over reactive mesothelium. Zuna et al. (1989a) demonstrated also the utility of monoclonal antibody B72.3 in peritoneal washing cytology in the categorization of difficult cases.

### 2.4.2 *Flow Cytometric Analysis*

Quantitative DNA measurement holds promise as a more objective method of diagnosis. However, attempts to improve the sensitivity using flow cytometric analysis of the DNA content alone upon fluids have been almost uniformly unsuccessful; in most cases the tumor cells are greatly outnumbered by reactive mesothelial cells and inflammatory cells, yielding data more representative of the reactive components than of the rare tumor cells. Single-parameter flow cytometric DNA analysis, though helpful in selected cases, is not sufficiently accurate in peritoneal washings in gynecological patients (Crosby et al. 1988). Recent data yielded by the multiparameter flow cytometric analysis approach utilizing dual staining demonstrate that dual labeling with keratin (or other specific monoclonal antibodies) in concert with other biologic parameters can expand the potential of flow cytometry in the analysis of effusions and can be used to increase the sensitivity of the cytologic analysis of body fluids (Kelsten and Chianese 1988).

## 3 Cytology of Nonneoplastic Cysts of the Ovary

An understanding of the cytologic features of nonneoplastic ovarian cysts may encourage aspiration as opposed to surgical removal, particularly in women of childbearing age. Follicular cysts show clusters of granulosa cells, some containing mitotic figures. Luteinized follicular cysts show granulosa cells admixed with luteinized cells. Hemorrhagic corpora lutea are characterized by fresh blood, hemosiderin-laden macrophages and luteinized cells. Hemorrhagic corpus luteal cysts show the presence of luteinized cells, fibroblasts, hemosiderin-laden macrophages, fresh blood, and abundant fibrin. Endometriotic cysts

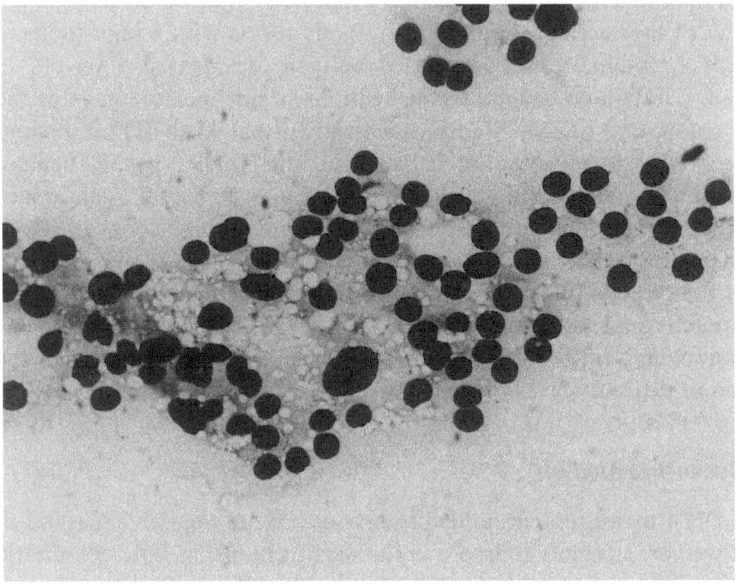

**Fig. 28.** Intraoperative smear of corpus luteum. Cluster of luteinized cells with vacuolated cytoplasm and variability in nuclear size. Diff-Quick, × 40

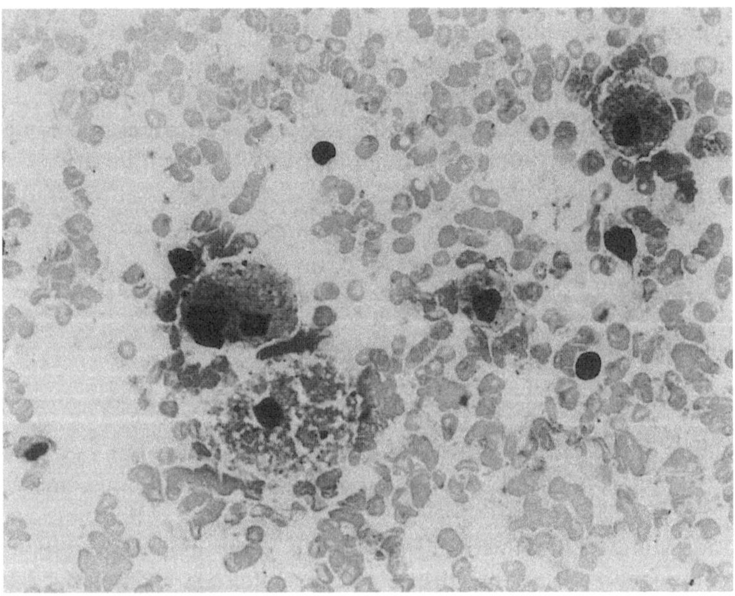

**Fig. 29.** Intraoperative smear of hemorrhagic endometriotic cyst shows red blood cells and several hemosiderin-laden macrophages. No endometrial cells are present. Diff-Quick, × 40

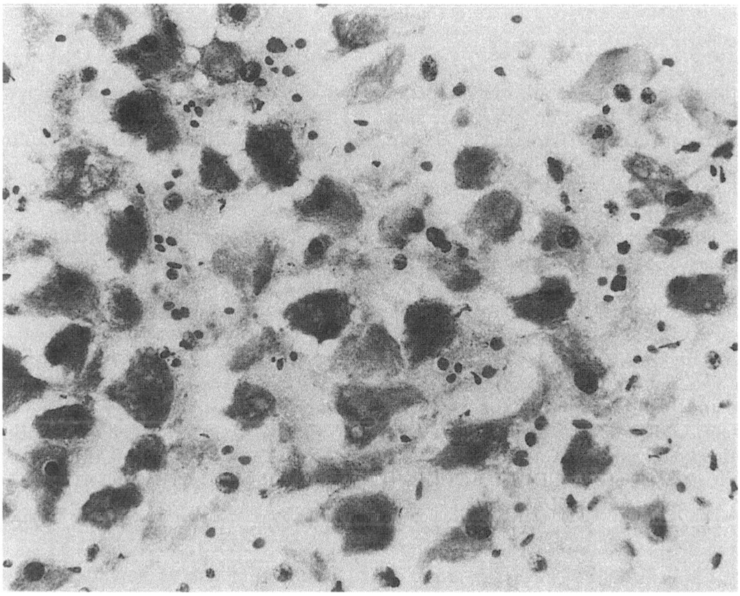

**Fig. 30.** Intraoperative smear of mature cystic teratoma shows anucleated and nucleated squamous cells. × 20

shows fresh blood, hemosiderin-laden macrophages, and scattered endometrial cells (SELVAGGI 1988).

Pathologists can achieve competence in interpreting cytologic material of various ovarian cysts by using the technique of intraoperative cytology as an adjunct to gross examination and frozen sections during intraoperative consultations (Figs. 28–30) (ABRAMS and SILVERBERG 1989).

## 4 Classification of Ovarian Cyst Fluid: Adjunct Studies

Measurements of CA-125, carcinoembryonic antigen, and α-fetoprotein in ovarian cyst fluid are recommended by some as a diagnostic adjunct to cytology for the classification of ovarian cysts (PINTO et al. 1988). Measuring the levels of the three antigens can be useful when fluid is obtained through laparoscopic puncture of ovarian cysts and tissue is unavailable for classification. All three antigens are very low in follicular/lutein cysts. Markedly elevated CA-125 and low carcinoembryonic antigen and α-fetoprotein levels are seen in serous neoplasms, both benign and malignant. Elevated carcinoembryonic antigen and CA-125 are seen in mucinous ovarian neoplasms (benign and malignant). Metastatic colonic carcinoma has elevated carcinoembryonic antigen and a normal CA-125. Malignant teratoma has elevated α-fetoprotein.

## References

Abrams J, Silverberg SG (1989) The role of intraoperative cytology in the evaluation of gynecologic disease. Pathol Annu 24:167–187

Abu-Ghazaleh S, Johnston WJ, Creasman ST (1984) The significance of peritoneal cytology in patients with carcinoma of the cervix. Gynecol Oncol 17:139–148

Allingham JD, King A (1985) Patient characteristics and endocervical cell recovery on Papanicolaou smears. J Fam Pract 20:185–190

Ayer B, Pacey F, Greenberg M, Bousfield L (1987) The cytologic diagnosis of adenocarcinoma in situ of cervix uteri and related lesions: I. Adenocarcinoma in situ. Acta Cytol 31:397–411

Ayer B, Pacey F, Greenberg M (1988) The cytologic diagnosis of adenocarcinoma in situ of the cervix and related lesions: II. Microinvasive adenocarcinoma. Acta Cytol 32:318–324

Barter RA, Waters ED (1970) Cyto and histomorphology of cervical adenocarcinoma in situ. Pathology 2:33–40

Boon ME, Baak JPA, Kurver PJH, Overdiep SH, Verdonk GW (1981) Adenocarcinoma in situ of the cervix: an underdiagnosed lesion. Cancer 48:768–773

Boon ME, deGraaff Guilloud JC, Rietveld WJ (1989) Analysis of five sampling methods for the preparation of cervical smears. Acta Cytol 33:843–848

Bosch BD, Davidson DD, Lanfeld CD, Fife KH (1989) Human papillomavirus features in cervical Papanicolaou smears. Acta Cytol 33:696–697

Burmeister RE, Fechner RE, Franklin RR (1969) Endosalpingiosis of the peritoneum. Obstet Gynecol 34:310–318

Covell JL, Corry TB, Feldman PS (1985) Peritoneal washings in ovarian tumors. Potential sources of error in cytologic diagnosis. Acta Cytol 29:310–316

Creasman WT, Rutledge F (1971) The prognostic value of peritoneal cytology in gynecologic malignant disease. Am J Obstet Gynecol 110:773–781

Crosby JH, Allsbrook WC Jr, Pantazis CG et al. (1988) Cytology and flow cytometric DNA evaluation of peritoneal washings in gynecologic patients. Acta Cytol 33:746

Crum C, Fu Y-S, Kurman RJ, Okagaki T, Twiggs LB, Silberberg SG (1989) Editorial board symposium. Practical approach to cervical human papillomavirus-related intraepithelial lesions. Int J Gynecol Pathol 8:388–399

Detweilder RE, Castilleja RM, Sneige N (1989) Endocervical columnar cells and adequacy of cervical samples: analysis of 43 discordant smears and cervical biopsies.Acta Cytol 33:730–731

Dorman AS, Danos LM, Caron BL et al. (1985) Detection of *Chalmydia trachomatis* in Papanicolaou stained smears by an indirect immunoperoxidase method. Acta Cytol 29:665–670

Duggan MA, Chang-Poon V, Gabos RS et al. (1988) Human papillomavirus DNA determination in cervical smears using dot-blot hybridization and biotinylated with cDNA probes. Acta Cytol 32:757

Fentanes de Torres E, Guevara EC (1981) Pleuritis by radiation. Acta Cytol 25:427–429

Friedell GH, McKay DG (1953) Adenocarcinoma in situ of the endocervix. Cancer 6:887–897

Gaudefroy M, Coliche D (1971) Deux cas de vaginite due a unparasite encore inconnu en pathologie gynecologique. J Sci Med Lille 89:301–302

Gershenson DM, Silver EG (1990) Serous ovarian tumors of low malignant potential with peritoneal implants. Cancer 65:578–585

Gondos B, Marshall D, Ostergad DR (1972) Endocervical cells in cervial smears. Am J Obstet Gynecol 114:833–834

Gupta PK, Lee EF, Erozan YS et al. (1979) Cytologic investigations in *Chlamydia* infection. Acta Cytol 23:315–329

Hart WR (1977) Ovarian epithelial tumors of borderline malignancy (carcinoma of low malignant potential). Hum Pathol 8:541–549

Henry MR, deMesy Jensen KL, Skoglund CD (1989) *Chlamydia trachomatis* in routine cervical smears: a microscopic and ultrastructural analysis. Acta Cytol 33:695

Hilding AC (1930) The common cold. Arch Otolaryngol 12:133–150

Hoffken H, Soost HJ (1981) Cervical cytology as a screening method. In: Dallenbach-Hellweg G (ed) Cervical cancer. Springer, Berlin Heidelberg New York (Current topics in pathology, vol. 70, pp 21–65)

Hollander DH, Gupta PK (1979) DCT, CCP and pseudoprotozoa. Acta Cytol 23:258–259

Imachi M, Tsukamoto N, Matsuyama T, Nakano H (1987) Peritoneal cytology in patients with carcinoma of the uterine cervix. Gynecol Oncol 26:202–207

Jabamoni R, Dodson MC, Blecka LJ, Jaskoski B, O'Leary J (1977) Unusual protozoal infestation of the cervical mucus. Obstet Gynecol 50:224–227

Jenson AB (1989) Historical perspectives and current perception of human papillomavirus infections. Focus on Human Papillomavirus 1:1–3

Katz RL, Ferre F, Sneige N et al. (1989) Comparison of the sensitivity of cytomorphology, slot-blot hybridization and polymerase chain reaction for the detection of human papillomavirus in cervical brushings. Acta Cytol 33:696

Kelsten ML, Chianese D (1988) Multiparamater flow cytometric analysis in the detection of malignant effusions. Acta Cytol 32:773

Kern WH (1969) Benign papillary structures with psammoma bodies in culdocentesis fluid. Acta Cytol 13:178–180

Killough BW, Clark AH, Garvin JB (1988) Correlation between cytodiagnosis and the presence of endocervical or squamous metaplastic cells in gynecologic smears. Acta Cytol 32:758

Kirk RS, Boon ME (1981) A comparison of the efficiency of diagnosis of early cervical carcinoma by general practitioners and cytology screening programs in the Netherlands. Acta Cytol 25:259–262

Kivlahan C, Ingram E (1986) Papanicolaou smears without endocervical cells: Are they adequate? Acta Cytol 30:258–260

Koss LG (1979a) Diagnostic cytology and its histopathologic bases, 3rd edn. Lippincott, Philadelphia.

Koss LG (1979b) Effusions in the absence of cancer. In: Koss LG (ed) Diagnostic cytology and its histopathologic bases, 3rd edn. Lippincott, Philadelphia, pp 229–230

Kristensen GB, Holund B, Grinsted P (1989) Efficacy of the Cytobrush versus the cotton swab in the collection of endocervical cells. Acta Cytol 33:849–851

Krumins I, Young Q, Pacey F, Boustfield L, Mulhearn L (1977) The cytologic diagnosis of adenocarcinoma in situ of the cervix. Acta Cytol 21:320–329

Lai-Goldman M, Nieberg RK, Wiesmeier E (1988) The Cytobrush (Zelsmyr) technique in the preparation of routine cervical-vaginal-endocervical smears. Acta Cytol 32:746

Lee KR (1988) False-positive diagnosis of adenocarcinoma in situ of the cervix. Acta Cytol 32:276–277

Lee KR, Manna E, Jones MA (1989) Comparative cytologic features of adenocarcinoma in situ of the cervix. Acta Cytol 33:697

Lindner LE, Geerling S, Nettum JA, Miller SL, Altman KH (1985) The cytologic features of chlamydial cervicitis. Acta Cytol 29:676–682

Masood S (1989) Use of monoclonal antibody B72.3 as an adjunct in the diagnosis of adenocarcinoma in malignant effusions. Acta Cytol 33:724–725

McGowan L (1989) Peritoneal fluid washings. Acta Cytol 33:414–415

McGrew EA, Nanos S (1983) The cytology of serous effusions. In: Keebler CM, Reagan JW (eds) A manual of cytotechnology, 6th edn. American Society of Clinical Pathologists, Chicago, pp 229–230

Mesonero CE, Garrett CT, Silverberg SG et al. (1991) Human papilloma virus in uterine cervix: A comparison of detection of HPV by morphology and dot blot hybridization. Int J Gynecol Pathol (in press)

Naib ZM (1970) Cytology of TRIC agent infection of the eye of newborn infants and their mother's genital tracts. Acta Cytol 14:390–395

Pacey F, Ayer B, Greenberg M (1988) The cytologic diagnosis of adenocarcinoma in situ of the cervix uteri and related lesions. III. Pitfalls in diagnosis. Acta Cytol 32:325–330

Papanicolaou GN (1956) Degenerative changes in ciliated cells exfoliating from the bronchial epithelium as a cytologic criterion in the diagnosis of diseases of the lung. NY State J Med 56:2647–2650

Papanicolaou GN, Traut HF (1943) Diagnosis of uterine cancer by the vaginal smear. Common Wealth Fund, New York

Pinto MM, Bernstein LH, Brogan DA (1988) Measurement of CA-125, carcinoembryonic antigen and alphafetoprotein in ovarian cyst fluids: diagnostic adjunct to cytology. Acts Cytol 32:747

Ravinsky E (1986) Cytology of peritoneal washings in gynecologic patients. Diagnostic criteria and pitfalls. Acta Cytol 30:8–16

Ries E (1897) Eine neue Operationsmethode des Uteruscarcinomas. Z Geburtshilfe Gynaekol 37:518–532

Rizzo T, Linker G, Schumann GB (1989) Cytologic pitfalls associated with microglandular endocervical hyperplasia. Acta Cytol 33:738
Roxby CM, Wood M, Martin AM, McHugh M (1986) Ciliated organisms seen in fluid following dialysis. Lancet I:916
Sampson JA (1930) Postsalpingectomy endometriosis (endosalpingiosis). Am J Obstet Gynecol 20:443–480
Selvaggi S (1988) Cytology of nonneoplastic cysts of the ovary. Acta Cytol 32:756
Selvaggi SM, Malviya V, Deppe G, Malone J Jr, Christensen C (1989) Efficacy of the modified Ayre spatula/Zelsmyr Cytobrush versus the modified Ayre spatula/bulb aspirator in the collection of cells from the uterine cervix. Acta Cytol 33:697–698
Shiina Y (1985) Cytomorphologic and immunocytochemical studies of chlamydial infections in cervical smears. Acta Cytol 29:683–691
Sidawy MK, Silverberg SG (1987) Endosalpingiosis in female peritoneal washings: a diagnostic pitfall. Int J Gynecol Pathol 6:340–346
Sidawy MK, Chandra P, Oertel YC (1987) Detached ciliary tufts in female peritoneal washings. A common finding. Acta Cytol 31:841–844
Sneige N, Fernandez T, Copeland LJ, Katz RL (1986) Müllerian inclusions in peritoneal washings: potential source of error in cytologic diagnosis. Acta Cytol 30:271–276
Spieler P, Gloor F (1985) Identification of types and primary sites of malignant tumors by examination of exfoliated tumor cells in serous fluid. Comparison with the diagnostic accuracy on small histologic biopsies. Acta Cytol 29:753–767
Szpak CA, Creasman WT, Vollmer RT, Johnston WW (1981) Prognostic value of cytologic examination of peritoneal washings in patients with endometrial carcinoma. Acta Cytol 25:640–646
Taylor PT Jr, Anderson WA, Barber SR et al. (1987) The screening Papanicolaou smear: contribution of the endocervical brush. Obstet Gynecol 70:734–738
The 1988 Bethesda system for reporting cervical/vaginal cytologic diagnoses. Developed and approved at the National Cancer Institute Workshop, Bethesda, Maryland, USA, 12-13 December 1988 (1989) Acta Cytol 33:567–574
Tutschka BG, Lauchlan SC (1980) Endosalpingiosis. Obstet Gynecol [Suppl] 55:57S–60S
Viciana AL, Mann WJ, Zuna RE (1989) Peritoneal washing cytology in ovarian malignancy: analysis of 211 cases. Acta Cytol 33:698
von Haam E (1990) Radiation cell changes. In: Weid GL, Keebler CM, Koss LG, Reagan JW (eds) Compendium on diagnostic cytology. Tutorials of cytology, Chicago, Ill, pp 239–253
Ward BE, Burkett B, Peterson C, Franquemont DW, Crum CP (1989) Cytological correlates of cervical papillomavirus infection. Mod Pathol 2:103A
Yazigi R, Piver MS, Blumenson L (1983) Malignant peritoneal cytology as prognostic indicator in stage I endometrial cancer. Obstet Gynecol 62:359-362
Zinsser KR, Wheeler JE (1982) Endosalpingiosis in the omentum: a study of autopsy and surgical material. Am J Surg Pathol 6:109–117
Ziselman EM, Harkavy SE, Hogan M, West W, Atkinson B (1984) Peritoneal washing cytology; uses and diagnostic criteria in gynecologic neoplasms. Acta Cytol 28:105–110
Zuna RE, Hansen K, Mann W (1988) Peritoneal washing cytology in cervical carcinoma: analysis of 108 patients. Acta Cytol 32:758–759
Zuna RE, Heimann A, Glantz L, Healy S (1989a) Utility of monoclonal antibody B72.3 in peritoneal washing cytology. Acta Cytol 33:727–728
Zuna RE, Mitchell ML, Mullick KA, Weijchert WM (1989b) Cytohistologic correlation of peritoneal washing cytology in gynecologic disease. Acta Cytol 33:327–336

# Impact of Human Papillomavirus Research on the Histopathologic Concepts of Genital Neoplasms

T. Okagaki



## 1 Introduction

Carcinoma of the uterine cervix is known to be closely associated with sexual promiscuity, age at first sexual experience, and multiple pregnancies (Stern et al. 1967; Kessler 1981). Based on the observed absence of cervical cancer among nuns, relationship between sexual intercourse and cervical cancer was suggested by the pioneering report of Rigoni-Stern in 1984. Since the nineteenth century many etiologic agents, mainly sexually transmitted diseases, have been proposed as causes or uterine cancer. Among them have been syphilis (Røjel 1953; Moghissi et al. 1968), gonorrhea (Sebastian et al. 1978; Furgyik and Astedt 1980), *Trichomonas vaginalis* (Bechtold and Reicher 1952; Hulka and Hulka 1967), cytomegalovirus (Fletcher et al. 1986), *Chlamydia tra-*

Current Topics in Pathology
Volume 85, Ed. N. Sasano

*chomatis* (HARE et al. 1982; SCHACHTER et al. 1982), semen (SINGER et al. 1976), and, more recently, herpes simplex hominis type 2 (HSV 2) virus (RAWLS et al. 1968; NAIB et al. 1969). Considerable research efforts have been made during the last two decades to prove the relationship between HSV 2 and cervical cancer. HSV 2 infection of the cervix has shown a high association with cervical cancer (RAWLS et al. 1968; NAIB et al. 1969; NAHMIAS et al. 1974; KESSLER 1974). Further, patients with cervical cancer have been found to have a higher incidence of antibodies in their blood against HSV 2 than controls (AURELIAN et al. 1973). However, neither integration of HSV 2 genomes to the host cancer cells nor molecular mechanisms of HSV 2 enhancing transcription of oncogenes of the host cells have been proven except in a few instances, and the "herpes theory" of cervical carcinogenesis has lost it supporters.

Human papillomavirus (HPV) is now widely regarded as an important factor in cervical carcinogenesis, if not its cause. Malignant transformation of condyloma acuminatum, a known sexually transmitted disease, has frequently reported in the literature (KOVI et al. 1974; SCHMAUZ et al. 1978). As we now know, condyloma acuminatum is mainly produced by type 6 or type 11 HPV (HPV 6 and HPV 11), and its malignant transformation is infrequent. A clinically less evident variant of condyloma of the uterine cervix, "flat condyloma," which was noted by MEISELS and FORTIN (1976) and PUROLA and SAVIA (1977), produced koilocytosis of the exfoliated cells in Papanicolaou smears, a unique cytologic change initially described by KOSS and DURFEE (1956). Its histologic resemblance to mild dysplasia of the uterine cervical epithelium (CIN I) gave rise to suspicion that HPV may be a causative agent of cervical cancer (MEISELS and FORTIN 1976). Later, frequent association of flat condyloma with cervical intraepithelial neoplasia (CIN) was reported by many authors (SYRJÄNEN 1979; LUDWIG et al. 1981; BOON and FOX 1981; NYEEM et al. 1982; SCHMAUZ et al. 1983; CRUM et al. 1983a; ZUNA 1984).

The development of Southern blot hybridization and DNA cloning in the 1970s revealed that more than one type of HPV exists, the different types causing various types of wart at various sites (KRZYZEK et al. 1980; DE VILLIERS et al. 1981). This led to the finding that HPV DNA can also be present in cervical cancer (ZUR HAUSEN 1977; GREEN et al. 1982) and its precursor lesion, CIN (GISSMANN et al. 1983; LANCASTER et al. 1983; MCCANCE et al. 1983; OKAGAKI et al. 1983). Using these new methods, HPV 6 was cloned from vulvar condyloma and HPV 16 and 18 from invasive cervical cancer (DE VILLIERS et al. 1981; DÜRST et al. 1983; BOSHART et al. 1984). Up until now HPV 6, 11, 16, 18, 31, 33, 35, 42, 43, 44, 45, 51, 52, and 56 have been identified in genital lesions ranging from condyloma to invasive carcinoma. HPV 16, 18, 31, 33, 35, and perhaps 52 are the frequently found types of HPV in premalignant lesions of high grade and in invasive carcinoma of the genitalia.

It is now apparent that cervical condyloma, dysplasia, and carcinoma in situ through the development of invasive squamous cell carcinoma in female and male external genitalia constitute a continuous spectrum with regard to the involvement of HPV. HPVs were initially reported in vulvar in situ and invasive carcinoma on the basis of electron microscopy (RASTKAR et al. 1982) and immunocytochemistry (CRUM et al. 1982), and were later confirmed by molecular biologic methods (ZACHOW et al. 1982; OKAGAKI 1984; BERGERON et al. 1987; TWIGGS et al. 1988).

## 2 Biology of HPV and Possible Mechanisms of Carcinogenesis

Human warts have been known for centuries. CIUFFO in 1907 first reported that a virus might be the causative agent of verruca vulgaris. His observation was subsequently confirmed (WILE and KINGERY 1919; SERRA 1924). Viral inclusion bodies were observed in the wart cell nuclei by light microscopy (LYELL and MILES 1951) and electron microscopy (STRAUSS et al. 1949; BUNTING 1953; ALMEIDA et al. 1962; DUNN and OGILVIE 1968).

Papillomaviruses (PVs) are found widely in many mammalian and avian species. Bovine papillomavirus of cattle (BPV) and Shope's papillomavirus or cotton tail rabbit papillomavirus (CRPV) have been studied as models of viral carcinogenesis (SHOPE 1933; KIDD and ROUS 1940; ITO and EVANS 1961; LANCASTER et al. 1976; also see the review by CHOW et al. 1987). PVs are placed in the Papovaviridae family together with polyoma viruses, SV40 virus, and BK and JC viruses. However, there is some disagreement on whether PVs should be placed in a separate genus. The mature virions of PVs are typically icosahedral and measure 55 nm in diameter. Although many different species of PVs share common capsid antigens (JENSON et al. 1980), the viruses show strong host specificity and organotropism. Their characteristic host specificity, their organotropism, and the molecular relatedness of the genetic structures among the species found in closely related hosts suggest that PVs are highly evolved in parallel with the evolution of the vertebrate animals. Because of host specificity, organotropism, and growth difficulty in a tissue culture environment, the biology and genetic structures of PVs were not elucidated until the late 1970s, and the biologic life cycles of many important types of HPV have yet to be clarified. Whether some of the HPV species, e.g., HPV 18, fail to mature to a vegetative state is not known.

The DNA structure of PV is circular and double stranded, consisting of 0.5 to 1 kb pairs. The types are defined as different when less than 50% of DNAs hybridize in a liquid phase. More than 65 types of HPV have been identified to date (Papillomavirus Workshop, Heidelberg, May 1990). PV DNAs contain several open reading frames (ORFs): two late transcribing regions ($L_1$ and $L_2$), and up to eight early transcribing regions ($E_1$–$E_8$). The sequences are homologous within $L_1$, $E_1$, and $E_2$ of many types of PV (PFISTER 1987). Thus, polyclonal antibodies developed from the pooled human warts or bovine papillomas cross-react with HPVs (JENSON et al. 1980). The latter is commercially available, and has been widely used for immunocytochemical demonstration of HPV in tissues. Recently transcription proteins of $E_6$ and $E_7$ of HPV 16 and 18 have been genetically engineered, and type-specific antibodies against $E_6$ and $E_7$ transcription proteins produced (Banks et al. 1987; Barbosa and Wettstein 1987; Schneider-Gadlicke et al. 1988).

Among 13 or so HPV types found in human genital lesions, types 16 and 18 are regarded as high-risk HPVs that produce genital neoplasms. HPV 31, 33, and 35 are considered to be of intermediate risk. These risk levels were deduced from the fact that HPV 16 and 18 were almost exclusively present in invasive cervical cancer while HPV 31, 33, and 35 were present in CIN of high grade (Crum et al. 1984; Meanwell et al. 1987). Also HPV 16-containing condylomas exhibit atypical mitoses; in turn, atypical mitoses and DNA aneuploidy are correlated with a poor prognosis (Fu et al. 1981; Crum et al. 1985; Bibbo et al. 1989). Although HPV 16 and HPV 18 are considered "high-risk types" of HPV as compared to HPV 6 and HPV 11, the probability that HPV 16- and HPV 18-infected women will develop cervical cancer is rather low (1:300).

Malignant transformation is known to occur when HPV is associated with epidermodysplasia verruciformis (EV) or with generalized papillomatosis in individuals with congenital immunodefficiency (Jablonska et al. 1979; Orth et al. 1979). Malignant transformation of bovine papillomas and Shope's papilloma has been known for many years. Transforming properties of oncogenic PVs have been widely studied. HPV 5, which is found in the lesions of EV, which frequently undergoes malignant transformation, has been shown to transform tissue cultured cells (Watts et al. 1984), and $E_5$ and $E_6$–$E_7$ regions of BPV have transforming activity (Yang et al. 1985; Schlegel et al. 1986; Neary and DiMaio 1989). In contrast, HPV 11 does not transform cells in vitro (Pater et al. 1988). HPV 16 and HPV 18 DNAs also show transforming activity in respect of cells in culture (Pirisi et al. 1987; Morgan et al. 1988; Watanabe and Yoshiike 1988; Hudson et al. 1990). Transforming properties of $E_6$–$E_7$ ORF regions of these HPV types have been demonstrated (Bedell et al. 1987; Cripe et al. 1987; Noda et al. 1988). The integration of parts of HPV 16 and 18 reportedly occurs in the vicinity of c-*src*-1, c-*raf*-1, Ki-*ras*-2, Ha-*ras*, and c-*myc* proto-oncogenes of the host cells (Dürst et al. 1987; Pelling et al. 1988). Recent works have demonstrated that the protein products of $E_6$ and $E_7$ ORFs bind to the retinoblastoma inhibiting gene product, which suppresses the cell-stimulating retinoblastoma gene (Dyson et al. 1989; Werness et al. 1990). Readers are referred to Chow et al. (1987), Gissmann et al. (1987), Pfister (1987), and Howley and Schlegel (1988) for more complete reviews.

The role of HPV in cervical carcinogenesis was further indicated by the demonstration of HPV 16 and HPV 18 DNA in three-quarters of established cell lines originating from human cervical cancer (Boshart et al. 1984; Yee et al. 1985; Schwarz et al. 1985; Pater and Pater 1985; Baker et al. 1987; Seedorf et al. 1987); Popescu et al. 1987; Shirasawa et al. 1987; Spence et al. 1988). The number of HPV copies varies from one to two in SiHa cell lines, to more than 600 in CaSki cell lines (Yee et al. 1985).

Despite strong evidence that HPV is the major factor in cervical carcinogenesis, the probability of cervical carcinogenesis among women who have HPV infection is not high. This led to the belief that another factor may be involved in carcinogenesis. As early as 1982 ZUR HAUSEN hypothesized that HPV may act synergistically with HSV 2. Association of HPV and HSV 2 among patients with cervical carcinoma has been shown (PRAKASH et al. 1985; KAUFMAN and ADAM 1986; BRANDT et al. 1987). Coexistence of HPV infection with chlamydia and with gardnerella has also been demonstrated (ALLERDING et al. 1985; SYRJÄNEN et al. 1986a; FALCO et al. 1987). In addition, cytomegalovirus enhances in vitro cell transformation by BPV (GOLDSTEIN et al. 1987). Nevertheless, all these studies stop short of directly demonstrating a biologic mechanism of synergistic carcinogenesis.

Association of immunosuppression with HPV-containing premalignant and malignant lesions of the uterine cervix and of the vulva has been noted (SHOKRI-TABIBZADEH et al. 1981; RASTKAR et al. 1982; SCHNEIDER et al. 1983; SYRJÄNEN 1983; SILLMAN et al. 1984; CARSON et al. 1986; HALPERT et al. 1986; TAY et al. 1987). The published data were initially interpreted as showing that the immunosuppression led to HPV infection, thus resulting in later development of premalignant and malignant neoplasms. Recent epidemiologic studies using detection methods of high sensitivity combining DNA amplification by polymerase chain reaction (PCR) with blot hybridization suggest that cervicovaginal HPV infection is widespread among healthy women. There is a likelihood that immunosuppression or reduce immunocompetence plays a more a direct role in carcinogenesis.

## 3 Methods of HPV Detection

Historically HPVs have been observed by a light microscopy, by electron microscopy, and, more recently, by immunocytochemistry. Cytopathic effects including koilocytosis have been described in various HPV types, and the cytopathic effect may vary from one HPV types to another. Yet histologic changes in the cells provide only circumstantial evidence of viral infection and its sensitivity and specificity is not high. Molecular methods using specific DNA probes have become the main method of HPV identification since the late 1970s. There are many variations on the HPV DNA hybridization methods. Some are tedious; others are simpler but less specific.

Growth or multiplication of HPVs using tissue cultured cells is at present still employed mainly for research purposes. HPVs grown in tissue cultured cells fail to mature unless the epithelial cells are grown half exposed to air. Only a few types of HPV have been shown to grow in human keratinocytes in culture, and the early contamination and tediousness of the method discourage the use of tissue cultures as a diagnostic tool for HPV detection. One interesting aspect is the successful transplantation of human condylomas to nude mice and the multiplication of HPV in this system (Kreider et al. 1987). This method, however, is limited to HPV 11-produced lesions; the lesions produced by other types of HPV have not proved "transplantable" in this system. Nevertheless, this model may serve as an important system for testing systemic therapies. Various methods of HPV identification will now be discussed.

### 3.1 Identification by Morphology

Koss and Durfee created the term "koilocytosis" for squamous epithelial cells seen in Papanicolaou smears which are characterized by nuclear atypia and a sharply marginated clear zone around the cell nuclei (Koss and Durfee 1956). Meisels and Fortin (1976) demonstrated that these changes are associated with cervical condyloma. They further reported that multinucleation, nuclear wrinkling, dyskaryosis, and epithelial spikes are characteristic cytologic features of cervical condylomas. These features can also be seen in tissue sections. Distinction of koilocytosis from glycogen vacuoles in squamous cells of women of reproductive age is at times difficult. The sensitivity of morphologic determination as compared to Southern blot DNA hybridization is not high; Sato et al. (1986) showed that the frequency of koilocytosis in lesions containing HPV ranged from 80% in condylomas to 20% in CIN III (Sato et al. 1986). Koilocytosis is usually not observed in invasive carcinomas that contain integrated HPV DNA in the most neoplastic cells. Because of frequent confusion of koilocytosis with perinuclear halo or other degenerative changes of the cervicovaginal cells, it may not be sufficiently specific for HPV infections. Koilocytosis is seen in routine gynecologic Papanicolaou smears of asymptomatic women at a frequency of 2% (Okagaki, unpublished data), whereas approximately 10% of cervicovaginal specimens of normal women are HPV DNA positive by Southern or dot hybridization (Wagner et al. 1984; McCance et al. 1985; Burk et al. 1986; Fuchs et al. 1988), and subclinical cervical lesions can be identified in the majority of them by colposcopy. Computing from these figures only 20% of women who have cervicovaginal HPV infection yield koilocytes in Papanicolaou smears. Koilocytosis in Papanicolaou smears and other morphologic features claimed to be characteristic of HPV infection are at best presumptive in predicting HPV infection. Although koilocytosis is one of several characteristic histologic features of HPV-related cervical lesions, its correlation with the result of biotin–avidin labeled in situ hybridization was shown to be low. Yet, many histopathologists have regarded koilocytosis as the principal diagnostic sign of HPV infection. Koilocytosis is also seen in HPV-related lesions of the vagina and vulva, and similar "cytopathic" cells were observed by Jablonska et al. (1989) in the skin lesions produced by HPV in EV patients.

## 3.2 Immunocytochemistry

The horseradish peroxidase–antiperoxidase (PAP) method using antibodies against the capsid antigens of HPV, mature HPV virions present in the tissue can be demonstrated. (KURMAN et al. 1981; WARHOL et al. 1984). Type-specific antibodies using $E_5$, $E_6$, and $E_7$ transcripts have been developed and some are commerically available (Triton Biosciences, Inc., Almeada, CA, USA). The sensitivity and specificity of the antibodies against these transcript products have yet to be tested. The positive reaction to immunocytochemistry probably requires at least a few hundred mature virions in a cell. This method at times may be convenient for the study of benign HPV-produced lesions in relation to histologic studies. The development of more sensitive in situ DNA hybridization has, however, made immunocytochemical methods practically obsolete.

## 3.3 Southern Blot DNA Hybridization

Rerearch into HPV has made significant progress since SOUTHERN, in 1975, developed a method to test DNA homology using a principle that two complementary DNAs form a pair when 85% of DNAs contain the same nucleotide sequences (homology) in a hybridization solution of high stringent condition created by addition of formamide (SOUTHERN 1975). DNAs of 50% homology pair under low stringency (relaxed) conditions. This method requires DNA to be extracted from a tissue sample, electrophoresed on agarose gel, and then transferred to a cellulose acetate film before actual hybridization is performed. The development of DNAs of known viral species ("probes") is achieved by DNA cloning and Nick translation. Under high stringency conditions, specific types of HPV are identified. Under low stringency conditions, one can detect both known and unknown types of HPV using a probe of a single type of HPV. The method is still considered to be the gold standard in the identification of the viral genuses or types. The disadvantage of this method is the fact that tissue must be homogenized and DNA extracted before the presence of HPV is tested. When the tissue consists of more than one cell type or more than one lesion (e.g., coexistence of adenocarcinoma and CIN), the localization of HPV will not be known. When HPV is present in a small focus of a tissue sample, HPV DNA may be diluted beyond the sensitivity of Southern blot hybridization. This method is sensitive to the degree that it can detect 0.1 to 1.0 copies of viral DNA per cell. For determining the localization of viral DNA, in situ hybridization is the method of choice.

## 3.4 Dot DNA Hybridization

Because Southern blot hybridization involves a tedious, labor-intensive process and because loss of DNA may occur during the process, dot hybridization became a popular method for mass screening of HPV. DNA is extracted from the cervical mucus or vaginal washing, placed on a cellulose acetate or a Nylon membrane, and then hybridized with radiolabeled DNA probes. After proper washings, hybridization is demonstrated on an autoradiograph in the same fashion as in Southern blot hybridization (Wickenden et al. 1985).

Plastic blocks made of Lucite with regularly placed wells are used so that many samples can be placed on a single membrane at regular spaces, and simultaneously protect dots of samples from coalescing each other. The final resutls can be viewed as multiple spots on an autoradiograph. Commercially available kits from Life Technologies, Inc. and others use this method, and are convenient for mass screening.

Because DNAs are not properly segregated into separate fractions by size in dot hybridization, it is not possible to determine nonspecific binding of the probe from specific binding. Consequently, the method tends to produce false-positive results. Conversely, a vigorous wash before autoradiography to eliminate false-positive binding may reduce the sensitivity. Nevertheless, studies that have compared this method with Southern blot hybridization have claimed acceptable sensitivity and specificity for practical mass screening uses. The sensitivity of the method is lower than that of Southern blot hybridization.

### 3.5 In Situ Dot Hybridization

Unlike dot blot hybridization, this method uses intact cell samples. It was developed and used for mass screening (Wagner et al. 1984; Schneider et al. 1985). Vaginal–cervical scrapings or washings are obtained. Cells are harvested with centrifugation, washed, and placed on a filter paper. After suitable treatment of the cells to increase DNA permeation, they are hybridized with radioisotope-labeled probes, and autoradiographed for interpretation. This method is simpler than dot hybridization because it does not require DNA extraction. The sensitivity of the method is low because the penetration of DNA probes through the cell and nuclear membranes is not always assured. It is believed to require more than 50 copies of HPV DNA per cell (L. Gissmann, personal communication).

### 3.6 In Situ Hybridization

The presence of HPV genomes can be demonstrated using fixed cells or tissue sections by in situ hybridization. Because the process requires vigorous washes and incubation of the samples at a relatively high temperature, the cell samples or tissue samples are best mounted on glass slides with glue (Emery's glue or polyalanine). When a paraffin-embedded tissue section is used, fixation of the tissue with a buffered formalin solution yields the best preservation of DNA (Nuovo and Richart 1989). The samples are initially treated with proteinase to increase the permeability of the cells and nuclear membranes, and then treated with labeled HPV DNA probes. Probes are radiolabeled with $^{35}S$ of $^{3}H$ (GUPTA et al. 1985; SYRJÄNEN et al. 1986b; OSTROW et al. 1987; SCHNEIDER et al. 1987c; TASE et al. 1988a; PILOTTI et al. 1989). After hybridization, the preparations are coated with a photographic emulsion and autoradiographed. The autoradiographs are examined under a microscope with a light or dark field illumination.

The exposure times are 1–3 days for $^{35}S$-labeled probes and 2–4 weeks for $^{3}H$-labeled probes. Because the energy of the beta particles of $^{35}S$ is more than ten times that of $^{3}H$, the resolution of autoradiographs using $^{35}S$ is poorer than that of $^{3}H$-labeled probes. Background is also high in situ hybridization using $^{35}S$ labeling. Its main advantage ovar $^{3}H$ is the shorter exposure time required.

STOLER and BROKER (1986) developed in situ hybridization using $^{3}H$-labeled antisense RNA. The sensitivity is comparable to that of $^{3}H$-labeled DNA in situ hybridization. The sensitivity of in situ hybridization using $^{3}H$-labeled DNA or antisense RNA is around three to five copies of DNA per cell.

To overcome the need for cumbersome microautoradiography and exposure of the emulsion for a few days to a few weeks, a number of nonradioactive DNA probes for in situ hybridization have been developed (BECKMAN et al. 1985; HEILES et al. 1988). Some have become commercially available. Biotin, digoxigenin, or peroxidase labeling are used. The probes are visualized with enzyme-labeled avidin (peroxidase or phosphatases) or enzyme-labeled antibodies against digoxigenin. The sensitivity of these products is at best 10–20 copies of DNA per cell (WALBOOMERS et al. 1988; GRUSSENDORF-CONEN and CREMER 1990). The advantage is that the samples can be processed without specialized laboratory facilities for radioisotopes and a dark room, and a short processing time is required.

In situ hybridization is an extremely useful tool for studying the target cells of HPV infection and histogenesis of human neoplasms in which the viral DNA is integrated. When a tissue consists of several different types of cells—a cervical biopsy, for example—in situ hybridization can be more sensitive than Southern blot hybridization performed on the extract of a homogenate of a mixture of heterogeneous cells because HPV DNA may be diluted in the latter.

### 3.7 Polymerase Chain Reaction as an Adjunct Method of DNA Detection

The recent development of the polymerase chain reaction (PCR) added a powerful tool for the detection of a small number of viral DNA molecules or genomes present in a sample (SAIKI et al. 1988). HPV DNA present in a sample acts as a template of new DNA synthesis with the presence of oligoprimers, nucleotides, and DNA polymerase. Twenty to 25 cycles of reaction are repeated, resulting in amplification of HPV DNA by a factor of more than $10^5$. Detection and typing of HPV DNA are then preformed by other conventional hybridization methods (TIDY et al. 1989a). The method has also proved capable of detecting

HPV genomes in paraffin-embedded tissues available in many surgical pathology laboratories (Shibata et al. 1988a).

A study by Tidy and co-workers revealed that HPV DNA is almost invariably present in the vaginal samples of women in Great Britain when PCR is combined with blot hybridization (Tidy et al. 1989b; Anonymous 1989). Their report has been later retracted. It appears that PCR assisted hybridization yields 20% of prevalence of HPV in normal women and 40% of prevalence in high risk women.

Oligoprimers of the major types of HPV have now become commercially available (Genemed Biotechnologies, Inc.). The equipment necessary for PCR is relatively inexpensive. It is expected that more clinical and epidemiologic studies using this method will appear in the literature.

## 4 Carcinomas and Their Precursor Lesions of the Lower Female Genitalia

Certain types of carcinoma of the uterine cervix, vagina, and vulva contain integrated or, quite frequently, episomal HPV DNA in the cells. The presence of HPV DNA in many cultured cell lines originated from carcinoma of the uterine cervix containing integrated HPV DNA provided strong supporting evidence for the role of HPV in carcinogenesis (Boshart et al. 1984; Yee et al. 1985). Tumors of the lower female genitalia containing HPV genomes thus far known are all epithelial tumors. There is no confirmed report that a particular connective tissue tumor is related to HPV in humans, although PV-produced benign and malignant connective tissue tumors (e.g., deer fibroma) are known to occur in other animals (Olson and Olson 1985).

Historically, skin warts of immunodeficient individuals known as epidermodysplasia verruciformis (EV) not infrequently progressed to invasive squamous cell carcinoma (Orth et al. 1979; Viac et al. 1987). HPV DNAs are found in premalignant lesions and malignant lesions of the conjunctiva, cornea, oral mucosa, nasal cavity, bronchus, esophagus, lungs, bladder, and bowels (Ostrow et al. 1985; Byrne et al. 1987; Nair et al. 1988; Trillo and Guha 1988; McDonnell et al. 1989; Bejui-Thivolet et al. 1990). Nevertheless, the frequency of detectable HPV DNA is highest in premalignant and malignant epithelial lesions of the external genitalia. Hence genital lesions became the focal point of investigations on HPV carcinogenesis in humans.

Most neoplasias in the external genitalia linked to HPV are squamous cell carcinoma and its precursors. CIN, vaginal intraepithelial neoplasia (VaIN), vulvar intraepithelial neoplasia (VIN; Bowen's disease, bowenoid atypia, and bowenoid papulosis), and penile intraepithelial neoplasia (PIN) constitute the precancerous lesions of the lower genitalia, and may develop through a stage of benign infectious disease of HPV—i.e., condyloma—or perhaps without clinically apparent condyloma. Because HPV is now believed to be a carcinogenic factor in these organs, some investigators regard condyloma acuminatum as a precursor lesion of cancer, and recommend treating condylomas as CIN, VaIN, or VIN.

Intraepithelial and invasive neoplasias of the lower female genitalia are frequently multicentric. Twenty percent of CINs are associated with VaIN or VIN. Likewise, 20% of VINs are associated with CIN or VaIN (Boutselis 1972; Choo and Morley 1980). Before HPV became implicated in these lesions, these associations were explained by the "field theory"; that is, the epithelia of the different parts of the lower female genitalia are under the influence of a single cancer-causing factor. The field theory was further used to explain a high recurrence rare among individuals with successfully treated intraepithelial neoplasia. However, multicentricity and multiorgan involvement are not limited to intraepithelial neoplasia. Any lesions in the spectrum from condyloma through invasive squamous cell carcinoma can occur in three organs of the lower female genitalia (cervix, vagina, and vulva) in various combinations synchronously or metachronously. The term "genital neoplasm papilloma syndrome" (GeNPS) was proposed for this frequently observed condition (Okagaki 1984). GeNPS may develop on a common ground of mild immunologic impairment of the host and resulting HPV infection, even though no other sings of immunosuppression may be clinically apparent (Carson et al. 1986).

HPV-produced lesions of the penis are believed to be an important factor from an epidemiologic standpoint. The frequencies of precancerous and cancerous lesions of the penis are much lower than the frequencies of such lesions of the external genitalia of women. Most penile lesions are subclinical or latent, yet they are believed to be the main source of sexual transmission. Specific genital lesions produced by HPV are discussed in the following section.

### 4.1 Squamous Cell Carcinoma of the Uterine Cervix and Its Precursor Lesions

Ayre in 1960 described a "perinuclear halo" in the squamous cells in Papanicolaou smears, and suggested viral infection as a possible cause. Koss and Durfee (1956) described a more morphologically specific change, kiolocytosis. Flat condyloma or "subclinical papillomavirus infection" (Reid et al. 1984) is histologically characterized by koilocytosis of the squamous epithelium, a "spiking" structure, elongated rete pegs, acanthosis, frequent multinucleation, wrinkling of the nuclear membranes at the basal and parabasal layers, dyskeratosis, cytoplasmic vacuolation, and the presence of kedratohyalin granules (Meisels and Fortin 1976; Reid et al. 1980, 1984; Ludwig et al. 1981; Kurman et al. 1982).

The subclassification of cervical condylomas may deserve some discussion. Meisels and Fortin (1976) proposed the term "flat condyloma" for the cervical lesion characterized by koilocytosis, dyskaryosis, and "unique" parabasal cells with multinucleation and nuclear wrinkling. Later the same authors proposed the term "inverted condyloma," for those lesions cytologically similar to flat condyloma, but with endophytic growth (MEISELS et al. 1977). The term "atypical condyloma" was given to condyloma containing marked nuclear atypia but otherwise similar to flat condyloma (MEISELS et al. 1981). The authors distinguished this lesion from dysplasia or carcinoma in situ of the cervix because, using immunocytochemistry to demonstrate HPV, "60% of condyloma with nuclear atypia contains HPV antigen while dysplasia, carcinoma in situ and invasive carcinoma do not." Their notion that atypical condyloma differed from dysplasia because of the presence of absence of HPV can be regarded as incorrect in the light of current knowledge. Their failure to demonstrate HPV in dysplasia and carcinoma in situ was due to a low sensitivity of immunocytoechemistry. Atypical condyloma is now considered to be identical to, or a subtype of, mild dysplasia by most pathologists. There is little need to separate flat condyloma from classic condyloma acuminatum of the cervix because these lesions share many features.

Inverted condyloma is a type of squamous metaplasia frequently associated with cervical condyloma. LANCASTER et al. (1983) demonstrated HPV by Southern blotting in two of seven of squamous metaplasia of the cervix. Another variant of squamous metaplasia containing HPV was reported by CRUM et al. (1983b), who applied the term "atypical immature metaplasia" (AIM) to this lesion. The lesion is represented by immature cells with "variable nuclear hypochromatism and mild pleomorphism with or without koilocytosis." AIM is frequently associated with CIN. However, AIM may be regarded as a form of gland involvement of low-grade CIN.

All subtypes of the lesions produced by HPV proposed in the past were based on the erroneous assumption that CIN is a "neoplasia," whereas "flat," "inverted," and "atypical" condyloma and "AIM" are infectious lesions caused by HPV. Molecular biologic studies demonstrated the presence of HPV in 90%–100% of all grades of CIN (GISSMANN et al. 1983; OKAGAKI et al. 1983; KURMAN et al. 1983; MCCANCE et al. 1983). Further, these findings concurred with the previous report that koilocytosis, a norphologic feature believed to be unique to condylomas, is present in all grades of CIN at various rates (KOMOROWSKI and CLOWRY 1976). A recent comparative study showed that different pathologists weigh pathognomonic features of cervical condyloma differently, and poor agreement between the diagnoses was observed (SPITZER et al. 1990).

Computing from the rate of HPV DNA positivity among healthy woman by in situ dot, dot blot, or Southern blot hybridization, less than 20% of those who have HPV infection of the cervix and the vagina produce "pathognomonic" cells for condylomas in smears when Papanicolaou smears are read without knowledge of HPV positivity. In contrast, case control studies in patients with known HPV infection detected by molecular methods have reported 70%–80% rates of cytologic manifestations (FALCONE and FERENCZY 1986). This discrepancy in detection rates with and without prior knowledge of HPV positivity may suggested that many cytologic features attributed to HPV infection are neither specific nor highly pathognomonic. Using in situ dot hybridization, 72% of patients with HPV infection of the cervix showed acetowhite lesions, punctation, mosaicism, etc. at the cervical squamocolumnar junction under colposcopic examinations, and histopathologic examinations confirmed cervical condylomas or lesions of higher grades (SCHNEIDER et al. 1988). Other studies on the accuracy of colposcopic detection reported 90% to 100% sensitivity (REID and SCALZI 1985; VAYRYNEN et al. 1985; FALCONE and FERENCZY 1986; FOLLEN et al. 1987; KREBS and SCHNEIDER 1987; MORIN et al. 1988). It appears that colposcopy is as good as or better than Papanicolaous smears in detecting cervical condylomas.

One of the items of circumstantial evidence that CIN might evolve from condylomatous lesions of the cervix was the presence of association of condylomas in 22.5%–91% of patients with CIN (SYRJÄNEN 1979; LUDWIG et al. 1981; BOON and FOX 1981; NYEEM et al. 1982; REID et al. 1982; CRUM et al. 1983a; SCHMAUZ et al. 1983; ZUNA 1984; FUJII et al. 1984; SAITO et al. 1987). CIN is usually located at the squamocolumnar junction of the uterine cervix, and the associated condylomas are found contiguously outside of the CIN.

The HPV capsid antigens are usually demonstrable in more than 50% in condylomas and low-grade CINs of the uterine cervix by means of immunocytochemistry using polyclonal or monoclonal antibodies and peroxidase–antiperoxidase amplification, and the positive rates steadily decline as the grade of CIN increases (KURMAN et al. 1982; SATO et al. 1986). The loss of immunocytochemically demonstrable HPV antigens is attributed to the failure of maturation and the reduction of copy numbers of HPV in high-grade CIN. In addition, immunocytochemistry is a relatively insensitive method; it may be negative even when virions are demonstrable by electron microscopy (SATO et al. 1986). The presence of immunoperoxidase-positive material is usually limited to the superficial layer of CIN, and multiple sections may be needed before a positive cell is found (KURMAN et al. 1982).

There have been several attempts to distinguish HPV-produced lesions that progress to severe CIN or invasive carcinoma from those that do not. One has involved the distinction between CIN with koilocytosis ("CINK") and other cases of CIN. FRANQUEMOUNT et al. (1989) concluded that CINK contained HPV 16 almost as frequently as CIN without koilocytosis. Whether benign condyloma can be distinguished from CIN by virtue of DNA contents as assessed by stationary and flow cytometry remains controversial (TSOU et al. 1984; REID et al. 1984; WINKLER et al. 1984; GÖPPINGER et al. 1987; WATTS et al. 1987; HUGHES et al. 1987; FU et al. 1989). The discrepancy may result from the fact that HPV DNA can take Feulgen stain (CHACHO et al. 1990), and also the fact that a false shift in the modal DNA may occur with increased S-phase cells in some of these lesions (OKAGAKI and IZUO 1978).

Unlike in CIN, the early reported rates of detectable HPV DNA present in invasive squamous cell carcinoma varied in a wide range from 10% to 90% (GREEN et al. 1982; DÜRST et al. 1983; GISSMANN et al. 1983; FUKUSHIMA et al. 1985; MCCANCE et al. 1985; PRAKASH et al. 1985; YOSHIKAWA et al. 1985; PATER et al. 1986; Meanwell et al. 1987; Mitrani-Rosenbaum et al. 1988; Tase et al. 1988a; also see the review by Koutsky et al. 1988). One reason for this wide variation was the probable geographic differences in HPV-related cervical cancer and the common types of HPV found in cancer. More importantly, unavailability of HPV DNAs of many newly discovered types resulted in the relatively low sensitivity of HPV detection in the early 1980s. At this point in time, precise comparison of the data reported in the literature is not meaningful because of the different sensitivities of the various methods employed. Recent applications of PCR amplification of HPV DNA have substantially increased detection rates of HPV DNA in both normal and cancerous tissues, and the full impact of PCR on our knowledge regarding HPV detectability is not reflected in the available publications.

Another sources of difficulty in achieving a fair comparison of the published data if the variability in the definition of "cervical cancer." Many early studies included CIN in cervical cancer and this led many molecular biologists to assume that CIN was a variant of "neoplasia." With our current knowledge, CIN is regarded as an infectious disease and not a true neoplasm. Many histologic types of cervical cancer have been grouped together as cervical cancer, yet the rates of different histologic types of cervical cancer show a wide geographic and temporal variability.

The proportion of the cases in which HPV genomes are detectable by Southern blot or dot blot methods on tissue homogenates is higher in CIN (90%–100%) than in invasive carcinoma. The copy numbers of HPV also appear much higher in CIN than in invasive squamous cell carcinoma. Although integration of HPV DNA into the host cell DNA has been observed in some cases of CIN (Lancaster et al. 1983; Shirasawa et al. 1986), others have reported that HPV DNA found in CIN is mostly episomal (Lehn et al. 1988; Fukushima et al. 1990). In invasive carcinoma of the cervix, 50% of cases contain the integrated form of HPV DNA, 25% both the integrated and the episomal form, and the rest the episomal form (Choo et al. 1987). It appears that HPV integration will not take place until CIN is of a high grade or until malignant transformation of the cells has taken place.

### 4.2 Adenocarcinoma, Adenosquamous Carcinoma, and Their Precursors

Many of the earlier studies of HPV and uterine cancer did not discriminate between various histologic types of cervical carcinoma. A few cases of undifferentiated carcinoma and adenocarcinoma containing HPV DNA were reported in 1985 (Fukushima et al. 1985; Yoshikawa et al. 1985). Smotkin et al. (1986) found HPV 16 DNA in a case of adenocarcinoma of the uterine cervix by filter hybridization. HPV 18 DNA was identified in four of five adenosquamous carcinomas in their study. Using in situ hybridization of high sensitivity on paraffin-embedded sections, Tase et al. (1988a) reported a preponderance of HPV 18 in adenocarcinoma and a preponderance of HPV 16 in squamous cell carcinoma. HPV 18 was also the most common type in adenocarcinoma among Japanese patients; thus the proponderance of HPV 18 does not seem to be limited to the North American population (TASE et al. 1988b). Adenocarcinoma and adenosquamous carcinoma contained HPV DNA almost as frequently as squamous cell carcinoma in the same series. WILCZYNSKI et al. (1988a, b) observed similar findings using Southern blot hybridization on fresh tissues. Further, associated CIN contained the same type of HPV as was found in adenocarcinoma or adenosquamous carcinoma. Findings of HPV 18 in adenocarcinoma in situ supported the theory that HPV 18 is primarily involved in carcinogenesis of adenocarcinoma of the uterine cervix (FARNSWORTH et al. 1989; TASE et al. 1989a). Adenocarcinoma in situ appears to contain unintegrated HPV 18 and can be regarded as the infectious lesion produced by HPV 18, analogous to CIN as the infectious lesion produced most commonly by HPV 16. Endocervical glandular dysplasia and microglandular endocervical hyperplasia, assumed to be the precursor lesions of adenocarcinoma of the uterine cervix by some, did not contain HPV DNA apart from a few exceptional cases (OKAGAKI et al. 1989; TASE et al. 1989b). It has for some time been known that 40% of adenocarcinomas of the cervix are associated with CIN in their vicinity (KOSS 1979; MAIER and NORRIS 1980). The observation of HPV DNA in CIN associated with three major histologic types of cervical carcinoma is not coincidental; instead, is an integral part of histologic lesions produced by HPV. Whether the higher proportion of adenocarcinoma and adenosquamous carcinoma in cervical cancer reported in the United States is related in any way to epidemiology of HPV 18 infection is not known (DAVIS and MOON 1975; PETERS et al. 1986; SCHWARTZ and WEISS 1986). However, it is interesting to note that the rates of two nonsquamous types of carcinoma of the uterine cervix and the rate of HPV 18 in cervicovaginal samples show considerable variability from one geographic area to another.

### 4.3 Squamous Cell Carcinoma of the Vagina and Its Precursor Lesions

Most of the research interest in HPV carcinogenesis has been directed to cervical carcinogenesis because cervical carcinoma is by far the most common malignancy of the lower female genital tract. In contrast, squamous cell carcinoma of the vagina is relatively rare, and the ratio of its frequency in comparison to that of cervical carcinoma is 1:25 to 1:55 (FRICK et al. 1968; KANBOUR et al. 1974; SMITH 1981). The histologic features of squamous cell carcinoma of the vagina and VaIN are similar to those of squamous cell carcinoma of the uterine cervix; thus, the histogenesis of these lesions is usually assumed to be the same. This notion is not quite correct because the vaginal mucosa typically lacks squamocolumnar junction, which is the site where cervical carcinoma develops. The earlier studies from our laboratory showed that the detection rate of HPV DNA in VaIN was comparable to that in CIN (OKAGAKI et al. 1983). Similar reports apeared later (BORNSTEIN et al. 1987; SCHNEIDER et al. 1987a). Our study by in situ DNA hybridization demonstrated that 40% of vaginal invasive squamous cell carcinomas contained HPV genomes, the majority of which were HPV 16 (Ostrow et al. 1988). The positive rate of HPV DNA in squamous cell carcinoma of the vagina was approximately the same as in squamous cell carcinoma of the cervix. VaIN developing in the vaginal mucosa of diethylstilbestrol (DES)-exposed progeny is believed to arise at the squamocolumnar junction similar to that of the uterine cervix. It was shown that HPV DNA was present in VaIN associated with vaginal adenosis among women who had been exposed to DES in utero (Fu et al. 1983). HPV DNA was also present at a high rate in postirradiation dysplasia of the vagina (Fujimura et al., unpublished data). No study has so far demonstrated the presence of HPV 18 in VaIN or squamous cell carcinoma of the vagina.

Because the vaginal mucosa lacks typical squamocolumnar junction, it is conceivable that the frequencies of various HPV types in vaginal lesions may be different from their frequencies in lesions of the cervix. The commonly used methods of detecting HPV, i.e., Southern blot or dot blot hybridization on exfoliated cells in the vagina or on vaginal wash specimens involve difficulties in discriminating HPV infection of the vagina from that of the cervix. From the rates of HPV types, HPV lesions of the vagina may be more comparable to erythroplasia of Queyrat (Kiryu and Ackerman 1990).

Two cases of verrucous carcinoma involving the vagina and the cervix contained HPV DNA (Okagaki et al. 1984); both cases showed HPV 6 by Southern blot hybridization, immunoperoxidase, and electron microscopy. One case also contained an unidentified type of HPV in addition to HPV 6 (presumably HPV 16). Like verrucous carcinoma or giant condyloma (Buskhke-Lüwenstein tumor) of the vulva, verrucous carcinoma of the vagina appears to be produced by HPV 6 or 11.

## 4.4 Squamous Cell Carcinoma of the Vulva and Its Precursor Lesions

The International Society of Vulvar Disease has now replaced older designations—Bowen's disease, bowenoid atypia, vulvar dysplasia, and vulvar dystrophy with cellular atypia—with "vulvar intraepithelial neoplasia of grades I through III" (VIN I, VIN II, VIN III) in correspondence with CIN I–III, the system used for the cervical cancer precursors (Ridley et al. 1989). This nomenclature unfortunately perpetuates the misnomer "neoplasia" at a time when studies of HPV increasingly support the view that CIN, VaIN, and VIN are infectious diseases rather than neoplasia.

Bowen's disease is typically a reddened scaling lesion of the skin; it shows cellular atypia under a microscope and has historically been considered as the precursor lesion of vulvar carcinoma. The term "bowenoid atypia" was used for lesions containing a lesser degree of cellular atypia for at least five decades (Skinner et al. 1973). A histologically similar disease of the penis characterized by multicentric pigmented papules was described by Lloyd in 1970. Because these lesions frequently disappear spontaneously, they have been considered to be different from Bowen's disease. WADE et al. (1978) applied the term "bowenoid papulosis" to such lesions of the penis in their report of 11 cases. Bowenoid papulosis usually involves multiple papules that are slightly raised and erythematous to brownish, whereas Bowen's disease typically involves a single erythematous lesion covered by a keratin layer. WADE et al. (1978) inferred that bowenoid papulosis is viral in origin, the causal agent being HPV or HSV 2; in contrast, Bowen's disease is neoplastic, although microscopically the lesions appear similar, i.e., they both show histologic features of carcinoma in situ. The term "bowenoid papulosis" was readily accepted by many histopathologists and applied to similar lesions of the vulva. Virus-like particles were observed in bowenoid papulosis of the penis (KATZ et al. 1978; ZELICKSON and PRAWER 1980). HPV antigen was also demonstrated (GUILLET et al. 1984). However, the presence of HPV virions was also demonstrated in Bowen's disease of the vulva by an electron microscopic study (RASTKAR et al. 1982) and by a molecular biologic study (ZACHOW et al. 1982). HPV capsid antigen was shown in Bowen's disease (PILOTTI et al. 1984). It appears that Bowen's disease, erythroplasia of Queyrat, bowenoid atypia, bowenoid papulosis, vulvar dysplasia, and VIN are essentially the same disease produced by HPV (BLAU and HYMAN 1955; GRAHAM and HELWIG 1973; ULBRIGHT et al. 1982; KIRYU and ACKERMAN 1990). The difference in the clinical courses of these two lesions may be due to the difference in host responses to the viral infection and chronicity. The detection rate of HPV DNA achieved using Southern blot hybridization was higher in bowenoid papulosis than in Bowen's disease (TWIGGS et al. 1988).

The histogenesis of squamous cell carcinoma of the vulva is not as clearly understood as that of cervical squamous cell carcinoma. Bowen's disease is generally regarded as a precursor of squamous cell carcinoma of the vulva, yet only 8% of patients with Bowen's disease eventually develop squamous cell carcinoma (FRIEDRICH et al. 1980). This contrasts with the 80% progression rate from CIN III to invasive squamous cell carcinoma in the uterine cervix. Some cases of invasive squamous cell carcinoma arise directly from clinically apparent vulvar condyloma (KOVI et al. 1974; SCHMAUZ et al. 1978; SHAFEEK et al. 1979), but the majority of vulvar squamous cell carcinomas are not associated with or preceded by condyloma acuminatum or Bowen's disease.

Vulvar carcinomas consist of several histologic subtypes although they are commonly diagnosed as squamous cell carcinoma (UNDERWOOD et al. 1978). Unlike invasive squamous cell carcinoma of the cervix, the majority of invasive squamous cell carcinomas of the vulva are well-differentiated or keratinized. Some are associated with a large condyloma acuminatum, and the focus of squamous cell carcinoma may be found in the midst of the condyloma. The term "condylomatous carcinoma" was applied to these lesions by JAPAZE et al. (1982). Most vulvar condylomas contain HPV 6 or HPV 11. Seventeen percent of HPVs found in vulvar condylomas are HPV 16 (GISSMANN et al. 1983). HPV 6 or HPV 16 was present in 55% of condylomatous carcinomas (DOWNEY et al. 1988). HPV DNA was found in 80% of cases of Bowen's disease or VIN (TWIGGS et al. 1988).

Sixty percent of HPVs found in high grade VIN were HPV 16 (BUSCEMA et al. 1988). The presence of HPV 18 in vulvar carcinoma has also been reported, though infrequently (SUTTON et al. 1987). Another variant of vulvar carcinoma is pseudoglandular squamous cell carcinoma. This lesion, although to a large extent resembling keratinizing squamous cell tumor, contains small gland-like nests of tumor cells infiltrating into the surrounding connective tissue, and has been shown to be adenosquamous carcinoma of the sweat gland in origin (UNDERWOOD et al. 1978). HPV DNA was not identified in pseudoglandular squamous cell carcinoma (CARSON et al. 1988). In a study by BORNSTEIN et al. (1988), all the cases of Paget's disease of the vulva, which is believed to be a variant of sweat gland adenocarcinoma, were shown to be negative for HPV 6, 11, and 16 by in situ hybridization using biotinated probes, a method has a relatively low sensitivity.

Other characteristic lesions related to condyloma are giant condyloma (Buschke-Löwenstein tumor) and verrucous carcinoma (DAWSON et al. 1965; FOYE et al. 1969; BOGOMOLETZ et al. 1985). A few studies of verrucous carcinoma and giant condyloma of the vulva confirmed HPV 6 or its variant in the cells (RANDO et al. 1986a; BOSHART and ZUR HAUSEN 1986; BUSCEMA et al. 1988). Some cases also involved associated invasive squamous cell carcinoma, suggesting that HPV 6 could produce invasive squamous cell carcinoma (RANDO et al. 1986b; DOWNEY et al. 1988; KASHER and ROMAN 1988).

### 4.5 Carcinoma and Precursor Lesions of Other Female Genital Organs

Human papillomavirus is not detected in adenocarcinoma of the endometrium or its precursor (BERGERON et al. 1988). KAUFMAN et al. (1987) reported the presence of HPV 6 in 10 out of 12 adenocarcinomas of the ovary. A later study, however, showed no significant association between HPV and ovarian carcinoma (LEAKE et al. 1989). Our study on endometrial and ovarian carcinoma also indicates that tumors of these organs do not contain HPV DNA (OKAGAKI, unpublished data).

### 4.6 Carcinomas and Precursor Lesions of the Male Genitalia

Compared to carcinoma of the external female genitalia, carcinoma of the penis is rare in North America and Europe. In contrast, penile cancer is more commonly seen in some parts of Africa and South America (SCHMAUZ et al. 1977; VILLA and LOPES 1986). HPV 16 and HPV 18 have been found in 25%–60% of cases of carcinoma of the penis (DÜRST et al. 1983; BOSHART et al. 1984; KREBS and SCHNEIDER 1987; BARRASSO et al. 1987). VILLA and LOPES (1986) observed that 9 of 18 cases (50%) of penile cancer in Brazil contained HPV 16. MCCANCE et al. (1986) reported that 49% of penile cacers contained HPV 16 and 9% HPV 18.

It has long been suspected that cervical carcinoma may be transmitted from male cohorts because of a high incidence of cervical cancer among wives of men with penile cancer (Kurihara and Asano 1956; Schmauz et al. 1977). On the other hand, a majority of male consorts of women with cervical cancer do not develop penile cancer. Papillomas of the male urethra also contain HPV (Dean et al. 1983). Papillomas of the male urethra or the penile skin are found in 53% of the male consorts of women with genital condylomas or CIN (Levine et al. 1984). Subsequent studies of the male consorts of HPV-infected women showed that 64%–76% of the males had HPV-related penile lesions ranging from condyloma and benign papules to penile intraepithelial neoplasia; a majority of the lesions were identifiable only with the aid of a colposcope or acetic acid application (Barrasso et al. 1987; Gal et al. 1989). In addition to HPV 16, HPV 6, 11, 33, and 42 were found in these lesions. HPV 16 and 33 were exclusively found in the lesions with cytologic atypia (Barrasso et al. 1987). It appears that HPV infection of the penile skin is more common than previously thought and that it is mostly subclinical, so that careful clinical examination using a colposcope is required to identify the lesions. For as yet unknown reason, these HPV-containing lesions of the penis seldomly evolve to invasive carcinoma, although so-called high-or intermediate-risk HPVs, HPV 16, and HPV 33, have often been found in these lesions.

The presence and extent of involvement of the prostate and the seminal vesicles are not well known. In view of the fact that HPV DNA was found in the semen of patients with chronic warty skin lesions, HPV DNA may be present in the prostate and seminal vesicles of certian men (Ostrow et al. 1985, 1986).

## 5 Epidemiology and Mode of Transmission

Human papillomavirus-related genital lesions are seen in every geographic area in the world. The link between cervical cancer and sexual promiscuity and the link between cervical cancer and penile cancer led researchers to suspect HPV as a causative agent of cervical cancer (Kurihara and Asano 1956; Martinez 1969; Kessler 1981; Reid et al. 1982; Tase et al. 1986). The types of HPV found in cervical cancer and its precursor lesions, however, vary from one geographic region to another (Koutsky et al. 1988). Whether these differences are actually attributable to climate, natural environment, social habits or race remains unanswered. A high rate of penile carcinoma in Africa, South America, and the South Pacific may be attributable to common extramarital sexual intercourse or frequent contacts with prostitutes by men in these areas, although some investigators have attributed it to "hygiene" (Boon et al. 1989). Given the high species specificity and organotropism of PVs, it is possible that some types of HPV may be found in specific races.

The sexual transmissibility of HPV was stressed by past investigators, which erroneously led to the notion that all HPV-related genital lesions are transmitted by sexual contact. This caused unnecessary anxiety, shame, and damage to patients with HPV-related genital lesions. In fact, 40%–60% of HPVs isolated from the sexual partners are of different types (McCANCE et al. 1986; BARRASSO et al. 1987). Moreover, children can develop HPV-related genital lesions without a history of sexual abuse (VALLEJOS et al. 1987; PADEL et al. 1990), and HPV can be transmitted to a neonate at the time of birth (SEDLACEK et al. 1989). All cases of juvenile laryngeal papillomatosis are believed to be due to infection during birth (QUICK et al. 1978; COSTA et al. 1981; MOUNTS et al. 1982; HALLDEN and MAJMUDAR 1986). HPV DNA has been found in vapor plumes of laser therapy for HPV-related genital lesions and on medical instruments after cold sterilization (GARDEN et al. 1988; FERENCZY et al. 1989; BERGERON et al. 1990). It is thus likely that a significant proportion of HPV infections occur without sexual contacts.

Using filter in situ hybridization, WAGNER et al. (1984) found that HPV DNA was present in 11% of cervicovaginal samples from normal women in Germany. Other European studies have shown similar results (WICKENDEN et al. 1985; ARMSTRONG et al. 1986; KJAER et al. 1988). HPV DNA appears in 28% of pregnant women according to SCHNEIDER et al. (1987b). Using Southern blot hybridization, HPV DNA was demonstrated in 5.5% of samples of hysterectomy specimens from patients with normal Papanicolaou smears (NUOVO et al. 1988). GERGELY et al. (1987) reported that, in a Hungarian papulation, in situ hybridization revealed 52% of negative cytology specimens to contain HPV DNA. HPV infection is not limited to young females: NUOVO et al. (1989) found that 12% of postmenopausal women harbor HPV in the cervical tissues.

Application of polymerase chain reaction (PCR) provided a higher sensitivity of HPV detection (SHIBATA et al. 1988). Using PCR HPV 16 DNA has been found in 80% of normal women (TIDY et al. 1989b; ANONYMOUS 1989). At the Papillomavirus Workshop held in May 1990 in Heidelberg it was reported that with the aid of PCR, HPV DNA can be detected in cervicovaginal samples in 20%–100% of normal women. Whether this extremely high rate of positivity of HPV in normal women was due to methodological errors in detection or whether HPV is a normal parasite of humans is unresolved at present. One may, however, conclude that a higher copy number of HPV is detected in premalignant and malignant lesions of the external genitalia than in controls.

## 6 Immunology and HPV-Related Lesions

Patients with HPV-related lesions frequently show common antibodies against HPV. Yet, apparently a substantial proportion of normal individuals have circulating antibodies detectable by enzyme-linked immunoabsorbent assay (BAIRD

1983). CUBIE and NORVAL (1988) reported that 48.8% of those with no known history of warts had detectable antibodies. The diagnosis of HPV infection by immunologic detection is at present of questionable value because of poor sensitivity and specificity. Further, the presence of common antibodies would simply indicate a past history of HPV infection including skin warts.

While the protective value of antibodies against repeat HPV infection is questionable, HPV infection can be precipitated by immunoincompetence of the host. The risk of developing cervical dysplasia is nearly five times higher among immunosuppressed patients (PORRECO et al. 1975; SZHORKI-TABIBZADEH et al. 1981; SCHNEIDER et al. 1983; KATZ et al. 1987; SILLMAN et al. 1987). HPV infection and CIN are more common among AIDS patients (HENRY et al. 1989).

Patients with squamous cell carcinoma of the cervix, Bowen's disease, and condyloma have lowered ability in respect of lymphocyte transformation in response to antigenic challenges or lower T4/T8 ratios (KHOO and MACKAY 1974; SESKI et al. 1978; CARSON et al. 1986). Whether immunosuppression is a cause or a result of HPV infection needs further clarification.

## 7 HPV Types, Clinical Course, and Therapy

HPV 6 and 11 are found in 40 % of benign condylomas of the cervix, and HPV 16 or HPV 18 in 17%. The proportion of HPV 16 or HPV 18 steadily rises with increasing grade of CIN (MITCHELL et al. 1986; FRANQUEMONT et al. 1989); HPV 16 and 18 are the major types of HPV in cervical carcinoma containing HPV DNA (DÜRST et al. 1983), whereas HPV 6 and 11 and only occasionally found in invasive carcinoma. CRUM et al. (1984) suggested that HPV 16 carries a high risk of carcinogenesis whereas HPV 6 and 11 carry a low risk. HPV 18 is also considered a high-risk type HPV as it is frequently found in invasive carcinoma (SYRJÄNEN and SYRJÄNEN 1985; CRUM and LEVINE 1984; REID et al. 1987). An extensive epidemiologic study showed that the risk of cervical cancer in HPV 16- or 18-positive women is four times that in controls; the risk ratio was only comparable to that of multiparity (REEVES et al. 1989). In other words, carcinogenesis by this high-risk HPV was not confirmed epidemiologically.

More recently, a number of other types of HPV have been isolated from CIN or invasive carcinoma of the cervix. HPV 31, 33, and 35 are now regarded as carrying a medium risk of carcinogenesis (WILLET et al. 1989). HPV 52 is probably a high-risk type because its variants, HPV 52a and HPV 52b, have been isolated from the tissues of invasive carcinoma in Latin America and Japan respectively. HPV 52b is reportedly the second most common type of HPV in cervical cancer in certain areas of Japan (SATO et al. 1989). The risk associated with HPV 42, 43, 44, 45, 51, and 56, isolated from premalignant or malignant cervical lesions, is unclear at present. As indicated above, HPV 6 and 11 are found in conylomas and low-grade CIN, and are not usually associated with invasive carcinoma. They have, however, occasionally been seen in association with verrucous carcinoma and invasive carcinoma of the vagina and the vulva (OKAGAKI et al. 1984; RANDO et al. 1986a, b; BOSHART and ZUR HAUSEN 1986; KASHER and ROMAN 1988).

The risk of cervical cancer among women infected with HPV 16 has been estimated as 1 in 300, while the risk among women infected with HPV 6 or 11 is around 1 in 2000–3000 (PFISTER 1987). One may conclude that the actual risk of developing cervical cancer with any type of HPV is small indeed. Possible implication of confounders such as HSV 2 infection and cigarette smoking complicates evaluation of the potential risk of developing carcinoma (TREVATHAN et al. 1983; WINKELSTEIN et al. 1984).

More recently several investigators have reported that cervical cancer containing HPV 18 is more aggressive than that containing HPV 16 (BARNES et al. 1988; KURMAN et al. 1988; WALKER et al. 1989). However, a study in which clinical stages and histologic types were matched in a large sample showed no statistically significant difference in prognosis between HPV 18- and HPV 16-containing cervical cancers (KING et al. 1989). The apparent poor prognosis of HPV 18-containing cancer may be due to the fact taht many poorly differentiated or undifferentiated carcinomas contain HPV 18 (KURMAN et al. 1988). The extremely high rate of HPV detected in the external genitalia of normal women by PCR shows how complex is the relationship between HPV infection and genital neoplasms. The further frustrates physicians in treating them. Because the diseases ranging from condyloma through invasive cancer are now believed to constitute a continuum of cervical carcinogenesis of the female external genitalia, it is the current trend to treat all HPV-related lesions of the external genitalia in women, including cervical condylomas. Since HPV-related genital lesions in men are, by contrast, mostly subclinical and asymptomatic and do not carry a substantial risk of invasive carcinoma, they are not always treated until they progress to the stage of carcinoma in situ. Whether destructive therapy (such as surgical excision, cryosurgery, or laser vaporization) for condylomas and CIN without eradication of the HPV infection is effective in the long term has not yet been conclusively established (BELLINA 1983). Treating all patients with cervical condyloma is not cost-effective because nearly 8% of women have cervical condylomas identifiable by colposcopic examination. Based on the premise that HPV must be eradicated in order to yield a complete cure, systemic therapy using interferon has been tested, but the results have not been an unqualified success (IKIC et al. 1981; MØLLER et al. 1983; GALL et al. 1985). In effect, current knowledge on HPV in relation to genital cancer has not resulted in any change in the therapeutic strategy employed in respect of the lesions in question. First, the mechanism of carcinogenesis by HPV must be established. Second, cofactors that act synergistically with HPV infection must be identified, if any exist. Currently postulated cofactors are at best deduced from a statistical association. Until these questions are resolved, logical and effective therapeutic methods may not be forthcoming.

## 8 Concluding Remarks

Although cloning of the high-risk type HPVs and subsequent demonstration of them in various carcinomas of the external genitalia strongly suggests that HPV might be a cause of cervical cancer, the cause and effect relationship of HPV and cervical cancer is far from proven. Recent observations using PCR have added more puzzling problems than answers. For one, not every woman with HPV 16 or 18 infection develops cervical cancer; the actual probability is in fact very small. If some of the preliminary data are confirmed, more than one-half of women may have HPV 16 in the cervicovaginal flora (Papillomavirus Workshop, Heidelberg, May 1990). Therefore, HPV does not satisfy Koch's postulates as the causative agent of cervical cancer. Also the relative risk of cervical cancer among HPV 16-positive women is not high enough to conclude that HPV 16 is a carcinogen.

Since the pioneering observations by Khoo and Mackay (1974), reduced immunoreactivity has been found in patients with invasive carcinoma of the cervix, CIN, VIN, and vulvar condyloma. These observations may be interpreted as indicating that reduced immunoreactivity is the main causative factor in cervical cancer, and that "overt" HPV infections such as CIN are only a confounder.

Nevertheless, HPV research during the past decade has yielded significant insights into the histopathology of premalignant lesions of the external genitalia in both males and females. It is now apparent that most forms of CIN, VaIN, and VIN are infectious diseases produced by HPV, similar to condyloma. Varieties of the lesions of the vulva, notably Bowen's disease (VIN III), bowenoid papulosis, and vulvar dysplasia (VIN I and VIN II) are essentially one disease with different clinical manifestations. From the types of HPV found, VaIN appears more closely related to erythroplasia of Queyrat of the glans penis than does to CIN. For the development of invasive carcinoma from CIN, VaIN, or VIN, other factors must be involved in addition to HPV. Why CIN has a higher probability of developing into invasive carcinoma than VaIN or VIN must be explained. Similarly, HPV research has shown that the development of cervical adenocarcinoma may be different from that of squamous cell carcinoma. One may not equate endocervical glandular dysplasia with CIN as the former is unrelated to HPV infection.

The detection of HPV in genital neoplasms and their precursor lesions has provided exciting new challenges to the conceptual foundation of histopathology of these lesions. This is one of the most exciting periods for pathologists interested in genital cancers.

## References


Allerding TJ, Jordan SW, Boardman RE (1985) Association of human papillomavirus and chlamydia infections with incidence of cervical neoplasia. Acta Cytol 29:653–660

Almeida JD, Howatson AF, Williams MG (1962) Electron microscope study of human warts; sites of virus production and nature of the inclusion bodies. J Invest Dermatol 38:337–345

Anonymous (1989) Human papillomaviruses and the polymerase chain reaction. Lancet I:1051–1952

Armstrong BK, Allen OV, Brennan BA et al. (1986) Time trends in prevalence of cervical cytological abnormality in women attending a sexually transmitted diseases clinic and their relationship to trends in sexual activity and specific infections. Br J Cancer 54:669–675

Aurelian L, Schumann B, Marcus RL, Davis HJ (1973) Antibody to HPV-2 included tumor specific antigens in serums from patients with cervical carcinoma. Science 181:161–164

Ayre JE (1960) Role of the halo cell in cervical carcinogenesis: a viral manifestation is premalignancy. Obstet Gynocol 15:481–491

Baird PJ (1983) Serological evidence for the association of papillomavirus and cervical neoplasia. Lancet II:17–18

Baker CJ, Phelps WC, Lindgren V, Braun MJ, Gonda MA, Howley PM (1987) Structural and transcriptional analysis of human papillomavirus type 16 sequences in carcinoma cell lines. J Virol 61:962–971

Banks K, Spence P, Androphy E, Hubbert N, Matlashewski G, Murray A, Crawford L (1987) Identification of human papillomavirus type 18 E6 polypeptide in cells derived from human cervical carcinomas. J Gen Virol 68:1351–1359

Barbosa MS, Wettstein FO (1987) Transcription of the cottontail rabbit papillomavirus early region and identification of two E6 polypeptides in COS–7 cells. J Virol 61:2938–2942

Barnes W, Delgado G, Kurman RJ et al. (1988) Possible prognostic significance of human papillomavirus type in cervical cancer. Gynecol Oncol 29:267–273

Barrasso R, de Brux J, Croissant O, Orth G (1987) High prevalence of papillomavirus-associated penile intraepithelial neoplasia in sexual partners of women with cervical intraepithelial neoplasia. N Engl J Med 317:916–923

Bechtold E, Reicher NB (1952) The relationship of trichomonas infestations to false diagnoses of squamous carcinoma of the cervix. Cancer 5:442–457

Beckman AM, Myerson D, Daling JR, Kiviat NB, Fenoglio CM, McDougall JK (1985) Detection and localization of human papillomavirus DNA in human genital condylomas by in situ hybridization with biotinylated probes. J Med Virol 16:265–273

Bedell MA, Jones RH, Laimins LA (1987) The E6–E7 region of human papillomavirus type 18 is sufficient for transformation of NIH 3T3 and rat-1 cells. J Virol 61: 3635–3640

Bejui-Thivolet F, Liagre N, Chignol MC, Chardonnet Y, Patricot LM (1990) Detection of human papillomavirus DNA in squamous bronchial metaplasia and squamous cell carcinomas of the lung by in situ hybridization using biotinylated probes in paraffin-embedded specimens. Hum Pathol 21:111–115

Bellina JH (1983) The use of carbon dioxide laser in the management of condyloma acuminatum with eight-year follow-up. Am J Obstet Gynecol 147:375–378

Bergeron C, Naghashfar Z, Canaan C, Shah K, Fu Y, Ferenczy A (1987) Human papillomavirus type 16 in intraepithelial neoplasia (Bowenoid papulosis) and the coexistent invasive carcinoma of the vulva. Int J Gynecol Pathol 6:1–11

Bergeron C, Shah K, Daniel R, Ferenczy A (1988) Search for human papillomaviruses in normal, hyperplastic, and neoplastic endometria. Obstet Gynecol 72:383–386

Bergeron C, Ferenczy A, Richart R (1990) Underwear: contamination by human papillomaviruses. Am J Obstet Gynecol 162:25–29

Bibbo M, Dytch HE, Alenghat E, Bartels PH, Wied GL (1989) DNA ploidy profiles as prognostic indicators in CIN lesions. Am J Clin Pathol 92:261–264

Blau S, Hyman AB (1955) Erythroplasia of Queyrat. Acta Derm Venereol (Stockh) 35:341–378

Bogomoletz WV, Potet F, Molos G (1985) Condylomata acuminata, giant condyloma acuminatum (Buschke-Loewenstein tumour) and verrucous squamous carcinoma of the perianal and anorectal region: a continuous precancerous spectrum? Histopathology 9:1155–1169

Boon ME, Fox CH (1981) Simultaneous condyloma acuminatum and dyspalsia of the uterine cervix. Acta Cytol 25:393–399

Boon ME, Susanti I, Tasche MJA, Kok LP (1989) Human papillomavirus (HPV)-associated male and female genital carcinomas in a Hindu population. Cancer 64:559–566
Bornstein J, Kaufman RH, Adam E, Adler-Storthz K (1987) Human papillomavirus associated with vaginal intraepithelial neoplasia in women exposed to diethylstilbestrol in utero. Obstet Gynecol 70:75–80
Bornstein J, Kaufman RH, Adam E, Burek J, Adler-Storthz K (1988) Paget's disease of the vulva: search for herpes simplex virus antigens and human papillomavirus antigens and DNA. Gynecol Oncol 31:384–388
Boshart M, zur Hausen H (1986) Human papillomaviruses in Buschke-Löwenstein tumor: physical state of the DNA and identification of a tandem duplication in the noncoding region of a human papillomavirus 6 subtype. J Virol 58:963–966
Boshart M, Gissmann L, Ikenberg H, Kleinheinz A, Scheurlen W, zur Hausen H (1984) A new type of papillomavirus DNA, its presence in genital cancer biopsies and in cell lines derived from cervical cancer. EMBO J 3:1151–1157
Boutselis JG (1972) Intraepithelial carcinoma of the vulva. Am J Obstet Gynecol 113:733–738
Brandt CR, McDougall JK, Galloway DA (1987) Synergistic interactions between human papillomavirus type-18 sequences, herpes simplex virus infection, and chemical carcinogen, treatment. In: Steinberg BM, Brandsma JL and Teichman LB (eds) Cancer Cells 5. Cold Spring Harbor Laboratory, New York, pp 179–186
Bunting H (1953) Close-packed array of virus-like particles within cells of a human skin papilloma. Soc Exp Biol Med 84:327–332
Burk RD, Kadish AS, Calderin S, Romney SL (1986) Human papillomavirus infection of the cervix detected by cervicovaginal lavage and molecular hybridization: correlation with biopsy results and Papanicolaou smear. Am J Obstet Gynecol 154:982–990
Buscema J, Naghashfar Z, Sawada E, Daniel R, Woodruff D, Shah K (1988) The predominance of human papillomavirus type 16 in vulvar neoplasia. Obstet Gystet Gynecol 71:601–606
Byrne JC, Tsao M-S, Fraser RS, Howley PM (1987) Human papillomavirus-11 DNA in a patient with chronic laryngotracheobronchial papillomatosis and metastatic squamous-cell carcinoma of the lung. N Engl J Med 317:873–878
Carson LF, Twiggs LB, Fukushima M, Ostrow RS, Faras AJ, Okagaki T (1986) Human genital papillomavirus infections: an evaluation of immunologic competence in the genital neoplasia-papilloma syndrome. Am J Obstet Gynecol 155:784–789
Carson LF, Twiggs LB, Okagaki T, Clark BA, Ostrow RS, Faras AJ (1988) Human papillomavirus DNA in adenosquamous carcinoma and squamous cell carcinoma of the vulva. Obstet Gynecol 72:63–67
Chacho MS, Eppich E, Wersto R, Koss LG (1990) Influence of human papillomavirus on DNA ploidy determination in genital condylomas. Cancer 65:2291–2294
Choo K-B, Pan C-C, Lui M-S et al. (1987) Presence of episomal and integrated human papillomavirus DNA sequences in cervical carcinoma. J Med Virol 21:101–107
Choo YC, Morley GW (1980) Double primary epidermoid carcinoma of the vulva and cervix. Gynecol Oncol 9:324–333
Chow LT, Hirochika H, Nasseri M et al. (1987) Human papillomavirus gene expression. In: Steinberg BM, Brandsma JL and Teichman LB (eds) Cancer Cells 5. Cold Spring Harbor Laboratory, New York, pp 55–72
Ciuffo G (1907) Innesto positivo con filtrato di verruca volgare. Gior Ital 48:12
Costa J, Howley PM, Bowling MC, Howard R, Bauer WC (1981) Presence of human papilloma viral antigens in juvenile multiple laryngeal papilloma. Am J Clin Pathol 75:194–197
Cripe TP, Haugen TH, Turk JP et al. (1987) Transcriptional regulation of the human papillomavirus-16 E6–E7 promoter by a keratinocyte-dependent enhancer, and by viral E2 trans-activator and repressor gene products: implications for cervical carcinogenesis. EMBO J 6:3745–3753
Crum CP, Levine RU (1984) Human papillomvirus infection and cervical neoplasia: new perspectives. Int J Gynecol Pathol 3:376–388
Crum CP, Braun LA, Shah KV et al. (1982) Vulvar intraepithelial neoplasia: correlation of nuclear DNA content and the presence of a human papilloma virus (HPV) structural antigen. Cancer 49:468–471
Crum CP, Egawa K, Barron B, Fenoglio CM, Levine RU, Richart RM (1983a) Human papilloma virus infection (condyloma) of the cervix and cervical intraepithelial neoplasia: a histopathologic and statistical analysis. Gynecol Oncol 15:88–94
Crum CP, Egawa K, Fu YS et al. (1983b) Atypical immature metaplasia (AIM): a subset of human papilloma virus infection of the cervix. Cancer 12:2214–2219

Crum CP, Ikenberg H, Richart RM, Gissmann L (1984) Human papilloma virus type 16 and early cervical neoplasia. N Engl J Med 310:880–883
Crum CP, Mitao M, Levine RU, Silverstein S (1985) Cervical papillomaviruses segregate within morphologically distinct precancerous lesions. J Virol 54:675–681
Cubie HA, Norval M (1988) Humoral and cellular immunity to papillomavirus in patients with cervical dysplasia. J Med Virol 24:85–95
Davis JR, Moon LB (1975) Increased incidence of adenocarcinoma of uterine cervix. Obstet Gynecol 45:79–82
Dawson DF, Duckworth JK, Bernhardt H, Young JM (1965) Giant condyloma and verrucous carcinoma of the genital area. Arch Pathol 79:225–231
Dean P, Lancaster WE, Chun B, Jenson AB (1983) Human papillomavirus structural antigens in squamous papillomas of the male urethra. J Urol 129: 873–875
de Villiers E, Gissmann L, zur Hausen H (1981) Molecular cloning of viral DNA from human genital warts. J Virol 40:932–935
Downey GO, Okagaki T, Ostrow RS, Clark BA, Twiggs LB, Faras AJ (1988) Condylomatous carcinoma of the vulva with special reference to human papillomavirus DNA. Obstet Gynecol 72:68–73
Dunn AEG, Ogilvie MM (1968) Intranuclear virus particles in human genital wart tissues: observations on the ultrastructure of the epidermal layer. J Ultrastruct Res 22:282–295
Dürst M, Gissmann L, Ikenberg H, zur Hausen H (1983) A papillomavirus DNA from a cervical carcinoma and its prevalence in cancer biopsy samples from different geographic regions. Proc Natl Acad Sci USA 80:3812–3815
Dürst M, Croce CM, Gissmann L, Schwarz E, Huebner K (1987) Pappillomavirus sequences integrate near cellular oncogenes in some cervical carcinomas. Proc Natl Acad Sci USA 84:1070–1074
Dyson N, Howley PM, Munger K, Harlow E (1989) The human papilloma virus-16 E7 oncoprotein is able to bid to the retinoblastoma gene product. Science 243:934–936
Falco JG, Madamba AMR, de la Fuente F, Aparicio LA, Chacon MJ, Harguindey S (1987) Cervical mosaic and an integrated pathophysiological approach to early cervical neoplasia. J Biol Response Mod 6:473–483
Falcone T, Ferenczy A (1986) Cervical intraepithelial neoplasia and condyloma: an analysis of diagnostic accuracy of posttreatment follow-up methods. Am J Obstet Gynecol 154:260–262
Farnsworth A, Laverty C, Stoler MH (1989) Human papillomavirus messenger RNA expression in adenocarcinoma in situ of the uterine cervix. Int J Gynecol Pathol 8:321–330
Ferenczy A, Bergeron C, Richart RM (1989) Human papillomavirus DNA in fomites on objects used for the management of patients with genital human papillomavirus infections. Obstet Gynecol 74:950–954
Fletcher K, Cordiner JW, Macnab JCM (1986) Detection of sequences that hybridize to human cytomegalovirus DNA in cervical neoplastic tissue. Disease Markers 4:219–229
Follen MM, Levine RU, Carillo E, Richart RM, Nuovo G, Crum CP (1987) Colposcopic correlates of cervical papillomavirus infection. Am J Obstet Gynecol 157:809–814
Foye G, Marsh MR, Minkowitz S (1969) Verrucous carcinoma of the vulva. Obstet Gynecol 34:484–488
Franquemont DW, Ward BE, Andersin WA, Crum CP (1989) Predictions of "high risk" cervical papillomavirus infection by biopsy morphology. Am J Clin Pathol 92:577–582
Frick HC, Jacox HW, Taylor HC (1986) Primary carcinoma of the vagina. Am J Obstet Gynecol 101:695–703
Friedrich Jr EG, Wilkinson EJ, Fu YS (1980) Carcinoma in situ of the vulva: a continuing challenge. Am J Obstet Gynecol 136:830–842
Fu YS, Reagan J, Richart RM (1981) Definition of precursors. Gynecol Oncol 12:5220–5231
Fu YS, Lancaster WD, Richart RM, Reagan JW, Crum CP, Levine RU (1983) Cervical papillomavirus infection in diethylstilbestrol-exposed progeny. Obstet Gynecol 61:59–62
Fu YS, Chang L, Huang I, Huang S, Wiesmeier E, Wettstein F, Weissman M (1989) DNA ploidy analysis of cervical condyloma and intraepithelial neoplasia in specimens obtained by punch biopsy. Anal Quant Cytol Histol 11:187–195
Fuchs PG, Girardi F, Pfister H (1988) Human papillomavirus DNA in normal, metaplastic, preneoplastic and neoplastic epithelia of the cervix uteri. Int J Cancer 41:41–45
Fujii T, Crum CP, Winkler B, Fu YS, Richart RM (1984) Human papillomavirus infection and cervical intraepithelial neoplasia: histopathology and DNA content. Obstet Gynecol 63:99–104

Fukushima M, Okagaki T, Twiggs LB, Clark BA, Zachow KR, Ostrow RS, Faras AJ (1985) Histological types of carcinoma of the uterine cervix and detectability of human papillomavirus DNA. Cancer Res 45:3252–3255

Fukushima M, Yamakawa Y, Shimano S, Sawada Y, Hashimoto M, Fujinaga K (1990) Status of HPV integration in invasive carcinoma of the uterine cervix and CIN. Cancer 66:2115–2161

Furgyik S, Astedt B (1980) Gonorrheal infection followed by an increased frequency of cervical carcinoma. Acta Obstet Gynecol Scand 59:521–524

Gal D, Friedman M, Mitrani-Rosenbaum S (1989) Transmissibility and treatment failures of different types of human papillomavirus. Obstet Gynecol 73:308–310

Gall SA, Hughes CE, Trofatter K (1985) Interferon for the therapy of condyloma acuminatum. Am J Obstet Gynecol 153:157–162

Garden JM, O'Banion MK, Shelnitz LS, Pinski KS, Bakus AD, Reichmann ME, Sundberg JP (1988) Papillomavirus in the vapor of carbon dioxide laser-treated verrucae. JAMA 259:1199–1202

Gergely L, Gzegledy J, Hernady Z (1987) Human papillomavirus frequency in normal cervical tissue. Lancet II:513

Gissmann L, Wolnik K. Ikenberg H, Koldovsky U, Schnurch HG, zur Hausen H (1983) Human papillomavirus types 6 and 11 DNA sequences in genital and laryngeal papillomas and in some cervical cancers. Proc Natl Acad Sci USA 80:560–563

Gissmann L, Dürst M, Oltersdorf T, von Knebel G, Doeberitz M (1987) Human papillomaviruses and cervical cancer. In: Steinberg BM, Brandsma JL and Teichman LB (eds) Cancer Cells 5. Cold Spring Harbor Laboratory, New York, pp 275–280

Goldstein SC, Byrne JC, Rabson AS (1987) Human cytomegalovirus (HCMV) enhances bovine papilloma virus (BPV) transformation in vitro. J Med Virol 23:157–164

Göppinger A, Birmelin G, Ikenberg H, Elmenthaler U, Hilgarth M, Hillemanns HG, Wied GL (1987) Human papillomavirus standardization and DNA cytophotometry in cervical intraepithelial neoplasia. J Reprod Med 32:609–613

Graham JH, Helwig EB (1973) Erythroplasia of Queyrat: a clinicopathologic and histochemical study. Cancer 23:1396–1414

Green M, Brackmann KH, Sanders PR, Loewenstein PM, Freel JH, Eisinger M, Switlyk SA (1982) Isolation of a human papillomavirus from a patient with epidermodysplasia verruciformis: presence of related viral DNA genomes in human urogenital tumors. Med Sci 79:4437–4441

Grussendorf-Conen E-I, Cremer S (1990) The demonstration of human papillomavirus 16 genomes in the nuclei of genital cancers using two different methods of in situ hybridization. Cancer 65:238–241

Guillet GY, Braun L, Masse R, Aftimos J, Geniaux M, Texier L (1984) Bowenoid papulosis: demonstration of human papillomavirus (HPV) with anti-HPV immune serum. Arch Dermatol 120:514–516

Gupta J, Gendelman HE, Naghashfar Z et al. (1985) Specific identification of human papillomavirus type in cervical smears and paraffin sections by in situ hybridization with radioactive probes: a preliminary communication. Int J Gynecol Pathol 4:211–218

Hallden C, Majmudar B (1986) The relationship between juvenile laryngeal papillomatosis and maternal condylomata acuminata. J Reprod Med 31:804–807

Halpert R, Fruchter RG, Sedlis A, Butt K, Boyce JG, Sillman FH (1986) Human papillomavirus and lower genital neoplasia in renal transplant patients. Obstet Gynecol 68:251–258

Hare MJ, Taylor-Robinson D, Cooper P (1982) Evidence for an association between *Chlamydia trachomatis* and cervical intraepithelial neoplasia. Br J Obstet Gynecol 89:489–492

Heiles HBJ, Genersch E, Kessler C, Neumann R, Eggers HJ (1988) In situ hybridization with digoxigenin-labeled DNA of human papillomaviruses (HPV 16/18) in HeLa and SiHa cells. Biotechniques 6:978–981

Henry MJ, Stanley MW, Cruikshank S, Carson L (1989) Association of human immunodeficiency virus-induced immunosuppression with human papillomavirus infection and cervical intraepithelial neoplasia. Am J Obstet Gynecol 160:352–353

Howley PM, Schelegel R (1988) The human papillomavirus. Am J Med 85:155–158

Hudson JB, Bedell MA, McCance DJ, Laimins LA (1990) Immortalization and altered differentiation of human keratinocytes in vitro by the E6 and E7 open reading frames of human papillomavirus type 18. J Virol 64:519–526

Hughes RG, Neill WA, Norval M (1987) Nuclear DNA analysis of koilocytic and premalignant lesions of the uterine cervix. Br Med J 294:267–269

Hulka BS, Hulka JF (1967) Dyskaryosis in cervical cytology and its relationship to trichomoniasis therapy. Am J Obstet Gynecol 98:180–187
Ikic D, Kirhmajer V, Maricic Z et al. (1981) Application of human leucocyte interferon in patients with carcinoma of the uterine cervix. Lancet I:1027–1030
Ito Y, Evans CA (1961) Induction of tumors in domestic rabbits with nucleic acid preparations from partially purified Shope papilloma virus and from extracts of the papillomas of domestic and cottontail rabbits. J Exp Med 114:485–500
Jablonska S, Orth G, Jarzabek-Chorzelska M et al. (1979) Epidermodysplasia verruciformis versus disseminated verrucae planae: Is epidermodysplasia verruciformis a generalized infection with wart verrus? J Invest Dermatol 72:114–119
Jablonska S, Orth G, Croissant O, Obalek S (1985) The clinical morphology, pathology and immunology of papillomavirus infection of the skin or related to the virus types. In: Howley PH, Broker TR (eds) Papillomaviruses: molecular and clinical aspects. Allen R Liss, New York, pp 69–84
Japaze H, Dinh TV, Woodruff JD (1982) Verrucous carcinoma of the vulva: study of 24 cases. Obstet Gynecol 60:462–466
Jenson AB, Rosenthal JD, Olson C, Pass F, Lancaster WD, Shah K (1980) Immunologic relatedness of papillomaviruses from different species. JNCI 64:495–500
Kanbour AI, Klionsky B, Murphy AI (1974) Carcinoma of the vagina following cervical cancer. Cancer 34:1838–1841
Kanbour MS, Roman A (1988) Characterization of human papillomavirus type 6b DNA isolated from an invasive squamous carcinoma of the vulva. Virology 165:225–233
Katz HI, Posalaky Z, McGinley D (1978) Pigmented penile papules with carcinoma in situ changes. Br J Dermatol 99:155–162
Katz RL, Veanattukalathil S, Weiss KM (1987) Human papillomavirus infection and neoplasia of the cervix and anogenital region in women with Hodgkin's disease. Acta Cytol 31:845–854
Kaufman RH, Adam E (1986) Herpes simplex virus and human papillomavirus in the development of cervical carcinoma. Clin Obstet Gynecol 29:678–692
Kaufman RH, Bornstein J, Gordon AN, Adam E, Kaplan AL, Adler-Storthz K (1987) Detection of human papillomavirus DNA in advanced epithelial ovarian carcinoma. Gynecol Oncol 27:340–349
Kessler II (1974) Perspectives on the epidemiology of cervical cancer with special reference to herpesvirus hypothesis. Cancer Res 34:1091–1110
Kessler II (1981) Etiological concepts in cervical carcinogensis. Gynecol Oncol 12:s7–s24
Khoo SK, Mackay EV (1974) Immunologic reactivity of female patients with genital cancer: status in preinvasive, locally invasive, and disseminated disease. Am J Obstet Gynecol 119:1018–1025
Kidd JG, Rous P (1940) Cancers deriving from the virus papillomas of wild rabbits under natural conditions. J Exp Med 71:469–492
King LA, Tase T, Twiggs LB et al. (1989) Prognostic significance of the presence of human papillomavirus DNA in patients with invasive carcinoma of the cervix. Cancer 63:897–900
Kiryu H, Ackerman AB (1990) A critique of current classification of vulvar diseases. Am J Dermatopathol 12:377–392
Kjaer SK, de Villiers E, Haugaard BJ et al. (1988) Human papillomavirus, herpes simplex virus and cervical cancer incidence in Greenland and Denmark. A population-based cross-sectional study. Int J Cancer 41:518–524
Komorowski RA, Clowry LJ Jr (1976) Koilocytotic atypia of the cervix. Obstet Gynecol 47:540–544
Koss LG (1979) Diagnostic cytology and its histopathologic bases, 3rd edn. JB Lippincott, Philadelphia, pp 406–409
Koss LG, Durfee GR (1956) Unusual patterns of squamous epithelium of the uterine cervix: cytologic and pathologic study of koilocytotic atypia. Ann NY Acad Sci 63:1245–1261
Koutsky LA, Galloway DA, Holmes KK (1988) Epidemiology of genital human papillomavirus infection. Epidemiol Rev 10:122–163
Kovi J, Tillman RL, Lee SM (1974) Malignant transformation of condyloma acuminatum. Am J Exp Pathol 61:702–705
Krebs H-B, Schneider V (1987) Human papillomavirus-associated lesions of the penis: colposcopy, cytology, and histology. Obstet Gynecol 70:299–304
Kreider JW, Howett MK, Leure-Dupree AE, Zaino RJ, Weber JA (1987) Laboratory production in vivo of infectious human papillomavirus type 11. J Virol 61:590–593

Krzyzek RA, Watts SL, Anderson DL, Faras AJ, Pass F (1980) Anogenital warts contain several distinct species of human papillomavirus. J Virol 36:236–244
Kurihara M, Asano K (1956) The correlation between cancer of uterus and cancer of penis. Tohoku J Exp Med 64:104
Kurman RJ, Shah KH, Lancaster WD, Jenson AB (1981) Immunoperoxidase localization of papillomavirus antigens in cervical dysplasia and vulvar condylomas. Am J Obstet Gynecol 140:931–935
Kurman RJ, Sanz LE, Jenson AB, Perry S, Lancaster WD (1982) Papillomavirus infection of the cervix. I. Correlation of histology with viral structural antigens and DNA sequences. Int J Gynecol pathol. 1:17–28
Kurman RJ, Jenson AB, Lancaster WD (1983) Papillomavirus infection of the cervix. II. Relationship to intraepithelial neoplasia based on the presence of specific viral structural proteins. Am J Surg Pathol 7:39–52
Kurman RJ, Schiffman MH, Lancaster WD, Reid R, Jenson AB, Temple GF, Lorincz AT (1988) Analysis of individual human papillomavirus types in cervical neoplasia: a possible role for type 18 in rapid progression. Am J Obstet Gynecol 156:293–296
Lancaster WD, Olson C, Meinke W (1976) Quantitation of bovine papilloma viral DNA in viral-induced tumors. J Virol 17:824–831
Lancaster WD, Kurman RJ, Sanz LE, Perry SM, Jenson AB (1983) Human papillomavirus: detection of viral DNA sequences and evidence for molecular heterogeneity in metaplasias and dysplasia of the uterine cervix. Intervirology 20:202–212
Leake JF, Woodruff JD, Searle C, Daniel R, Shah KV, Currie JL (1989) Human papillomavirus and epithelial ovarian neoplasia. Gynecol Oncol 34:268–273
Lehn H, Villa LL Marziona F, Hilgarth M, Hillemans H-G, Sauer G (1988) Physical state and biological activity of human papillomavirus genomes in precancerous lesions of the female genital tract. J Gen Virol 69:187–196
Levine RU, Crum CP, Herman E, Silvers D, Ferenczy A, Richart RM (1984) Cervical papillomavirus infection and intraepithelial neoplasia: a study of male sexual partners. Obstet Gynecol 64:16–20
Lloyd KM (1970) Multicentric Bowen's disease of the groin. Arch Dermatol 101:48–51
Ludwig ME, Lowell DM, LiVolsi VA (1981) Cervical condylomatous atypia and its relationship to cervical neoplasia. Am J Clin Pathol 76:255–262
Lyell A, Miles JAR (1951) The myrmecia: a study of inclusion bodies in warts. Br Med J I:912–915
Maier RC, Norris HJ (1980) Coexistence of cervical intraepithelial neoplasia with primary adenocarcinoma of the endocervix. Obstet Gynecol 56:361–364
Martinez I (1969) Relationship of squamous cell carcinoma of the cervix uteri to squamous cell carcinoma of the penis among Puerto Rical women married to men with penile carcinoma. Cancer 24:777–780
McCance DJ, Walker PG, Dyson JL, Coleman DV, Singer A (1983) Presence of human papillomavirus DNA in cervical intraepithelial neoplasia (CIN). Br J Med 287:784–788
McCance DJ, Campion MJ, Clarkson PK, Chesters PM, Jenkins D, Singer A (1985) Prevalence of human papillomavirus type 16 DNA sequences in cervical intraepithelial neoplasia and invasive carcinoma of the cervix. Br J Obstet Gynecol 92:1101–1105
McCance DJ, Kalache A, Ashdown K, Andrade L, Menezes F, Smith P, Doll R (1986) Humanpapillomavirus types 16 and 18 in carcinomas of the penis from Brazil. Int J Cancer 37:55–59
McDonnell JM, Mayr AJ, Martin WJ (1989) DNA of human papillomavirus type 16 in dysplastic and malignant lesions of the conjuctiva and cornea. N Engl J Med 320:1442–1445
Meanwell CA, Blackledge G, Cox MF, Maitland NJ (1987) HPV 16 DNA in normal and malignant cervical epithelium: implications for the aetiology and behaviour of cervical neoplasia. Lancet I:703–707
Meisels A, Fortin R (1976) Condylomatous lesions of the cervix and vagina. I. Cytologic patterns. Acta Cytol 20:505–509
Meisels A, Fortin R, Roy M (1977) Condylomatous lesions of the cervix. II. Cytologic, colposcopic and histopathologic study. Acta Cytol 21:379–390
Meisels A, Roy M, Fortier M, Morin C, Cases-Cordero M, Shah KV, Turgeon H (1981) Human papillomavirus infection of the cervix. Acta Cytol 25:7–16
Mitchell H, Drake M, Medley G (1986) Prospective evaluation of risk of cervical cancer after cytological evidence of human papillomavirus infection. Lancet I:573–575

Mitrani-Rosenbaum S, Gal D, Friedman M, Kitron N, Tsvieli R, Mordel N, Anteby SO (1988) Papillomaviruses in lesions of the lower genital tract in Israeli patients. Eur J Cancer Clin Oncol 24:725–731
Moghissi KS, Mack HC, Porzak JP (1968) Epidemiology of cervical cancer: study of a prison population. Am J Obstet Gynecol 100:607–614
Møller BR, Johannesen P, Osther K, Ulmsteen U, Hastrup J, Berg K (1983) Treatment of dysplasia of the cervical epithelium with an interferon gel. Obstet Gynecol 62:625–629
Morgan D, Pecoraro G, Rosenberg I, Defendi V (1988) Transformation of C127 mouse fibroblasts by human papillomavirus 16. Cancer Res 48:2505–2511
Morin C, Bouchard C, Fortier M, Levesque R, Meisels A (1988) A colposcopical lesion of the uterine cervix frequently associated with papillomavirus type 16 as detected by in situ and southern blot hybridization: a cytohistological correlation study. Int J Cancer 41:531–536
Mounts P, Shah KV, Kashima H (1982) Viral etiology of juvenile-and adult-onset squamous papilloma of the larynx. Proc Natl Acad Sci USA 79:5425–5429
Nahmias HJ, Naib ZM, Josey W (1974) Epidemiological studies relating genital herpes infection to cervical carcinoma. Cancer Res 43:1111–1117
Naib ZM, Nahmias AJ, Josey WE, Kramer JH (1969) Genital herpetic infection: associations with cervical dysplasia and carcinoma. Cancer 23:940–945
Nair MK, Sankaranarayanan R, Pedmanabhan TK, Maduhu CS (1988) Oral verrucous carcinoma: treatment with radiotherapy. Cancer 61:458–461
Neary K, DiMaio D (1989) Open reading frames E6 and E7 of bovine papillomavirus type 1 are both required for full transformation of mouse C127 cells. J Virol 63:259–266
Noda T, Yajima H, Ito Y (1988) Progression of the phenotype of transformed cells after growth stimulation of cells by a human papillomavirus type 16 gene function. J Virol 62:313–324
Nuovo GJ, Richart RM (1989) Buffered formalin is the superior fixative for the detection of HPV DNA by in situ hybridization analysis. Am J Pathol 134:837–842
Nuovo GJ, Nuovo MA, Cottral S, Gordon S, Silverstein SJ, Crum CP (1988) Histological correlates of clinically occult human papillomavirus infection of the uterine cervix. Am J Surg Pathol 12:198–204
Nuovo GJ, Cottral S, Richart RM (1989) Occult human papillomavirus infection of the uterine cervix in postmenopausal women. Am J Obstet Gynecol 160:340–344
Nyeem R, Wilkinson EJ, Grover LJ (1982) Condylomata acuminata of the cervix: histopathology and association with cervical neoplasia. Int J Gynecol Pathol 1:498–501
Okagaki T (1984) Female genital tumors associated with human papillomavirus infection, and the concept of genital neoplasm-papilloma syndrome (GENPS). Pathol Annu 19:31–62
Okagaki T, Izuo M (1978) Correction of the model DNA values obtained by microscopophotomedy and tests for their shifts. JNCI 60:1251–1258
Okagaki T, Twiggs LB, Zachow KR, Clark BA, Ostrow RS, Faras AJ (1983) Identification of human papillomavirus DNA in cervical and vaginal intraepithelial neoplasia with molecularly cloned virus specific DNA probes. Int J Gynecol Pathol 2:153–159
Okagaki T, Clark B, Zachow KR, Twiggs LB, Ostrow RS, Pass F, Faras AJ (1984) Presence of human papillomavirus in verrucous carcinoma (Ackerman) of the vagina. Arch Pathol Lab Med 108:567–570
Okagaki T, Tase T, Twiggs LB, Carson LF (1989) Histogenesis of cervical adenocarcinoma with reference to human papillomavirus-18 as a carcinogen. J Reprod Med 34:639–644
Olson C, Olson O (1985) Transmissible animal papillomas. In: Howley PM, Broker TR (eds) Papillomaviruses: molecular and clinical aspects. Alan R Liss, New York, pp 279–298
Orth G, Jablonska S, Jarzabek-Chorzelska M, Obalek S, Rzesa G, Favre M, Croissant O (1979) Characteristics of the lesions and risk papillomavirus involved in epidermodysplasia verruciformis. Cancer Res 39:1074–1082
Ostrow RS, Zachow K, Webber D et al. (1985) Presence and possible involvement of HPA DNA in premalignant and malignant tumors. In: Howley PM, Broker TR (eds) Papillomaviruses: molecular and clinical aspects. Alan R Liss, New York, pp 101–124
Ostrow RS, Zachow KR, Niimura M, Okagaki T, Muller S, Bender M, Faras AJ (1986) Detection of papillomavirus DNA in human semen. Science 231:731–733
Ostrow RS, Manias DA, Clark BA, Okagaki T, Twiggs LB, Faras AJ (1987) Detection of human papillomavirus DNA in invasive carcinomas of the cervix by in situ hybridization. Cancer Res 47:649–653

Ostrow RS, Manias DA, Clark BA, Fukushima M, Okagaki T, Twiggs LB, Faras AJ (1988) The analysis of carcinomas of the vagina for human papillomavirus DNA. Int J Gynecol Pathol 7:308–314

Padel AF, Venning VA, Evans MF, Quantrill AM, Fleming KA (1990) Human papillomaviruses in anogenital warts in children: typing by in situ hybridisation. Br Med J 300:1491–1494

Pater MM, Pater A (1985) Human papillomavirus types 16 and 18 sequences in carcinoma cell lines of the cervix. Virology 145:313–318

Pater MM, Dunne J, Hogan G, Ghatage P, Pater A (1986) Human papillomavirus types 16 and 18 sequences in early cervical neoplasia. Virology 155:13–18

Pater MM, Hughes GA, Hyslop DE, Nakshatri H, Pater A (1988) Glucocorticoid-dependent oncogenic transformation by type 16 but not type 11 human papilloma virus DNA. Nature 335:832–835

Pelling JC, Neades R, Strawhecker J (1988) Epidermal papillomas and carcinomas induced in uninitiated mouse skin by tumor promoters alone contain a point mutation in the 61st codon of the Ha-*ras* oncogene. Carcinogenesis 9:665–667

Peters RK, Chao A, Mack TM, Thomas D, Bernstein L, Henderson BE (1986) Increased frequency of adenocarcinoma of the uterine cervix in young women in Los Angeles Country. JNCI 76:423–428

Pfister H (1987) Human papillomaviruses and genital cancer. Adv Cancer Res 48:113–147

Pilotti S, delle Torre G, Rilke F, de Palo G, Shah KV (1984) Immunohistochemical and ultrastructural evidence of papilloma virus infection associated with in situ and microinvasive squamous cell carcinoma of the vulva. Am J Surg Pathol 8:751–761

Pilotti S, Gupta J Stefanon B, de Palo G, Shah KV, Rilke F (1989) Study of multiple human papillomavirus-related lesions of the lower female genital tract by in situ hybridization. Hum Pathol 20:118–122

Pirisi L, Yasumoto S, Feller M, Doniger J, DiPaolo JA (1987) Transformation of human fibroblasts and keratinocytes with human papillomavirus type 16 DNA. J Virol 61:1061–1066

Popescu NC, Amsbaugh SC, DiPaolo JA (1987) Human papillomavirus type 18 DNA is integrated at a single chromosome site in cervical carcinoma cell line SW756. J Virol 51:1682–1685

Porreco R, Penn I, Droegemueller W, Greer B, Makowski E (1975) Gynecologic malignancies in immunosuppressed organ homograft recipients. J Obstet Gynecol 45:359–364

Prakash SS, Reeves WC, Sissor GR et al. (1985) Herpes simplex virus type 2 and human papillomavirus type 16 in cervicitis, dysplasia and invasive cervical carcinoma. Int J Cancer 35:51–57

Purola E, Savia E (1977) Cytology of gynecologic condyloma acuminatum. Acta Cytol 21:26–31

Quick CA, Faras A, Krzysek R (1978) The etiology of laryngeal papillomatosis. Laryngoscope 88:1789–1795

Rando RF, Sedlacek TV, Hunt J, Jenson AB, Kurman RJ, Lancaster WE (1986a) Verrucous carcinoma of the vulva associated with an unusual type 6 human papillomavirus. Obstet Gynecol 67:71s–74s

Rando RF, Groff DE, Chirikjian JG, Lancaster WD (1986b) Isolation and characterization of a novel human papillomavirus type 6 DNA from an invasive vulvar carcinoma. J Virol 57:353–356

Rastkar G, Okagaki T, Twiggs LB, Clark BA (1982) Early invasive and in situ warty carcinoma of the vulva: clinical, histologic, and electron microscopic study with particular reference to viral association. Am J Obstet Gynecol 143:814–820

Rawls WE, Laurel D, Melnick JL, Glicksman JM, Kaufman RH (1968) A search for viruses in smegma, premalignant and early malignant cervical tissues. The isolation of herpesviruses with distinct antigenic properties. Am J Epidemiol 87:647–655

Reeves WC, Brinton LA, Garcia M et al. (1989) Human papillomavirus infection and cervical cancer in Latin America. N Engl J Med 320:1437–1440

Reid R, Scalzi P (1985) Genital warts and cervical cancer. VII. An improved colposcopic index for differentiating benign papillomaviral infections from high-grade cervical intraepithelial neoplasia. Am J Obstet Gynecol 153:611–618

Reid R, Laverty CR, Coppleson M, Isarangkul W, Hills E (1980) Condylomatous cervical wart virus infection. Obstet Gynecol 55:476–483

Reid R, Stanhope CR, Herschman BR, Booth E, Phibbs GD, Smith JP (1982) Genital warts and cervical cancer I. Evidence of an association between subclinical papillomavirus infection and cervical malignancy. Cancer 50:377–387

Reid R, Crum CP, Herschman BR et al. (1984) Genital warts and cervical cancer. III. Subclinical papillomaviral infection and cervical neoplasia are linked by a spectrum of continuous morphologic and biologic change. Cancer 53:943–953
Reid R, Greenburg M, Jenson AB et al. (1987) Sexually transmitted papillomavirus infections. I. The anatomic distribution and pathologic grade of neoplastic lesions associated with different viral types. Am J Obstet Gynecol 156:212–222
Ridley CM, Frankman O, Jones ISC et al. (1989) Correspondence. Hum Pathol 20:495–496
Rigoni-Stern (1942) Falli statistici relativi alle mellattie cancerose. Gior Servire Progr Path Terep 2:507
Røjel J (1953) Previous clinical and experimental investigations into the relations between cancer and syphilis. Acta Pathol Microbiol Scand suppl 97:13–25
Saiki RK, Gelfand DH, Stoffel S et al. (1988) Primer-directed enzymatic amplification of DNA with a thermostable DNA polymerase. Proc Natl Acad Sci USA 85:4869–4873
Saito K, Saito A, Fu YS, Smotkin D, Gupta J, Shah K (1987) Topographic study of cervical condyloma and intraepithelial neoplasia. Cancer 59:2064–2070
Sato S, Okagaki T, Clark BA, Twiggs LB, Fukushima M, Ostrow RS, Faras AJ (1986) Sensitivity of koilocytosis, immunocytochemistry, and electron microscopy as compared to DNA hybridization in detecting human papillomavirus in cervical and vaginal condyloma and intraepithelial neoplasia. Int J Gynecol Pathol 5:297–307
Sato S, Yajima A, Tase T, Okagaki T (1989) Human papillomavirus infection and uterine cervical carcinoma. Therapy in Gynecol 59:375–381
Schachter J, Hill EC, King EB, Heilbron DC, Ray RM, Margolis AJ, Greenwood SA (1982) *Chlamydia trachomatis* and cervical neoplasia. JAMA 248:2134–2138
Schlegel R, Wade-Glass M, Rabson MS, Yang Y-C (1986) The E5 transforming gene of bovine papillomavirus encodes a small, hydrophobic polypeptide. Science 233:464–468
Schmauz R, Findlay M, Lalwak A, Katsumbira N, Buxton E (1977) Variation in appearance of giant condyloma in a Ugandan series of cases of carcinoma of the penis. Cancer 40:1686–1696
Schmauz R, Elsasser E, Lalwak A, Cordes B (1978) Spitze Kondylome und Karzinome der Vulva, Vagina und des Penis. Geburtshilfe Frauenheilkd 38:342–351
Schmauz R, Claussen CP, Cordes B, Owor R (1983) Condylomata acuminata and their possible relation to cancer of the uterine cervix: case report and geographic observations. Acta Cytol 27:533–539
Schneider A, Kraus H, Schumann R, Gissmann L (1985) Papillomavirus infection of the lower genital tract: detection of viral DNA in gynecological swabs. Int J Cancer 35:443–448
Schneider A, de Villiers E-M, Schneider V (1987a) Multifocal squamous neoplasia of the female genital tract: significance of human papillomavirus infection of the vagina after hysterectomy. Obstet Gynecol 70:294–298
Schneider A, Holz M, Gissmann L (1987b) Increased prevalence of human papillomaviruses in the lower genital tract of pregnant women. Int J Cancer 40:198–201
Schneider A, Oltersdorf T, Schneider V, Gissmann L (1987c) distribution pattern of human papilloma virus 16 genome in cervical neoplasia by molecular in situ hybridization of tissue sections. Int J Cancer 39:717–721
Schneider A, Sterzik K, Buck G, de Villiers E-M (1988) Colposcopy is superior to cytology for the detection of early genital human papillomavirus infection. Obstet Gynecol 71:236–241
Schneider V, Kay S, Lee HM (1983) Immunosuppression as a high-risk factor in the development of condyloma acuminatum and squamous neoplasia of the cervix. Acta Cytol 27:220–224
Schneider-Gädlicke A, Kaul S, Schwarz E, Gausepohl H, Frank R, Bastert G (1988) Identification of the human papillomavirus type 18 E6* and E6 proteins in nuclear protein fractions from human cervical carcinoma cells grown in the nude mouse or in vitro. Int J Cancer 48:2969–2974
Schwartz SM, Weiss NS (1986) Increased incidence of adenocarcinoma of the cervix in young women in the United States. Am J Epidemiol 124:1045–1047
Schwarz E, Freese UK, Gissmann L, Mayer W, Roggenbuck B, Stremlau A, zur Hausen H (1985) Structure and transcription of human papillomavirus sequences in cervical carcinoma cells. Nature 314:111–114
Sebastian JA, Leeb BO, See R (1978) Cancer of the cervix—a sexually transmitted disease: cytologic screening in a prostitute population. Am J Obstet Gynecol 131:620–622
Sedlacek TV, Lindheim S, Eder C, Hasty L, Woodland M, Ludomirsky A, Rando RF (1989) Mechanism for human papillomavirus transmission from birth. Am J Obstet Gynecol 161:55–58

Seedorf K, Oltersdorf T, Krammer G, Rowekamp W (1987) Identification of early proteins of the human papilloma viruses type 16 (HPV 16) and type 18 (HPV 18) in cervical carcinoma cells. EMBO J 6:139–144
Serra A (1924) Studi sul virus della verruca, del papilloma, del condiloma acuminato. Giorn Ital Mal Venereal 65:1808–1814
Seski JC, Reinhalter ER, Silva J (1978) Abnormalities of lymphocyte transformation in women with condylomata acuminata. Obstet Gynecol 51:188–192
Shafeek MA, Osman MI, Hussein MA (1979) Carcinoma of the vulva arising in condylomata acuminata. Obstet Gynecol 54:120–124
Shibata DK, Arnheim N, Martin WJ (1988a) Detection of human papilloma virus in paraffin-embedded tissue using the polymerase chain reaction. J Exp Med 167:225–230
Shibata DK, Fu YS, Gupta JW, Shah KV, Arnheim N, Martin WJ (1988b) Detection of human papillomavirus in normal and dysplastic tissue by the polymerase chain reaction. Lab Invest 59:555–559
Shirasawa H, Tomita Y, Kubota K, Kasai T, Sekiya S, Takamizawa H, Simizu B (1986) Detection of human papillomavirus type 16 and evidence for integration into the cell DNA in cervical dysplasia. J Gen Virol 67:2011–2915
Shirasawa H, Tomita Y, Sekiya S, Takamizawa H, Simizu B (1987) Integration and transcription of human papillomavirus type 16 and 18 sequences in cell lines derived from cervical carcinomas. J Gen Virol 68:583–591
Shokri-Tabibzadeh S, Koss LG, Molnar J, Romney S (1981) Association of human papillomavirus with neoplastic processes in the genital tract of four women with impaired immunity. Gynecol Oncol 12:s129
Shope RE (1933) Infectious papillomatosis of rabbits. J Exp Med 58:606–624
Sillman FH, Sedlis A (1987) Anogenital papillomavirus infection and neoplasia in immunodeficient women. Obstet Gynecol Clin North Am 14:537–558
Sillman FH, Stanek A, Sedlis A et al. (1984) The relationship between human papillomavirus and lower genital intraepithelial neoplasia in immunosuppressed women. Am J Obstet Gynecol 150:300–308
Singer A, Reid BL, Coppleson M (1976) A hypothesis: the role of a high-risk male in the etiology of cervical carcinoma. Am J Obstet Gynecol 126:110–114
Skinner MS, Sternberg WH, Ichinose H, Collins J (1973) Spontaneous regression of Bowenoid atypia of the vulva. Obstet Gynecol 42:40–46
Smith WG (1981) Invasive cancer of the vagina. Clin Obstet Gynecol 24:503–515
Smotkin D, Berek JS, Fu YS, Hacker NF, Major FJ, Wettstein FO (1986) Human papillomavirus deoxyribonucleic acid in adenocarcinoma and adenosquamous carcinoma of the uterine cervix. Obstet Gynecol 68:241–244
Southern EM (1975) Detection of specific sequences among DNA fragments separated by gel electrophoresis. J Mol Biol 98:503–520
Spence RP, Murray A, Banks L, Kelland LR, Crawford L (1988) Analysis of human papillomavirus sequences in cell lines recently derived from cervical cancers. Cancer Res 48:324–328
Spitzer M, Chernys AE, Hirschfield L et al. (1990) Assessment of criteria used in the histologic diagnosis of human papillomavirus-related disease of the female lower genital tract. Gynecol Oncol 38:105–109
Stern E, Lachenbruch PA, Dixon WJ (1967) Cancer of the uterine cervix. II. A biometric approach to etiology. Cancer 20:190–200
Stoler MH, Broker TR (1986) In situ hybridization detection of human papillomavirus DNAs and messenger RNAs in genital condylomas and a cervical carcinoma. Hum Pathol 17:1250–1258
Strauss MJ, Shaw EW, Bunting H, Melnick JL (1949) "Crystalline" virus-like particles from skin papillomas characterized by intranuclear inclusion bodies. Soc Exp Biol Med 72:46–50
Sutton GP, Stehman FB, Ehrlich CE, Roman A (1987) Human papillomavirus deoxyribonucleic acid in lesions of the female genital tract: evidence for type 6/11 in squamous carcinoma of the vulva. Obstet Gynecol 70:564–568
Syrjänen KJ (1979) Morphologic survey of the condylomatous lesions in dysplastic and neoplastic epithelium of the uterine cervix. Arch Gynecol 227:153–161
Syrjänen KJ (1983) Immunocompetent cells in uterine cervical lesions of human papillomavirus origin. Gynecol Obstet Invest 16:327–340
Syrjänen KJ, Syrjänen SM (1985) Human papilloma virus (HPV) infections related to cervical intraepithelial neoplasia (CIN) and squamous cell carcinoma of the uterine cervix. Ann Clin Res 17:45–56

Syrjänen K, Mantyjarvi R, Vayrynen M et al. (1986a) Coexistent chlamydial infections related to natural history of human papillomavirus lesion in uterine cervix. Genitourin Med 62:345–351
Syrjänen S, Syrjänen K, Mantyjarvi R, Parkkinen S, Vayrynen M, Saarikoski S, Castren O (1986b) Human papillomavirus (HPV) DNA sequences demonstrated by in situ DNA hybridization in serial paraffin-embedded cervical biopsies. Arch Gynecol 239:39–48
Tase T, Oikawa N, Toki T, Wada T, Yajima A (1986) Interrelations between vulvar condylomata and cervical pathology, and a study of the sexual partners. J Jpn Soc Clin Cytol 25:683–689
Tase T, Okagaki T, Clark BA, Manias DA, Ostrow RS, Twiggs LB, Faras AJ (1988a) Human papillomavirus types and localization in adenocarcinoma and adenosquamous carcinoma of the uterine cervix: a study by in situ DNA hybridization. Cancer Res 48:993–998
Tase T, Sato S, Wada Y, Yajima A, Okagaki T (1988b) Prevalence of human papillomavirus type 18 DNA in adenocarcinoma and adenosquamous carcinoma of the uterine cervix occurring in Japan. Tohoku J Exp Med 156:47–53
Tase T, Okagaki T, Clark BA, Twiggs LB, Ostrow RS, Faras AJ (1989a) Human papillomavirus DNA in adenocarcinoma in situ, microinvasive adenocarcinoma of the uterine cervix, and coexisting cervical squamous intraepithelial neoplasia. Int J Gynecol Pathol 8:8–17
Tase T, Okagaki T, Clark BA, Twiggs LB, Ostrow RS, Faras AJ (1989b) Human papillomavirus DNA in glandular dysplasia and microglandular hyperplasia: presumed precursors of adenocarcinoma of the uterine cervix. Obstet Gynecol 73:1005–1008
Tay SK, Jenkins D, Maddox P, Singer A (1987) Lymphocyte phenotypes in cervical intraepithelial neoplasia and human papillomavirus infection. Br J Obstet Gynecol 94:16–21
Tidy JA, Mason WP, Farrell PJ (1989a) A new and sensitive method of screening for human papillomavirus infection. Obstet Gynecol 74:410–413
Tidy JA, Parry GCN, Ward P, Coleman DV, Peto J, Malcolm ADB, Farrell PJ (1989b) High rate of human papillomavirus type 16 infection in cytologically normal cervices. Lancet I:434
Trevathan E, Layde P, Webster LA, Adams JB, Benigno BB, Ory H (1983) Cigarette smoking and dysplasia and carcinoma in situ of the uterine cervix. JAMA 250:499–502
Trillo A, Guha A (1988) Solitary condylomatous papilloma of the bronchus. Arch Pathol Lab Med 112:731–733
Tsou K-C, Hong D-H, Varello M et al. (1984) Flow cytometric DNA analysis as a diagnostic aid for cervical condyloma and cancer. Cancer 54:1778–1787
Twiggs LB, Okigaki T, Clark B, Fukushima M, Ostrow R, Faras AJ (1988) A clinical, histopathologic, and molecular biologic investigation of vulvar intraepithelial neoplasia. Int J Gynecol Pathol 7:48–55
Ulbright TM, Stehman FB, Roth LM, Ehrlich CE, Ransburg RC (1982) Bowenoid dysplasia of the vulva. Cancer 50:2910–2919
Underwood JW, Adcock LL, Okagaki T (1978) Adenosquamous carcinoma of skin appendages (adenoid squamous cell carcinoma, pseudoglandular squamous cell carcinoma, adenoacanthoma of sweat gland of Lever) of the vulva; clinical and ultrastructural study. Cancer 42:1851–1858
Vallejos H, del Mistro A, Kleinhaus S, Braunstein JD, Halwar M, Koss LG (1987) Characterization of human papilloma virus types in condylomata acuminata in children by in situ hybridization. Lab Invest 56:611–615
Vayrynen M, Syrjänen K, Castren O, Saarikoski S, Mantyjarvi R (1985) Colposcopy in women with papillomavirus lesions of the uterine cervix. Obstet Gynecol 65:409–414
Viac J, Chardonnet Y, Gilgenkrantz H, Leval J, Thivolet J (1987) Effect of human papillomavirus infection of epithelial antigen expression in cutaneous and mucosal lesions. Epithelia 1:5–16
Villa LL, Lopes A (1986) Human papillomavirus DNA sequences in penile carcinomas in Brazil. Int J Cancer 37:853–855
Wade TR, Kopf AW, Ackerman AB (1978) Bowenoid papulosis of the penis. Cancer 42:1890–1903
Wagner D, Ikenberg H, Boehm N, Gissmann L (1984) Identification of human papillomavirus in cervical swabs by deoxyribonucleic acid in situ hybridization. Obstet Gynecol 64:767–772
Walboomers JMM, Melchers WJG, Mullink H et al. (1988) Sensitivity of in situ detection with biotinylated probes of human papilloma virus type 16 DNA in frozen tissue sections of squamous cell carcinomas of the cervix. Am J Pathol 131:587–594
Walker J, Bloss JD, Liao S-Y, Berman M, Bergen S, Wilczynski SP (1989) Human papillomavirus genotype as a prognostic indicator in carcinoma of the uterine cervix. Obstet Gynecol 74:781–785
Warhol MJ, Pinkus GS, Rice RH, El-Tawil GH, Lancaster WD, Jenson AB, Kurman RJ (1984) Papillomavirus infection of the cervix. III. Relationship of the presence of viral structural proteins to the expression of involucrin. Int J Gynecol Pathol 3:71–81

Watanabe S, Yoshiike K (1988) Transformation of rat 3YI cells by human papillomavirus type-18 DNA. Int J Cancer 41:896–900
Watts KC, Husain OAN, Campion MJ et al. (1987) Quantitative DNA analysis of low grade cervical intraepithelial neoplasia and human papillomavirus infection by static and flow cytometry. Br J Med 295:1090–1092
Watts SL, Phelps WC, Ostrow RS, Zachow KR, Faras AJ (1984) Cellular transformation by human papillomavirus DNA in vitro. Science 225:634–636
Werness BA, Levine AJ, Howley PM (1990) Association of human papillomavirus types 16 and 18 E6 proteins with p53. Science 248:76–80
Wickenden C, Malcolm ADB, Steele A, Coleman DV (1985) Screening for wart virus infection in normal and abnormal cervices by DNA hybridization of cervical scrapes. Lancet I:65–67
Wilczynski SP, Bergen S, Walker J, Liao S-Y, Pearlman LF (1988a) Human papillomaviruses and cervical cancer: analysis of histopathologic features associated with different viral types. Hum Pathol 19:697–704
Wilczynski SP, Walker J Liao S-Y, Bergen S, Berman M (1988b) Adenocarcinoma of the cervix associated with human papillomavirus. Cancer 62:1331–1336
Wile UJ, Kingery LB (1919) The etiology of common warts. JAMA 73:970–973
Willet GD, Kurman RJ, Reid R, Greenberg M, Jenson AB, Lorincz AT (1989) Correlation of the histologic appearance of intraepithelial neoplasms of the cervix with human papillomavirus types. Int J Gynecol Pathol 8:18–25
Winkelstein W, Shillitoe EJ, Brand R, Johnson KK (1984) Further comments on cancer of the uterine cervix, smoking, and herpesvirus infection. J Epidemiol 119:1–7
Winkler B, Crum CP, Fujii T et al. (1984) Koilocytotic lesions of the cervix: the relationship of mitotic abnormalities to the presence of papillomavirus antigens and nuclear DNA content. Cancer 53:1081–1087
Yang Y-C, Okayama H, Howley PM (1985) Bovine papillomavirus contains multiple transforming genes. Proc Natl Acad Sci USA 82:1030–1034
Yee C, Krishnan-Hewlett I, Baker CC, Schlegel R, Howley PM (1985) Presence and expression of human papillomavirus sequences in human cervical carcinoma cell lines. Am J Pathol 119:361–366
Yoshikawa H, Matsukura T, Yamamoto E, Kawana T, Mizuno M, Yoshiike K (1985) Occurrence of human papillomavirus types 16 and 18 DNA in cervical carcinomas from Japan: age of patients and histological hype of carcinomas. Jpn J Cancer Res 76:667–671
Zachow KR, Ostrow RS, Bender M, Watts S, Okagaki T, Pass F, Faras AJ (1982) Detection of human papillomavirus DNA in anogenital neoplasms. Nature 300:771–773
Zelickson AS, Prawer SE (1980) Bowenoid papulosis of the penis: demonstration of intranuclear viral-like particles. Am J Dermatopathol 2:305–308
Zuna R (1984) Association of condylomas with intraepithelial and microinvasive cervical neoplasia: histopathology of conization and hysterectomy specimens. Int J Gynecol Pathol 2:364–372
zur Hausen H (1977) Human papillomavirus and their possible role in squamous cell carcinomas. Curr Top Microbiol Immunol 78:1–30
zur Hausen H (1982) Human genital cancer: synergism between two virus infections or synergism between a virus infection and initiation events? Lancet II:1370–1372

# Neuroendocrine Carcinoma of the Uterus

G. UEDA and M. YAMASAKI



## 1 Introduction

The production of hormones by cervical carcinomas has been reported, albeit infrequently, since 1961 (BERTHELOT et al. 1961); these tumors are now considered to be neuroendocrine carcinomas. Until now, more than 140 cases have been described in case reports or in clinicopathologic analyses. Similar neuroendocrine tumors are also known to develop in the endometrium.

Adenocarcinomas with neuroendocrine cells have been reported quite frequently in the endometrium, but only occasionally in the cervix. Although it is questionable to include them in the spectrum of neuroendocrine carcinomas, these tumors will also be reviewed in this chapter.

## 2 Nomenclature

There has been some confusion about the terminology of cervical neuroendocrine carcinomas. They have been variously named according to characteristic morphologic features defined by light and electron microscopy, argyrophil stainability, and expression of neuroendocrine markers.

Current Topics in Pathology
Volume 85, Ed. N. Sasano

The term “carcinoid” was first suggested in 1972 by ALBORES-SAAVEDRA et al. (1979) in respect of a small cell carcinoma with neuroendocrine differentiation, and has frequently been used in later papers. The term “carcinoid” was coined by OBERNDORFER in 1907 to describe gastrointestinal tract tumors, most often in the appendix, which to some extent resemble carcinomas but which rarely metastasize. Histologically, these tumors exhibit the classical architecture of solid cellular clusters and/or ribbons, minimal pleomorphism of cells, and rare mitosis. It subsequently became apparent that some of the tumors resembling carcinoids architecturally behave in an aggressive fashion. The term “atypical carcinoid” (ARRIGONI et al. 1972) was introduced to designate such tumors of the lung, which are characterized histologically by increased mitotic activity, organoid (carcinoid-like) architecture, and the absence or limited extent of necrosis. However, “carcinoid” tumors of the cervix are much less differentiated than classical carcinoid tumors even in well-differentiated variants, as has already been pointed out by ALBORES-SAAVEDRA et al. (1979). In addition, the majority of the cervical tumors thus far reported have been highly aggressive, as will be discussed later. Therefore, the term “carcinoid” seems misleading clinically and pathologically for most neuroendocrine carcinomas of the cervix.

“Argyrophil cell carcinoma” and “apudoma” were introduced by TATEISHI et al. in 1975. These or similar names such as “argyrophilic carcinoma” (STASSART et al. 1982) and “argyrophil small cell carcinoma” (YAMASAKI et al. 1984) were used quite frequently in subsequent literature. Argyrophilia is considered to be one of the most reliable indicators of neuroendocrine cells that store neuropeptides and/or biogenic amines, but it is not highly sensitive and at times may not even be specific (GRIMELIUS and WILANDER 1980). Argyrophilia is known to be related nonspecifically to lipofuscin (WAXMAN et al. 1979), lactalbumin (CLAYTON et al. 1982), mucin (AGUIRRE et al. 1984; BANNATYNE et al. 1983; SATAKE et al. 1982), and glycogen (AGUIRRE et al. 1984; INOUE et al. 1984b; UEDA et al. 1984b). Moreover, some neuroendocrine cells lack argyrophilia (GRIMELIUS and WILANDER 1980). Therefore, we cannot rely solely on argyrophil reactions to diagnose neuroendocrine carcinomas of the cervix.

“Small cell carcinoma” is a term applied simply from a morphologic viewpoint and used with or without accompanying descriptions which explain the nature of the tumor in more detail (JONES et al. 1976; MACKAY et al. 1979; GROBEN et al. 1985; GERSELL et al. 1988). “Oat cell carcinoma” (JACOBS et al. 1980) may be included in this category. These terms were employed because neuroendocrine carcinomas of the cervix display histologic and biologic similarities to small cell or oat cell carcinomas of the lung. The classification of small cell lung cancer has been changing, and subdivision into the following three subtypes has recently been proposed: small cell carcinoma including the previous oat cell intermediate types, mixed small cell/large cell carcinoma, and combined small cell carcinoma (HIRSCH et al. 1988). However, the term "small cell carcinoma" has been generally used to refer to the samll cell nonkeratinizing type of squamous cell carcinoma of the cervix in the widely used classification originally proposed by REAGAN et al. in 1957, although one-third of such carcinomas have been reported to be neuroendocrine in nature (VAN NAGELL et al. 1988). In addition to neuroendocrine tumors, small cell carcinomas may include various nonneuroendocrine tumors such as basaloid carcinoma (FERRY and SCULLY 1988) and reserve cell carcinoma (GROBEN et al. 1985) or small cell undifferentiated carcinoma without neuroendocrine differentiation (ALBORES-SAAVEDRA et al. 1979; FUJII et al. 1986). On the other hand, neuroendocrine carcinoma has actually be diagnosed as small cell nonkeratinizing carcinoma (JONES et al. 1976). Furthermore, tumors diagnosed initially as adenosquamous carcinoma (MILES et al. 1982) or even squamous cell carcinoma (STAHL et al. 1981) have been revealed to be neuroendocrine in nature. Therefore, morphologic terms may not be adequate for the tumors under discussion.

The terms "neuroendocrine carcinoma" (PAZDUR et al. 1981; TURNER et al. 1986; SHEETS et al. 1988; WALKER et al. 1988; CHAN et al. 1989) and "endocrine carcinoma" (JOHANNESSEN et al. 1980; SILVA et. al. 1984) are major designations of function rather than morphology. In the gastrointestinal tract, "neuroendocrine carcinoma" was defined as a malignant epithelial neoplasm whose predominant pattern of differentiation is neuroendocrine, but excluding carcinoids, atypical carcinoids, and adenocarcinomas with neuroendocrine cells (GOULD et al. 1984). In the lung, the similarities of oat cell carcinomas with bronchial carcinoids were first pointed out in 1968 by BENSCH et al. GOULD et al. (1983) proposed a classification of the spectrum of neuroendocrine pulmonary neoplasms, dividing them into four categories, namely, carcinoids, well-differentiated neuroendocrine carcinomas, neuroendocrine carcinomas of intermediate cell type, and neuroendocrine carcinomas of small cell type. Neuroendocrine carcinomas of intermediate and small cell type were similarly aggressive and differed only in size and tumor cell arrangement, but the well-differentiated types were distinct entities and distinguishable from intermediate/small cell neuroendocrine carcinomas by virtue of their consistently recognizable organoid architecture as well as the absence or limited extent of necrosis (WARREN et al. 1988). Since the neuroendocrine characteristics were made evident in pulmonary small cell carcinomas, the term "neuroendocrine carcinoma" has been widely used for this type of lung tumor, although the descriptive designations continue to prevail. The term "endocrine carcinoma" of the cervix, as opposed to "carcinoid", has been used owing to the more benign connotation of the latter term (SILVA et al. 1984). Actually, the majority of cervical tumors are highly aggressive and seem to correspond to either gastrointestinal neuroendocrine carcinoma or pulmonary neuroendocrine carcinoma of intermediate/small cell sub-type; hence the term "neuroendocrine carcinoma" has been applied to such cervical tumors.

In the endometrium, only a few such cases have been reported and all have been referred to as "small cell carcinoma" (OLSON et al. 1982; BANNATYNE et al. 1983; KUMAR 1984; PAZ et al. 1985; MANIVEL et al. 1986).

"Adenocarcinoma with neuroendocrine cells" is the name which has been given to the usual adenocarcinomas with neuroendocrine cells found in the cervix and endometrium. The term “argyrophil cell adenocarcinoma” (UEDA et al. 1977, 1979) was first applied to such tumors of the endometrium, but this has not been generally accepted because they appear to differ substantially in many respects from the neuroendocrine carcinomas of the cervix. A broad spectrum of tumors ranging from carcinoid to adenocarcinoma has been well documented in the gastrointestinal tract (LEWIN 1987). In some cases, it may be difficult to differentiate between neuroendocrine carcinoma and adenocarcinoma with neuroendocrine cells. Actually, atypical carcinoids were initially diagnosed as poorly differentiated gastric adenocarcinomas (SWEENEY and McDONNELL 1980). However, it became recognized as questionable whether adenocarcinomas with neuroendocrine cells should be included in the spectrum of neuroendocrine carcinomas because their biologic behavior is identical to that of other adenocarcinomas (BONAR and SWEENEY 1986; SMITH and HAGGITT 1984).

## 3 Histogenesis

Carcinoid tumors are known to develop in any site, including the gastrointestinal and bronchopulmonary tracts (DELELLIS et al. 1984). They may arise directly from mature neuroendocrine cells, which were first considered to originate from the neural crest (PEARSE 1969) but were later proved to arise from the endodermal cells in the gastrointestinal tract (PICKET et al. 1976; FONTAINE and LE-DOURAIN 1977; COX and PIERCE 1982). On the other hand, the occurrence of mixed neuroendocrine and nonneuroendocrine tumors is a well-known phenomenon (LEWIN 1987), and nonneuroendocrine carcinomas have been reported to contain isolated neuroendocrine cells (AZZOPARDI and POLLACK 1963). Conversely, neuroendocrine carcinomas often show evidence of nonneuroendocrine differentiation (GOULD et al. 1983). This phenomenon supports the hypothesis that neuroendocrine cells and their tumors develop through multidirectional differentiation of primitive stem cells, which differentiate in endoderm to either epithelial cells or Kulchitsky cells (GOULD et al. 1983). This stem cell theory, however, cannot adequately explain the difference in the kinds of endocrine cell and their relative frequency between carcinomas and classical carcinoids. An alternative postulation may be that the precursor cells of the classical carcinoid are immature endocrine cells or immatue neoplastic cells already destined to differentiate into particular kinds of endocrine cell (IWAFUCHI et al. 1987).

In the cervix, neuroendocrine carcinoma was initially proposed by ALBORES-SAAVEDRA et al. (1979) to arise from argyrophil cells which normally inhabit the cervical mucosa (FOX et al. 1964; TATEISHI et al. 1975) and were considered to be a part of the APUD cell system by PEARSE (1969). Subsequently, however, an increasing number of mixed tumors were also reported in the cervix, casting doubt on this histogenetic proposal. MATSUYAMA et al. (1979) reported a case of neuroendocrine carcinoma of the cervix which was composed of anaplastic carcinoma, adenocarcinoma, and squamous cell carcinoma, and discussed the possibility that the tumor had developed from totipotent, immature epithelial cells of the cervix which not are argyrophilic. In subsequent reports, a tumor of similar morphology (TSUKAMOTO et al. 1989), a tumor associated with adenocarcinoma, adenocarcinoma in situ, and squamous cell carcinoma in situ (CHAN et al. 1989), and even a tumor associated with adenocarcinoma, squamous cell carcinoma, adenocarcinoma in situ, and squamous cell carcinoma in situ (GERSELL et al. 1988) have been described. Other types of tumor associated with neuroendocrine carcinoma include adenocarcinoma (SILVA et al. 1984; MURAOKA et al. 1987; GERSELL et al. 1988; WALKER et al. 1988; HUSAIN et al. 1989), adenosquamous carcinoma (WALKER et al. 1988), squamous cell carcinoma (ALBORES-SAAVEDRA et al. 1979; STAHL et al. 1981; GERSELL et al. 1988; WALKER et al. 1988), adenocarcinoma in situ and severe squamous dysplasia (MULLINS and HILLARD 1981), and squamous cell carcinoma in situ or dysplasia (WARNER 1978; MILES et al. 1982; STASSART et al. 1982; GERSELL et al. 1988). Neuroendocrine cells were frequently found in adenocarcinoma components (MATSUYAMA et al. 1979; SILVA et al. 1984; MURAOKA et al. 1987; CHAN et al. 1989), but not in others. Also, pure cervical adenocarcinomas with neuroendocrine cells have been reported (AZZOPARDI and HOU 1965; KAKU and ENJOJI 1983; SCULLY et al. 1984; UEDA et al. 1984a). All these phenomena may be explained by the stem cell theory, as in the gastrointestinal and bronchopulmonary tracts. However, whether classical carcinoid could ever arise from immature endocrine cells in the cervix requires further investigation.

The cellular origin of both neuroendocrine carcinomas and neuroendocrine cells in adenocarcinomas of the endometrium is considered to be a common stem cell, although some other possibilities have been discussed (UEDA et al. 1979). The common stem cell theory seems to be further supported by a unique case of mixed müllerian tumor containing small cell neuroendocrine carcinoma (MANIVEL et al. 1986), because this kind of tumor is generally believed to develop from the immature müllerian cells with the potential for mesenchymal or epithelial differentiation. However, SCULLY et al. (1984) applied the term "neometaplasia" to the appearance of neuroendocrine cells in mesodermal tumors, the term initially having been introduced to explain the development of glioma in the uterus. They postulated that the common stem cell theory may not adequately explain the presence of neuroendocrine cells in mesodermal tumors which arise from organs in which these cells are normally not apparent; these cells have been identified only occasionally in specimens of normal cervix (FOX et al. 1964; TATEISHI et al. 1975) and endometrium (SATAKE and MATSUYAMA 1987).

## 4 Clinical Features

Characteristic endocrine syndromes have been described in a few cases of neuroendocrine carcinoma of the cervix. Cushing's syndrome due to excessive ACTH production has been most frequently encountered (BERTHELOT et al.

1961; JONES et al. 1976; MATSUYAMA et al. 1979; LOJEK et al. 1980); others include carcinoid syndrome due to oversecretion of serotonin (DRIESSENS et al. 1964; STOCKDALE et al. 1986) and hypoglycemia associated with elevated levels of insulin (KIANG et al. 1973). Although not related to clinical symptoms, the production of β-MSH, serotonin, histamine, and amylase was reported in one case of Cushing's syndrome due to ACTH secretion (MATSUYAMA et al. 1979), and that of calcitonin in another case (TSUKAMOTO et al. 1989). However, the majority of cases showed no specific symptoms and were indistinguishable from invasive squamous cell carcinomas. Similarly, no endocrine symptoms have been described so far in patients with neuroendocrine small cell carcinomas of the endometrium.

With regard to adenocarcinomas with neuroendocrine cells in the cervix and endometrium, it was likewise not possible to distinguish them clinically from usual adenocarcinomas in these sites.

## 5 Pathology

Macroscopically, neuroendocrine carcinomas of the cervix differ little from squamous cell carcinomas; that is, there is progression from erosion in the earliest stage to tumor formation with or without ulceration in the later stages. They are first diagnosed histologically as small cell or undifferentiated carcinoma in most cases, but as adenosquamous or squamous cell carcinoma of large cell type in rare cases.

The tumors were microscopically subgrouped into two types by ALBORES-SAAVEDRA et al. (1979): poorly differentiated carcinoids and well-differentiated carcinoids. The former are quite comparable to the oat cell carcinomas of the lung, but the latter are less differentiated than classical carcinoid tumors of the gastrointestinal tract. Poorly differentiated variants were composed of small round to oat or spindle-shaped cells with hyperchromatic nuclei and scanty cytoplasm. Mitotic figures were usually numerous. These cells were arranged to form solid sheets, nests, cords, and trabecular patterns. Peripheral palisading and foci of squamous differentiation may be seen. On the other hand, the well-differentiated types were composed of medium sized, round to polygonal cells with a more prominent cytoplasm and less hyperchromatic nuclei. Mitoses were less frequent. They showed variable arrangements such as insular, trabecular, glandular, and spindle patterns. Some of these were similar to the poorly differentiated variants, but ribbon-like structures and glandular patterns were characteristic of the well-differentiated tumors. The poorly differentiated tumors have subsequently occasionally been called either undifferentiated (small cell) carcinoma or oat cell carcinoma, and the well-differentiated variants either intermediate cell type or carcinoid type.

The Grimelius stain revealed the presence of tumor cells containing argyrophil granules in their cytoplasm, although the frequency varied greatly in different tumors and even within different areas of the same tumor (TATEISHI et al. 1975). The Fontana-Masson stain was, however, positive only in rare cases (MATSUYAMA et al. 1979; JOHANNESSEN et al. 1980; KATSUBE et al. 1984; BARRETT et al. 1987; MURAOKA et al. 1987).

Small cell carcinomas of the endometrium have not been reported sufficiently often (OLSON et al. 1982; BANNATYNE et al. 1983; KUMAR 1984; PAZ et al. 1985; MANIVEL et al. 1986) to permit comment on their pathologic characteristics, but focal argyrophilia was seen with the Grimelius stain in some tumors (PAZ et al. 1985; MANIVEL et al. 1986).

Adenocarcinomas with and without argyrophilia of the cervix and endometrium are reported not to differ macroscopically or histologically. Argyrophil cells of cervical adenocarcinomas are very similar to enterochromaffin cells of the gastrointestinal tract (AZZOPARDI and HOU 1965; KAKU and ENJOJI 1983; SCULLY et al. 1984; UEDA et al. 1984a). When the argyrophil cells were first found in endometrial adenocarcinomas, it was not realized that they are heterogeneous (UEDA et al. 1977). Later, however, only the triangular cells similar to enterochromaffin cells were proven to have the capacity for amine precursor uptake and decarboxylation (INOUE et al. 1982). The heterogeneous populations of argyrophil cells were also ascertained by subsequent investigations (BANNATYNE et al. 1983; AGUIRRE et al. 1984; INOUE et al. 1984b). Presently, at least two types of argyrophil cell are observed in endometrial adenocarcinomas. We have classified them as follows: type I cells are triangular and similar to the enterochromaffin cells, whereas type II cells are the same as glandular tumor cells in shape and loaded with argyrophilic granules in the apical portion or whole cytoplasm. Type II cells may, however, comprise heterogeneous populations.

## 6 Electron Microscopy

Neurosecretory type granules are ultrastructurally the most characteristic feature in neuroendocrine tumor cells of the cervix. They consist of an electron-dense core enclosed by a limiting membrane. The granules vary from 60 to 600 nm in size and are mostly round to oval, but infrequently pleomorphic (ALBORES-SAAVEDRA et al. 1979). Their numbers vary greatly in different tumors, and even in cells within the same tumor (TATEISHI et al. 1975). They may be too few to find in some tumors, which may render it difficult to differentiate them from more primitive tumors without neuroendocrine differentiation (FUJII et al. 1986). They are said to be generally more densely and evenly distributed in well-differentiated carcinoids than in poorly differentiated carcinoids. According to ALBORES-SAAVEDRA et al. (1979), round granules tend to be found in the former, whereas pleomorphic granules are found only in the latter. Actually, pleomorphic granules were later described only in a few poorly differentiated tumors (Johannessen et al. 1980; Miles et al. 1982). An attempt was made by Black (1968) to correlate granule morphology with the content of specific hormones in carcinoid tumors of the gastrointestinal tract, but it proved extremely difficult to generalize. This seems also to be the case with regard to neuroendocrine tumors of the cervix. A diagnosis of neuroendocrine tumor should not be made by solely relying on the presence of secretory granules, since they may be too few to find even in neuroendocrine tumor cells, as already described. Moreover, similar electron-dense granules may be found in various nonneuroendocrine cells (Taxy et al. 1981; Aguirre et al. 1984).

Other ultrastructural features include variable development of microfibrils, microtubules, free ribosomes, endoplasmic reticulum, and mitochondria in the cytoplasm. Microvilli and a few poorly developed desmosomes may also be observed.

Small cell carcinomas of the endometrium have been described as containing only a few small round neurosecretory granules (Olson et al. 1982; Bannatyne et al. 1983; Kumar 1984; Paz et al. 1985; Manivel et al. 1986). Neurosecretory type granules are also found in the argyrophil cells of adenocarcinoma of the endometrium (Ueda et al. 1979; Okudaira et al. 1980; Bannatyne et al. 1983), although whether they are limited to a specific cell type, namely our type I cells, is a matter of controversy.

## 7 Immunohistochemistry

Recent progress in immunohistochemistry has made it possible to detect a variety of neuroendocrine markers directly in the cells. This has played an important role in the diagnostic establishment of neuroendocrine carcinomas in various organs. Neuroendocrine carcinoma of the cervix was reviewed by Scully et al. 1984 and found to be only infrequently studied by immunohistochemistry. Since then, several neuroendocrine markers have been investigated, as well as serotonin and peptide hormones.

Serotonin was most frequently detected in the cells of neuroendocrine carcinoma of the cervix (Scully et al. 1984; Silva et al. 1984; Ulich et al. 1986; Muraoka et al. 1987). Peptide hormones identified by immunohistochemistry include ACTH (Lojek et al. 1980; Pazdur et al. 1981), gastrin (Yamasaki et al. 1984), somatostatin, substance P, vasointestinal polypeptide, pancreatic polypeptide (Silva et al. 1984), and calcitonin (Albores-Saavedra et al. 1979).

Neuron-specific enolase (NSE) is a neural form of the glycolytic enzyme enolase and is used as a marker for neuroendocrine cells. NSE is related to neuroendocrine differentiation and cellular function, in contrast to argyrophilia in which neurosecretory granules are present (Lundqvist et al. 1985). NSE has been reported to be strongly positive in most of the neuroendocrine carcinomas of the cervix (INOUE et al. 1985; ULICH et al. 1986; UEDA et al. 1989). NSE may not be entirely specific, but the intense and diffuse reactivity is considered to be highly suggestive of endorcine differentiation in small cell carcinomas of the cervix.

Chromogranin, a specific endorcine marker, was shown to be intimately associated with argyrophilia in neuroendocrine cells of pancreatic carcinoma (LLOYD et al. 1984), but not in small cell carcinoma of the lung (SAID et al. 1985). In neuroendocrine carcinoma of the cervix, chromogranin reactivity was reported in one publication to be present in only half of the tumors (ULICH et al. 1986), although the reported frequency was much higher in another study (GERSELL et al. 1988). In our study, chromogranin reactivity paralleled argyrophilia if the antibody used was sufficiently sensitive (UEDA et al. 1989).

Synaptophysin is an integral membrane glycoprotein originally isolated from bovine neuronal presynaptic vesicles and considered to be a significant neuroendocrine marker expressed more broadly than chromogranin (GOULD et al. 1987). Many neuroendocrine carcinomas of the cervix were found to be positive for synaptophysin (GERSELL et al. 1988).

Leu-7 is an antigen expressed originally by a subset of lymphocytes with natural killer activity, but also shared by normal and neoplastic cells derived from the neuroendocrine system (CAILLAUD et al. 1984). Nearly half of the small cell neuroendocrine carcinomas have been reported to express Leu-7 (UEDA et al. 1986; MICHELS et al. 1987; GERSELL et al. 1988).

Immunohistochemical studies of adenocarcinomas of the cervix with neuroendocrine cells have only infrequently been reported; so far they have demonstrated serotonin, neurotensin (SCULLY et al. 1984), gastrin, somatostatin, and ACTH (UEDA et al. 1984a) in some of the argyrophil cells.

A few cases of small cell neuroendocrine carcinoma of the endometrium have been reported, but immunohistochemistry was successfully applied only in two cases (MANIVEL et al. 1986), demonstrating NSE, Leu-7, and chromogranin.

Endometrial adenocarcinomas with argyrophilia have been studied extensively by immunohistochemistry, so that the nature of heterogeneous populations of argyrophil cells could be better clarified, although our type I cells were proved to contain dopamine by the formaldehyde-induced fluorescence method (INOUE et al. 1982). Serotonin (AGUIRRE et al. 1984) and peptide hormones such as somatostatin (AGUIRRE et al. 1984; INOUE et al. 1984b) and ACTH (AGUIRRE et al. 1984) have so far been detected in type I cells of the endometrial carcinoma with argyrophilia. Similarly, serotonin and somatostatin were localized in this type of argyrophil cell in the normal endometrium, where it is rarely observed (SATAKE and MATSUYAMA 1987). Some cells of endometrial carcinoma with argyrophilia were immunohistochemically positive for gastrin (INOUE et al. 1984b; WICK et al. 1986) and substance P (WICK et al. 1986), but they did not usually correspond with the argyrophil cells (INOUE et al. 1984b). Some cells of this kind of tumor were also positive for NSE (INOUE et al. 1985; WICK et al.

1986), but they were not argyrophilic except for a few cases in which type I argyrophil cells were weakly positive. On the other hand, all type I argyrophil cells and also many type II argyrophil cells were strongly positive for chromogranin (UEDA et al. 1985, 1987b; INOUE et al. 1986). The immunohistochemical demonstration of chromogranin in the cytoplasm of type II argyrophil cells supported for the first time the neuroendocrine nature of these cells. Leu-7 was demonstrated in some type I argyrophil cells, but also in tumor cells without argyrophilia (UEDA et al. 1986).

Markers of epithelial differentiation such as epithelial membrane antigen tend to be expressed inversely to the neuroendocrine markers in neuroendocrine carcinomas of the cervix (UEDA et al. 1989), although both markers have been reported to be coexpressed frequently in this kind of tumor (SILVA et al. 1984; ULICH et al. 1986; GERSELL et al. 1988). The same tendency was observed in endometrial carcinoma with argyrophilia, regardless of the type (UEDA et al. 1987a). In addition, it is interesting that in endometrial carcinomas with argyrophilia, nonargyrophil cells of a gland containing argyrophil cells did not express the epithelial marker, in sharp contrast to its expression in the cells of adjacent glands without argyrophilia (UEDA et al. 1987a).

## 8 Biologic Behavior

Neuroendocrine carcinomas of the cervix are relatively rare and their biologic behavior has not yet been elucidated in detail, but they are generally believed to be highly aggressive. ALBORES-SAAVEDRA et al. (1976) presented follow-up information on four of six well-differentiated and five of six poorly differentiated carcinoids. Two patients with the well-differentiated carcinoids died 5 and 6 years later, whereas in three patients with the poorly differentiated type the interval until death was 3, 7, and 24 months. Later, they reported the follow-up information on 8 of 13 patients with poorly differentiated carcinoid; only two were alive, one after 2 years and one after 3 years (ALBORES-SAAVEDRA et al. 1979). Therefore, they inferred that well-differentiated carcinoid of the cervix is a low-grade malignancy similar to classical carcinoids in other locations, and that poorly differentiated carcinoid behaves more aggressively. In fact, however, the well-differentiated carcinoid type of tumor can likewise be aggressive and fatal (SILVA et al. 1984; GROBEN et al. 1985). Such tumors appear to correspond morphologically with the intermediate cell type of lung tumor. Neuroendocrine tumors thus far described in case reports or clinicopathologic analyses of a number of cases are listed in Table 1, but seven cases of ALBORES-SAAVEDRA et al. (1979) and 14 cases of SHEETS et al. (1988) are not included due to the lack of individual data. The majority of neuroendocrine carcinomas of the cervix reported have been poorly differentiated and aggressive in nature. Some patients with a more differentiated type of tumor seem to be in the earlier

**Table. 1.** A list of neuroendocrine carcinomas of the uterine cervix together with the main clinicopathologic features

| Case | Age | Histology[a] | Stage | Treatment[b] | Metastasis/Recurrence[c] | Follow-up[d] | Other remarks | Author |
|---|---|---|---|---|---|---|---|---|
| 1 | 52 | UDSC | IV | XRT | Liver | DOD, 2 mo | Cushing's syndrome | BERTHELOT et al. (1961) |
| 2 | 34 | Basel cell | IV | NT | Liver, lung | DOD, 12 d | Carcinoid syndrome | DRIESSENS et al. (1964) |
| 3 | 25 | Small cell | Ib? | Cone, XRT | Lung | DOD, 1 yr 1 mo | Hypoglycemia | KIANG et al. (1973) |
| 4 | 38 | PD carcinoid | I | RH | Pelvic LN | DOC | | ALBORES-SAAVEDRA et al. (1976) |
| 5 | 72 | PD carcinoid | IIb | RH | NM | DOD, 2 yr | | ALBORES-SAAVEDRA et al. (1976) |
| 6 | 50 | PD carcinoid | I | RH | Parametrium | A&W, 2 yr | | ALBORES-SAAVEDRA et al. (1976) |
| 7 | 47 | PD carcinoid | I | RH, XRT | Parametrium | DOD, 7 mo | | ALBORES-SAAVEDRA et al. (1976) |
| 8 | 64 | PD carcinoid | IV | NT | Pelvic LN | DOD, 3 mo | | ALBORES-SAAVEDRA et al. (1976) |
| 9 | 52 | PD carcinoid | III | RH | r. tube | Lost | | ALBORES-SAAVEDRA et al. (1976) |
| 10 | 47 | WD carcinoid | III | RH | Pelvic, LN, r. ovary | DOD, 6 yr | | ALBORES-SAAVEDRA et al. (1976) |
| 11 | 34 | WD carcinoid | IIa | TAH, XRT, TPE | Rectovag. septum, Inguinal, Supraclav, LN | DOD, 5 yr | | ALBORES-SAAVEDRA et al. (1976) |
| 12 | 72 | WD carcinoid | IIb | RH | NM | A&W, 1 yr | | ALBORES-SAAVEDRA et al. (1976) |
| 13 | 66 | WD carcinoid | IIb | RH | NM | A&W, 9 mo | | ALBORES-SAAVEDRA et al. (1976) |
| 14 | 39 | WD carcinoid | I | RH | Tube, ovary | Lost | | ALBORES-SAAVEDRA et al. (1976) |
| 15 | 33 | WD carcinoid | IIa | RH | NM | Lost | | ALBORES-SAAVEDRA et al. (1976) |
| 16 | 40 | Small cell | IIa | XRT, PL, Chemo | Liver, bone | DOD, 4 mo | Cushing's syndrome | JONES et al. (1976) |
| 17 | 29 | Small cell | Ib | CS, RH | Widespread | DOD, 6 mo | Pregnancy 28 wk | KODOUSEK et al. (1976) |
| 18 | 50 | Carcinoid | Ib | TAH-BSO | NM | A&W, 1 yr | | DAW (1977) |
| 19 | 64 | Carcinoid, CIS, DYS | IIb | PL, XRT | Widespread | DOD, 23 d | | WARNER (1978) |
| 20 | 59 | Oat cell | ? | TAH | Vagina, perineum, inguinal region | DOD, 28 mo | | TUJI et al. (1978) |
| 21 | 48 | Small cell | IV | Chemo | Pelvic LN, pancreas | ? | | MACKAY et al. (1979) |
| 22 | 63 | Small cell | IV | XRT | Para-aortic LN, liver | ? | | MACKAY et al. (1979) |
| 23 | 38 | Small cell, AC, SC | Ib | RH, Chemo | Skin, lung, mediastinum | DOD, 2 yr 3 mo | Cushing's syndrome | MATSUYAMA et al. (1979) |
| 24 | 33 | Carcinoid | Ib | RH-RSO | NM | A&W, 2.5 mo | | HABIB et al. (1979) |
| | (37) | Carcinoid | Ib | RH-RSO | Lung, brain | DOD, 4 yr | | SEIDEL and STEINFELD (1988) |
| 25 | 25 | PD SC | Ib | Chemo, RH, XRT | Widespread | DOD, 24 mo | Pregnancy 10 wk | JACOB et al. (1980) |
| 26 | 28 | Small cell | IIa | CS, XRT | Chest wall to pleura , spine | DOD, 32 mo | Cushing's syndrome Pregnancy 25 wk | LOJEK et al. (1980) |

**Table 1.** *(Continued)*

| Case | Age | Histology[a] | Stage | Treatment[b] | Metastasis/Recurrence[c] | Follow-up[d] | Other remarks | Author |
|---|---|---|---|---|---|---|---|---|
| 27 | 21 | Oat cell | IIIb | XRT | Local | DOD, 4 mo | | Johannessen et al. (1980) |
| 28 | 62 | Carcinoid | Ib | XRT | NM | A&W 8 mo | | Hus et al. (1981) |
| 29 | 37 | Carcinoid | Ib | RH | NM | A&W, 1 yr 1 mo | | Stahl et al. (1981) |
| 30 | 27 | Carcinoid, AC | IVb | Chemo | Liver | DOD 1 yr | | Miwa et al. (1981) |
| 31 | 29 | Carcinoid | Ib | RH | NM | A&W 1 yr 6 mo | | Mullins and Hillard (1981) |
| 32 | 48 | Small cell | III | XRT, Chemo | Supraclav, LN, brain | DOD 13 mo | | Pazdur et al. (1981) |
| 33 | 32 | Small cell | IIa | XRT, Chemo | Para-aortic, supraclav, LN, liver, bone | DOD, 7 mo | | Pazdur et al. (1981) |
| 34 | 79 | Small cell | III | XRT | Para-aortic, supraclav, LN, liver, bone | DOD, 5 mo | | Pazdur et al. (1981) |
| 35 | 39 | Small cell | IV | Chemo | Lung, liver, bone | DOD, 1 wk | | Pazdur et al. (1981) |
| 36 | 58 | PD SC | IIIb | NT | Bladder, rectum, diaphragm | DOD, 9 mo | | Ouchi et al. (1981) |
| 37 | 30 | Small cell | IIIb | PL, Chemo | Pelvic, para-aortic LN, bone | DOD, 4 mo | | Louka et al. (1982) |
| 38 | 52 | Oat cell | IIIb | PL, Chemo, XRT | Pelvic, para-aortic LN | AWD, 4 mo | | Louka et al. (1982) |
| 39 | 49 | Small cell | IIa | RH, XRT, Chemo | Supraclav, LN, lung,brain | DOD, 11 mo | | Sakamoto et al. (1982) |
| 40 | 54 | ASC, DYS | IIb | XRT, Chemo, Lobectomy | Lung | AWD, 1 yr 8 mo | | Miles et al. (1982) |
| 41 | 37 | Small cell, CIS | Ib | RH, Chemo, XRT | Pelvic LN | A&W, 14 mo | Postpartum 4 mo | Stassart et al. (1982) |
| 42 | 60 | Carcinoid | Ib? | RH | NM | A&W, 11 mo | | Hariri et al. (1983) |
| 43 | 38 | Carcinoid | Ib | XRT, TAH-BSO | NM | A&W, 12 yr | | Silva et al. (1984) |
| 44 | 55 | Carcinoid | IIb | XRT | Retroperic, LN, bone, Liver lung, spleen, meninges | DOD, 2 mo | | Silva et al. (1984) |
| 45 | 66 | Carcinoid | Ib | XRT | NM | A&W, 16 mo | | Silva et al. (1984) |
| 46 | 42 | Carcinoid | IIb | XRT, TPE | Local | DOD, 3 yr | | Silva et al. (1984) |
| 47 | 76 | Carcinoid | Ib | XRT, TAH-USO | Lung | DOD, 3 yr | | Silva et al. (1984) |
| 48 | 65 | Carcinoid | Ib | TAH-BSO | Lung | DOD, 27 mo | | Silva et al. (1984) |
| 49 | 23 | Carcinoid, AC | Ib | TAH-USO, XRT, Chemo | Pelvic, mediast, LN, lung, local | DOD, 15 mo | | Silva et al. (1984) |
| 50 | 62 | Carcinoid, AC | IIIb | XRT | Lung, bladder | DOD, 1 yr | | Silva et al. (1984) |

| | | | | | | | | | |
|---|---|---|---|---|---|---|---|---|---|
| 51 | 57 | Carcinoid, AC | IV | XRT, chemo | Lung, brain | DOD, 6 mo | | SILVA et at. (1984) |
| 52 | 46 | Small cell | IIb | RH | NM to LN | DOD, 11 mo | | YAMASAKI et al. (1984) |
| 53 | 35 | Small cell | Ib | RH | Pelvic LN | A&W, 10 yr | | YAMASAKI et al. (1984) |
| 54 | 50 | Small cell | IIb | RH | NM to LN | DOD, 4 yr 11 mo | | YAMASAKI et al. (1984) |
| 55 | 38 | Small cell | Ib | RH, XRT | NM to LN | DOD 1 yr 1 mo | | YAMASAKI et al. (1984) |
| 56 | 58 | Small cell | III | P[illegible] | ? | DOD, 1 mo | | YAMASAKI et al. (1984) |
| 57 | 36 | Small cell | IIa | RH | NM to LN | DOD, 6 mo | | YAMASAKI et al. (1984) |
| 58 | 53 | Small cell | Ib | RH | ? | DOD, 1 yr 8 mo | | YAMASAKI et al. (1984) |
| 59 | 52 | Small cell | Ib | RH | NM to LN | A&W, 7 yr | | YAMASAKI et al. (1984) |
| 60 | 33 | Small cell | Ib | RH, XRT | NM to LN | DOD, 3 yr 4 mo | | YAMASAKI et al. (1984) |
| 61 | 46 | Small cell | IIb | RH, XRT | Pelvic LN | DOD, 1 yr | | YAMASAKI et al. (1984) |
| 62 | 46 | Small cell | Ib | RH | NM to LN | A&W, 2 yr | | YAMASAKI et al. (1984) |
| 63 | 50 | Small cell | IIb | RH | NM to LN | A&W, 1 yr | | YAMASAKI et al. (1984) |
| 64 | 38 | Small cell | Ib | RH, XRT | Pelvic LN | DOD, 1 yr | | YAMASAKI et al. (1984) |
| 65 | 46 | Carcinoid | Ib | TAH-BSO, XRT | NM | A&W, 5 yr 10 mo | | KATSUBE et al. (1984) |
| 66 | 76 | Carcinoid | IVb | XRT, Chemo | Lung | DOD, 8 mo | | YOSHIDA et al. (1984) |
| 67 | 40 | Small cell | Ib | RH, XRT | Pelvic LN, widespread | DOD, 4 mo | | INOUE et al. (1984a) |
| 68 | 50 | Small cell | III | XRT, Chemo | Local, bone, liver | DOD, 12 mo | | GROBEN et al. (1985) |
| 69 | 78 | Small cell | IV | XRT, Chemo | Local, liver | DOD, 16 mo | | GROBEN et al. (1985) |
| 70 | 58 | Small cell | Ib | XRT, Chemo | Bone, lung, leptomeninges | DOD, 24 mo | | GROBEN et al. (1985) |
| 71 | 68 | Small cell | Ib | XRT, Chemo | Para-aortic LN | A&W, 8 mo | | GROBEN et al. (1985) |
| 72 | 38 | Small cell | IV | XRT, Chemo | Local, lung | DOD, 4 mo | | GROBEN et al. (1985) |
| 73 | 40 | Carcinoid | Ib | RH, Chemo | Local, lung | DOD, 20 mo | | GROBEN et al. (1985) |
| 74 | 26 | Small cell | Ib | CS, RH, Chemo | Liver, bone, lung | DOD, 9 mo | Pregnancy 26 wk | TURNERet al. (1986) |
| 75 | 38 | Carcinoid | Ib | TAH, Chemo | Pelvic, para-aortic LN, ovary, omentum | DOD, 18 mo | Carcinoid syndrome | STOCKDALA et al. (1986) |
| 76 | 44 | Small cell | IVa | XRT, Chemo | Bladder | DOD, 6 mo | | KAMIYA et al. (1986) |
| 77 | 31 | Small cell | Ib | TAH, LND | NM | A&W, 14 mo | | IWAOK et al. (1986) |
| 78 | 38 | Carcinoid, AC | Ia | TAH-BSO | NM | A&W, 1 yr | | MURAOKA et al. (1987) |
| 79 | 33 | PD SC | Ib | Chemo | Liver | DOD, 5 mo | | BARRETT et al. (1987) |
| 80 | 30 | PD SC | Ib | RH | NM | DOD, 20 mo | | BARRETT et al. (1987) |
| 81 | 32 | PD ASC | Ib | NT | NM | DOD, 24 mo | | BARRETT et al. (1987) |
| 82 | 62 | Small cell | Ib | RH | NM | Lost, 6 mo | | BARRETT et al. (1987) |
| 83 | 38 | Small cell | Ib | RH, XRT | Pelvic LN | DOD, 11 mo | | BARRETT et al. (1987) |
| 84 | 70 | Small cell | IIIb | SAH | Peritoneum, diaphragm, liver, bowel serosa | DOD, 5 mo | | BARRETT et al. (1987) |
| 85 | 77 | PD SC | IVb | XRT | Lung | DOD, 10 mo | | BARRETT at al. (1987) |

**Table 1.** *(Continued)*

| Case | Age | Histology[a] | Stage | Treatment[b] | Metastasis/Recurrence[c] | Follow-up[d] | Other remarks | Author |
|---|---|---|---|---|---|---|---|---|
| 86 | 31 | Small cell | Ib | RH, Chemo | Brain | DOD, 2 yr | | Ichimura et al. (1988) |
| 87 | 33 | Small cell | IIb | RH, XRT | Pelvic LN, liver, lung, bone | DOD, 7 mo | | Ueda (1988) |
| 88 | 26 | Small cell, CIS | Ib | RH | NM | A&W, 78 mo | | Gersell et al. (1988) |
| 89 | 74 | Small cell | Ib | XRT | | DOD, 19 mo | | Gersell et al. (1988) |
| 90 | 39 | Small cell | Ib | RH, XRT | LN, bladder, lung, bone, dura, pancreas | DOD, 9 mo | | Gersell et al. (1988) |
| 91 | 32 | Small cell, SC AC, CIS, AIS | Ib | XRT | Lung | DOD, 71 mo | | Gersell et al. (1988) |
| 92 | 74 | Small cell, SC | Ib | XRT | Lung | AWD, 10 mo | | Gersell et al. (1988) |
| 93 | 33 | Small cell | Ib | XRT | Lung, meninges, spinal cord | DOD, 11 mo | | Gersell et al. (1988) |
| 94 | 50 | Small cell | Ib | XRT, Chemo | Brain | DOD, 15 mo | | Gersell et al. (1988) |
| 95 | 34 | Small cell, CIS | Ib | RH, Chemo, XRT | Brain | AWD, 4 mo | | Gersell et al. (1988) |
| 96 | 87 | Small cell, SC | Ib | XRT | | A&W, 11 mo | | Gersell et al. (1988) |
| 97 | 51 | Small cell, AC | IIa | XRT | Liver | DOD, 12 mo | | Gersell et al. (1988) |
| 98 | 42 | Small cell | IIb | XRT, Chemo | | A&W, 5 mo | | Gersell et al. (1988) |
| 99 | 65 | Small cell | IIb | XRT | Bone | DOD, 4 mo | | Gersell et al. (1988) |
| 100 | 60 | Small cell | IIIb | XRT, Chemo | Liver | DOD, 9 mo | | Gersell et al. (1988) |
| 101 | 25 | Small cell, AC | IIIb | XRT, Chemo | Liver | DOD, 11 mo | | Gersell et al. (1988) |
| 102 | 28 | Small cell | IV | XRT | Bone | DOD, 3 mo | | Gersell et al. (1988) |
| 103 | 29 | IC-NEC | Ib | RH, Chemo | | DOD, 16 mo | | Walker et al. (1988) |
| 104 | 51 | IC-NEC | IV | XRT, Chemo | Lung | DOD, 7 mo | | Walker et al. (1988) |
| 105 | 74 | Small cell, IC-NEC | IV | XRT | | DOD, 16 mo | | Walker et al. (1988) |
| 106 | 75 | Small ceil, IC-NEC | IIIb | XRT | | DOD, 6 mo | | Walker et al. (1988) |
| 107 | 67 | Small cell | IIIb | XRT | | DOD, 4 mo | | Walker et al. (1988) |
| 108 | 65 | Small cell | IIa | XRT | | DOD, 26 mo | | Walker et al. (1988) |
| 109 | 82 | Small cell | IIa | XRT | | DOD, 33 mo | | Walker et al. (1988) |
| 110 | 27 | Small cell | IIb | Chemo | | DOD, 12.5 mo | | Walker et al. (1988) |

| | | | | | | | | |
|---|---|---|---|---|---|---|---|---|
| 111 | 26 | Small cell | Ib | RH, Chemo | Pelvic LN | DOD, 11.5 mo | Pregnancy | WALKER et al. (1988) |
| 112 | 75 | Small cell | IV | XRT | | DOD, 4.5 mo | | WALKER et al. (1988) |
| 113 | 32 | Small cell | Ib | XRT | | A&W, 10.5 yr | | WALKER et al. (1988) |
| 114 | 83 | Small cell, SC | IIa | XRT | | DOC, 24 mo | | WALKER et al. (1988) |
| 115 | 81 | Small cell, ASC | IIa | XRT | | DOD, 20.5 mo | | WALKER et al. (1988) |
| 116 | 36 | Small cell, AC | Ib | TAH, XRT | | AWD, 12 mo | | WALKER et al. (1988) |
| 117 | 49 | Small cell, AC | Ib | RH | NM | A&W, 7 mo | | HUSAIN et al. (1989) |
| 118 | 67 | Small cell, carcinoid, AC, SC | Ib | RH | Lung | DOD, 4 yr 6 mo | Calcitonin producing | TSUKAMOTO et al. (1989) |
| 119 | 33 | Small cell, AC, AIS, CIS | Ia | RH, Chemo | NM | A&W 6 mo | | CHAN et al. (1989) |

[a] UD, undifferentiated; PD, poorly differentiated; WD, well differentiated; SC, squamous cell carcinoma; AC, adenocarcinoma; ASC, adenosquamous carcinoma; CIS, carcinoma in situ; DYS, dysplasia; AIS, adenocarcinoma in situ; IC-NEC, intermediate cell neuroendocrine carcinoma

[b] XRT, radiotherapy; Chemo, chemotherapy; RH, radical hysterectomy with bilateral pelvic lymphadenectomy; TAH, total abdominal hysterectomy; SAH, subtotal abdominal hysterectomy; TPE, total pelvic exenteration; PL, probe laparotomy; BSO, bilateral salpingo-oophorectomy; USO, unilateral salpingo-oophoretomy; RSO, right salpingo-oophorectomy; LND, lymph node dissection; CS, cesarean section; NT, no treatment.

[c] NM, no metastasis; LN, lymph node; r, right

[d] DOD, died of disease; DOC, died of other causes; A&W, alive and well; AWD, alive with disease

stages and to have had a better prognosis when reported, but, the follow-up periods are considered insufficiently long to evaluate. Although it is not clear whether the biologic behavior is related to the anaplasia or the neuroendocrine differentiation, it was shown by MATSUYAMA et al. (1979) that patients with anaplastic carcinoma with neuroendocrine differentiation had a poorer prognosis than those without such differentiation. Also, in a recent study, the presence of neurosecretory granules was correlated with decreased survival in poorly differentiated carcinomas of the cervix (BARRETT et al. 1987). The development of carcinoid tumor of low-grade malignancy seems to be extremely rare, and perhaps unknown, in the cervix.

Endocrine symptoms were noted in seven patients. Six patients were pregnant while one had given birth, but full data were not supplied for one of the pregnant patients (SHEETS et al. 1988). All six patients associated with pregnancy died despite adequate treatment at an early stage

The presence of neuroendocrine cells is probably of little or no prognostic significance in the case of female genital tract adenocarcinomas (BANNATYNE et al. 1983; UEDA et al. 1984a; SATO et al. 1986). However, their presence in gastrointestinal tumors may well be of prognostic significance (RADI et al. 1986), although this claim is not supported by others (SMITH and HAGGITT 1984; BONAR and SWEENEY 1986; OOI et al. 1988). Moreover, it is noteworthy that prostatic adenocarcinoma with a few neuroendocrine cells recurred after hormonal treatment as a tumor consisting predominantly of neuroendocrine cells (STRATTON et al. 1986), suggesting a subpopulation of cells with neuroendocrine differentiation which are hormone insensitive (DISANT'AGNESE and DEMESY JENSEN 1987).

## 9 Treatment

Stage I and II neuroendocrine cervical carcinomas have mostly been treated by surgery or radiation therapy with or without adjuvant therapy, while more advanced or recurrent cases have been treated by chemotherapy, in exactly the same way as other histologic variants. Some patients have reportedly been successfully treated by surgery alone (DAW 1977; ALBORES-SAAVEDRA et al. 1979; HABIB et al. 1979; STAHL et al. 1981; HARIRI et al. 1983; MURAOKA et al. 1987; HUSAIN et al. 1989), but many cases recur owing to a tendency toward dissemination even in the early stages. Radiation therapy has also been described as effective in some tumors (JONES et al. 1976; ALBORES-SAAVEDRA et al. 1979; JOHANNESSEN et al. 1980; HUS et al. 1981; MILES et al. 1982). Combination chemotherapy has been advocated for neuroendocrine carcinomas of the cervix because they are analogous to pulmonary neuroendocrine tumors in which this method of treatment has been proven to be very effective (SHEETS et al. 1988; VAN NAGELL et al. 1988). Complete remission of some tumors has indeed been achieved at least temporarily by this treatment (PAZDUR et al. 1981; LOUKA et al. 1982). However, the optimal treatment remains to be further defined.

Adenocarcinomas with neuroendocrine cells in the cervix (UEDA et al. 1984a) and endometrium (BANNATYNE et al. 1983; SATO et al. 1986) are not significantly different biologically from the usual adenocarcinomas of these sites. Therefore, they should be treated in a similar manner.

## 10 Case Report and Experimental Study

### 10.1 Case Report

A 29-year-old Japanese married woman attended the outpatient clinic of the Department of Obstetrics and Gynecology in Kure National Hospital on February 15, 1985 because of genital bleeding. Adenocarcinoma of the cervix was diagnosed by histologic examination. The patient was admitted to the hospital on March 22. On 30 May she underwent a semiradical hysterectomy, left adnexectomy, and pelvic lymph node dissection under the diagnosis of Ib adenocarcinoma of the cervix.

The pathologic diagnosis was small cell carcinoma with a focus of adenocarcinoma. There was an invasion into the stroma of less than 5 mm and no lymph node metastasis. Postoperative radiation therapy was given to the pelvis in a dose of 50 Gy. The patient was discharged on 20 August.

The patient was readmitted and treated because of fever due to infection from a pelvic lymphocyst from 9 September to 4 October. After discharge, the patient was followed up once or twice a month. No problems arose until 10 December 1986, when the patient complained of nausea and dizziness and was found to have metastases in the brain and bones by computed tomography of the brain and bone scintigraphy. Serum assays for polypeptide hormones and amines revealed that NSE, insulin, and somatostatin were elevated to 15.0 ng/ml (normal values, <10.0 ng/ml), 71 mcu/ml (normal values, 2–19 mcu/ml), and 66.0 pg/ml (normal values, 1.0–2.2 pg/ml), respectively. ACTH, epinephrine, norepinephrine, dopamine, cortisol, and glucagon were within normal ranges. In the urine, 5-hydroxyindoleacetic acid was found to be slightly elevated, up to 7.7 mg/day (normal values, <5 mg/day), but epinephrine, norepinephrine, dopamine, vanillylmandelic acid, 17-hydroxycorticosteroids, and 17-ketosteroids were all within normal values.

Osteoplastic craniotomy and total removal of the brain and skull bone tumors were performed on 15 December. Radiation therapy was applied to the spine, trochanter, brain, and chest to relieve pain. The patient was given 100 mg cisplatin on 17 February and 50 mg etoposide on 18 and 20 February. The patient received a second course of cisplatin and etoposide from 24 to 27 March.

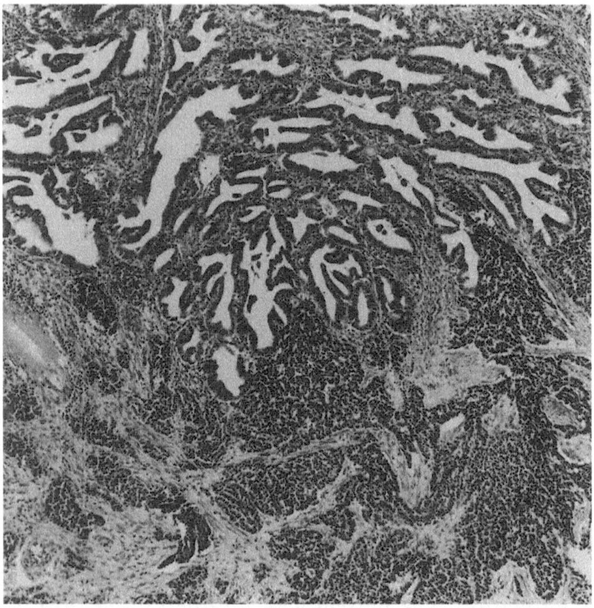

**Fig. 1.** Low-power view of primary tumor of the cervix shows that adenocarcinoma and small cell carcinoma are proliferating separately. H&E, × 40

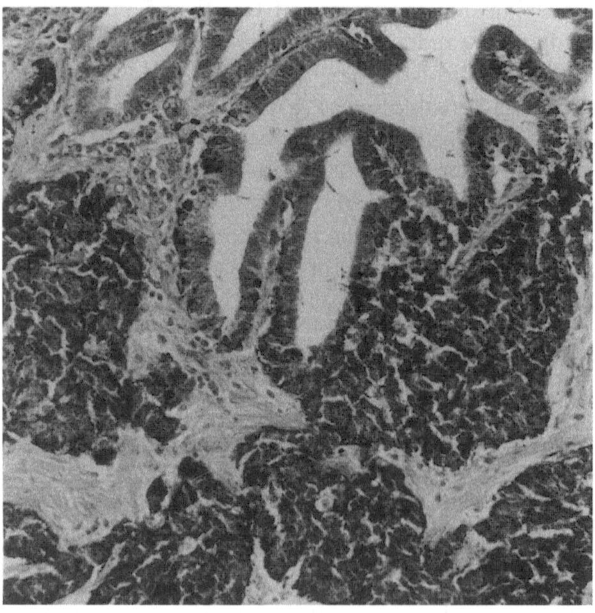

**Fig. 2.** A few cells of adenocarcinoma and most cells of small cell carcinoma in this primary tumor of the cervix are filled with argyrophil granules. Grimelius, × 100

Despite radiation and chemotherapy, the patient died of widespread metastases on 27 June 1987.

*Autopsy Findings.* Small cell carcinoma was found to have affected mediastinal, para-aortic, pulmonary hilar, paracholedochal, and subclavicular lymph nodes. Widespread involvement of liver, pancreas, kidneys and adrenals, skull, ribs, and vertebrae was also found. Lung metastases were not found.

*Histologic and Immunohistologic Findings.* Histologic examination of a primary uterine cervical tumor showed that small cell carcinoma and a small focus of adenocarcinoma had proliferated separately, so admixed in one area (Fig. 1). Tumor cells consisted of small round cells with hyperchromatic nuclei and scanty cytoplasm. The growth pattern showed a streaming pattern, solid nests, and well-defined intercellular spaces. Argyrophil granules stained by the Grimelius method were positive in a few adenocarcinoma cells and in most of the small cell carcinoma cells (Fig. 2).

Tumor cells in small cell carcinoma were positive immunohistochemically for NSE, chromogranin, and serotonin, but negative for ACTH, somatostatin, cytokeratin, and carcinoembryonic antigen.

## 10.2 Experimental Study

Metastatic lesions from the brain were cut into small pieces in Eagle's minimal essential medium (MEM) and transplanted subcutaneously into the back of nude mice (BALB/c, female nude, Clea Japan Inc., Japan). The xenografts have been subpassaged successfully 11 times and designated as YIK-1. Metastatic tumors to the brain (Fig. 3) and YIK-1 (Fig. 4) were similar histologically to the primary cervical tumor except for the absence of the adenocarcinoma component. Electron microscopic examination of YIK-1 showed neurosecretory type granules (Fig. 5).

For Southern blot analysis, genomic DNAs were extracted from tumor tissues. They were digested with Bam HI and Bgl II supplied by Toyobo Co, Ltd., Japan. The digested DNAs were electrophoresed in 0.6%–1.5% agarose gels, transferred to nylon membranes, and hybridized to $^{32}P$-labeled HPV 6, 11, 16 and 18 probes. Autoradiographs were prepared on Fuji x-ray films. DNAs from metastatic brain lesions and YIK-1 at the fourth subpassage contained more than 1000 copies of HPV 16 DNA per diploid cell and comigrated with cellular DNA (Fig. 6) (Ichimura et al. 1988). HPV 6, 11, and 18 DNAs were not detected. There was no difference in the integration profiles of HPV 16 DNA between metastatic carcinoma to the brain and YIK-1.

For the cytogenetic studies, single cell suspensions were prepared from the transplanted tumors by mincing and digesting with collagenase. They are cultured at a seed density of 0.5–1.0 X $10^6$ per 25 $cm^2$ in MEM supplemented with 20% FBS, penicillin, streptomycin, and nystatin. The cells were incubated at 37 °C in a humidified atmosphere of 5% $CO_2$/95% air. The cells were

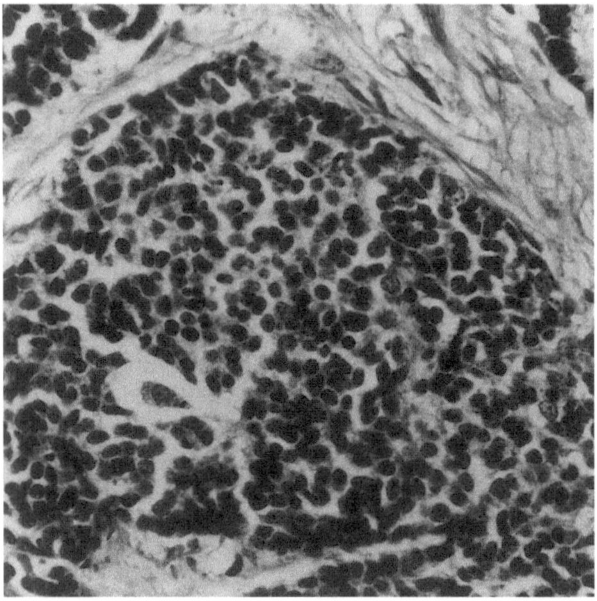

**Fig. 3.** Metastatic tumor to the brain consisting exclusively of small cell carcinoma. H&E, × 200

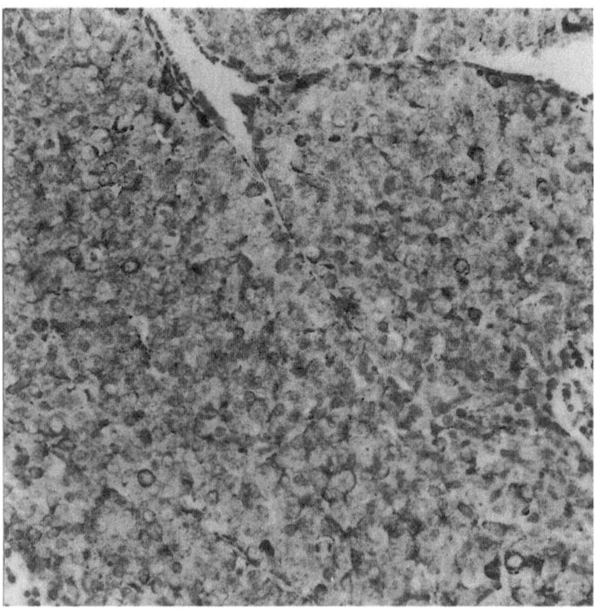

**Fig. 4.** Transplanted tumor to nude mouse (YIK-1) showing similar histologic characteristics to the metastatic lesion to the brain. Grimelius, × 100

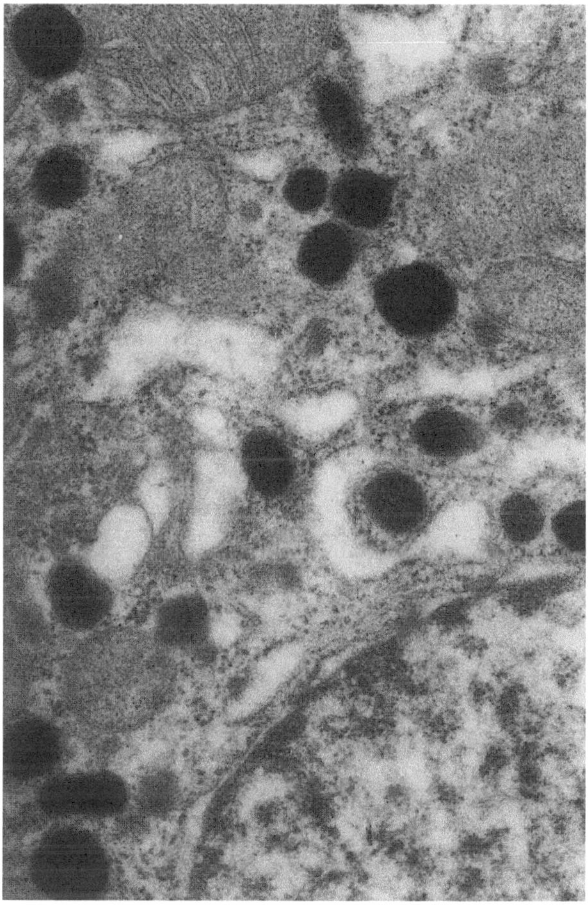

**Fig. 5.** Dense-core membrane-bound granules are seen in the cytoplasm of YIK-1 tumor cells. Electron micrograph, × 15 000

harvested for cytogenetic analysis after overnight exposure to Colcemid (Wake et al. 1981). Giemsa-trypsin G band analysis was performed. Fifty cells were karyotyped. There was a broad spectrum of karyotypic abnormalities, ranging from 47 to 54 chromosomes. A deletion of 4q and 9q was present in all cells examined. A deletion of 14q was present in most cells examined (Fig. 7). However, chromosome 3p deletion could not be demonstrated in YIK-1 by Giemsa-trypsin G band analysis, although small cell lung carcinoma cells were demonstrated to have the 3p deletion (Graziano et al. 1987) and both HPV integration and loss of 3p were suggested to be necessary to convert normal cervical epithelial cells into malignant cells (Yokota et al. 1989).

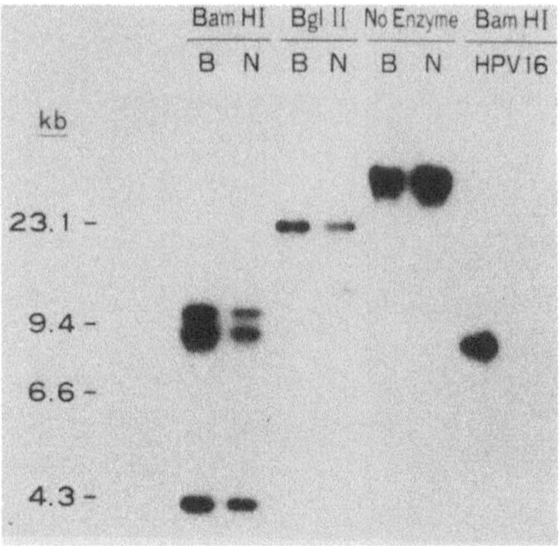


**Fig. 6.** Blot hybridization of $^{32}$P-labeled HPV-16 DNA to DNAs from metastatic small cell carcinoma to the brain (*B*) and from YIK-1 (*N*), showing more than 1000 copies of HPV-16 per diploid cell and no difference in the integration profiles

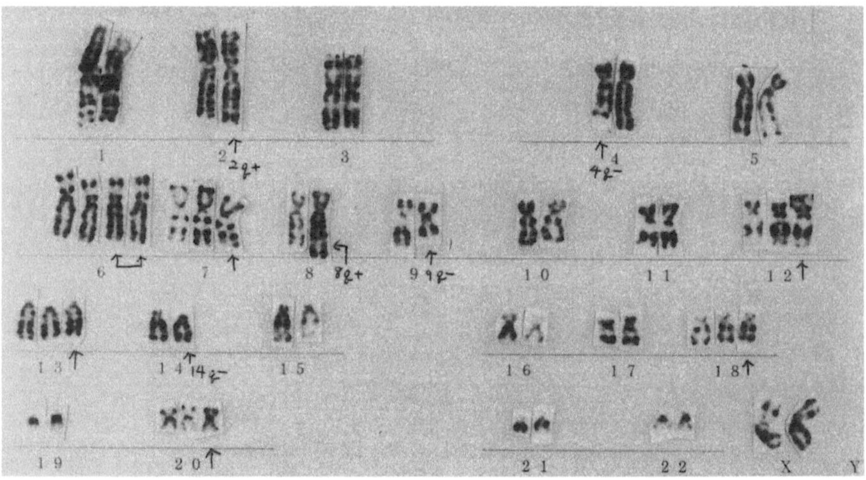

**Fig. 7.** Karyology of YIK-1 shows deletion of chromosomes 4q, 9q, and 14q

## 11 Summary

Neuroendocrine carcinomas of the cervix and endometrium were reviewed. They have been variously designated as carcinoid, argyrophil cell carcinoma, apudoma, small cell carcinoma, oat cell carcinoma, endocrine carcinoma, and neuroendocrine carcinoma, the last-mentioned term being preferred in this chapter. Adenocarcinomas with neuroendocrine cells are occasionally encountered in the cervix and endometrium. It is generally questioned whether they should be included in the spectrum of neuroendocrine carcinomas, although differential diagnosis between some such tumors of the gastrointestinal tract and neuroendocrine carcinoma is reported to be difficult.

Since the majority of neuroendocrine carcinomas of the cervix are highly aggressive, it is important to establish the neuroendocrine nature in the cervical carcinomas. In addition to the characteristic histologic features and argyrophil stainability, immunohistochemical demonstration of several neuroendocrine markers may be helpful in diagnosing neuroendocrine carcinoma of the cervix. Ultrastructural demonstration of neurosecretory granules is almost decisive in establishing the tumor's neuroendocrine nature, but it is not applicable in all cases.

Neuroendocrine carcinomas of the cervix have been treated by surgery, radiation therapy, and chemotherapy, but optimal treatment methods have not yet been established because of the rarity of the tumor.

Finally, we have described a typical neuroendocrine carcinoma of the cervix and reported some data regarding its experimental study.

## References


Aguirre P, Scully RE, Wolfe HJ, DeLellis RA (1984) Endometrial carcinoma with argyrophil cells. Hum Pathol 15:210–217

Albores-Saavedra J, Larraza O, Poucell S, Rodríguez-Martínez HA (1976) Carcinoid of the uterine cervix. Additional observation on a new tumor entity. Cancer 38:2328–2342

Albores-Saavedra J, Rodríguez-Martínez HA, Larraza-Hernández O (1979) Carcinoid tumors of the cervix. Pathol Annu 14:273–291

Arrigoni MG, Woolner LB, Bernatz PE (1972) Atypical carcinoid tumors of the lung. J Thorac Cardiovasc Surg 64:413–421

Azzopardi JG, Hou LT (1965) Intestinal metaplasia with argentaffin cells in cervical adenocarcinoma. J Pathol Bacteriol 90:686–690

Azzopardi JG, Pollack DJ (1963) Argentaffin and argyrophil cells in gastric carcinoma. J Pathol Bacteriol 86:443–452

Bannatyne P, Russell P, Wills E (1983) Argyrophilia and endometrial carcinoma. Int J Gynecol Pathol 2:235–254

Barrett RJ II, Davos I, Leuchter RS, Lagasse LD (1987) Neuroendocrine features in poorly differentiated and undifferentiated carcinomas of the cervix. Cancer 60:2325–2330

Bensch KG, Corrin B, Pariente R, Spencer H (1968) Oat-cell carcinoma of the lung: its origin and relationship to bronchial carcinoid. Cancer 22:1163–1172

Berthelot P, Benhamou JP, Fauvert R (1961) Hypercorticisme et cancer de l'utérus. Presse Med 69:189–190

Black WC (1968) Enterchromaffin cell types and corresponding carcinoid tumors. Lab Invest 19:473–486

Bonar SF, Sweeney EC (1986) The prevalence, prognostic significance and hormonal content of endocrine cells in gastric cancer. Histopathology 10:53–63

Caillaud J-M, Benjelloun S, Bosq J, Braham K, Lipinski M (1984) HNK-1-defined antigen detected in paraffin-embedded neuroectoderm tumors and those derived from cells of the amine precursor uptake and decarboxylation system. Cancer Res 44:4432–4439

Chan JKC, Tsui WMS, Tung SY, Ching RCT (1989) Endocrine cell hyperplasia of the uterine cervix. A precursor of neuroendocrine carcinoma of the cervix? Am J Clin Pathol 92:825–830

Clayton F, Sibley RK, Ordonez NG, Hansson G (1982) Argyrophilic breast carcinomas: evidence of lactational differentiation. Am J Surg Pathol 6:323–333

Cox WF, Pierce GB (1982) The endodermal origin of the endocrine cells of an adenocarcinoma of the colon of rat. Cancer 50:1530–1538
Daw E (1977) Carcinoid tumour of the cervix. Postgrad Med J 53:272–273
DeLellis RA, Dayal Y, Wolfe HJ (1984) Carcinoid tumors. Changing concepts and new perspectives. Am J Surg Pathol 8:295–300
DiSant'Agnese PA, DeMesy Jensen KL (1987) Neuroendocrine differentiation in prostatic carcinoma. Hum Pathol 18:849–856
Driessens J, Clay A, Adenis L, Demaille A (1964) Tumeur cervico-utérine et syndrome biologique de carcinoïdose. Arch Anat Pathol 12:200–203
Ferry JA, Scully RE (1988) "Adenoid cystic" carcinoma and adenoid basal carcinoma of the uterine cervix. A study of 28 cases. Am J Surg Pathol 12:134–144
Fontaine J, LeDourain NM (1977) Analysis of endoderm formation in the avian blastderm by the use of quail-chick chimeras: the problem of the neuroectodermal origin of the cells of the APUD series. J Embryol Exp Morphol 41:209–222
Fox H, Kazzaz B, Langley FA (1964) Argyrophil and argentaffin cells in the female genital tract and in ovarian mucinous cysts. J Pathol Bacteriol 88:479–488
Fujii S, Konishi I, Ferenczy A, Imai K, Okamura H, Mori T (1986) Small cell undifferentiated carcinoma of the uterine cervix: histology, ultrastructure, and immunohistochemistry of two cases. Ultrastruct Pathol 10:337–346
Gersell DJ, Mazoujian G, Mutch DG, Rudloff MA (1988) Small-cell undifferentiated carcinoma of the cervix. Am J Surg Pathol 12:684–698
Gould VE, Linnoila RI, Memoli VA, Warren WH (1983) Neuroendocrine cells and neuroendocrine neoplasms of the lung. Pathol Annu 18:287–330
Gould VE, Jao W, Chejfec G, Banner BF, Bonomi P (1984) Neuroendocrine carcinomas of the gastrointestinal tract. Semin Diagn Pathol 1:13–18
Gould VE, Wiedenmann B, Lee I et al. (1987) Synaptophysin expression in neuroendocrine neoplasms as determined by immunocytochemistry. Am J Pathol 126:243–257
Graziano SL, Gowan BY, Carney DN et al. (1987) Small cell lung cancer cell line derived from a primary tumor with a characteristic deletion of 3p. Cancer Res 47:2148–2155
Grimelius L, Wilander E (1980) Silver stains in the study of endocrine cells of the gut and pancreas. Invest Cell Pathol 3:3–12
Groben P, Reddick R, Askin F (1985) The pathologic spectrum of small cell carcinoma of the cervix. Int J Gynecol Pathol 4:42–57
Habib A, Kaneko M, Cohen CJ, Walker G (1979) Carcinoid of the uterine cervix. A case report with light and electron microscopic study. Cancer 43:535–538
Hariri J, Rasmussen EA, Hage E (1983) Carcinoid tumor of the uterine cervix. Acta Obstet Gynecol Scand 62:539–540
Hirsch FR, Matthews MJ, Aisner S et al. (1988) Histopathologic classification of small cell lung cancer. Changing concepts and terminology. Cancer 62:973–977
Hus C, Wong LC, Chan CW (1981) Nonendocrine carcinoid tumor of the uterine cervix. Aspects of diagnosis and treatment. Case report. Br J Obstet Gynecol 88:1056–1060
Husain AN, Gattuso P, Abraham K, Castelli MJ (1989) Synchronous adenocarcinoma and carcinoid of the uterine cervix: immunohistochemical study of a case and review of literature. Gynecol Oncol 33:125–128
Ichimura H, Yamasaki M, Yamane T, Shimizu H, Katsumoto T, Kurimura O, Kurimura T (1988) Heterotransplantation of argyrophil small cell carcinoma of the uterine cervix integrating HPV16DNA into nude mice. Jpn J Cancer Res (Gann) 79:1255–1258
Inoue M, Ueda G, Yamasaki M et al. (1982) Endometrial argyrophil cell adenocarcinoma with indole- or catecholamine precursor uptake and decarboxylation. Int J Gynecol Pathol 1:47–58
Inoue M, Inafuku S, Okano K, Minagawa J, Mori H (1984a) Cervical carcinoid associated with adenocarcinoma and squamous cell carcinoma. J Jpn Soc Clin Cytol 23:455–460
Inoue M, Ueda G, Yamasaki M, Tanaka Y, Hiramatsu K (1984b) Immunohistochemical demonstration of peptide hormones in endometrial carcinomas. Cancer 54:2127–2131
Inoue M, Ueda G, Nakajima T (1985) Immunohistochemical demonstration of neuron-specific enolase in gynecologic malignant tumors. Cancer 55:1686–1690
Inoue M, DeLellis RA, Scully RE (1986) Immunohistochemical demonstration of chromogranin in endometrial carcinomas with argyrophil cells. Hum Pathol 17:841–847
Iwafuchi M, Watanabe H, Ishihara N, Enjoji M, Iwashita A, Yanaihara N, Ito S (1987) Neoplastic endocrine cells in carcinomas of the small intestine: histochemical and immunohistochemical studies of 24 tumors. Hum Pathol 18:185–194

Iwaoki Y, Nogawa T, Katsube Y, Fujiwara A (1986) A case of the cervical carcinoid tumor. Cytologic, histologic, and electronmicroscopic study. J Jpn Soc Clin Cytol 25:150–156
Jacobs AJ, Marchevsky A, Gordon RE, Deppe G, Cohen CJ (1980) Oat cell carcinoma of the uterine cervix in a pregnant woman treated with cis-diamminedichloroplatinum. Gynecol Oncol 9:405–410
Johannessen JV, Davy M, Capella C, Sobrinho-Simoes M, Solcia E (1980) Endocrine cell carcinoma of the uterine cervix. Diagn Gynecol Obstet 2:127–134
Jones HW III, Plymate S, Gluck FB, Miles PA, Greene JF Jr (1976) Small cell nonkeratinizing carcinoma of the cervix associated with ACTH production. Cancer 38:1629–1635
Kaku T, Enjoji M (1983) Extremely well-differentiated adenocarcinoma ("adenoma malignum") of the cervix. Int J Gynecol Pathol 2:28–41
Kamiya H, Nagai S, Sakai K, Kudo R (1986) A case report of so called "carcinoid tumor of the uterine cervix". J Jpn Soc Clin Cytol 25:808–815
Katsube Y, Teramoto H, Nomura K, Miyagawa K, Ifuji H, Namba K (1984) A case of carcinoid tumor of the uterine cervix containing serotonin. Jpn J Cancer Clin 38:198-204
Kiang DT, Bauer GE, Kennedy BJ (1973) Immunoassayable insulin in carcinoma of the cervix associated with hypoglycemia. Cancer 31:801–805
Kodousek R, Gazarek F, Dusek J, Dostal S (1976) Malignant "apudoma" (argyrophil cell cancer) of the uterine cervix in a 24-year old woman in pregnancy. Cs Patol 12:37–44
Kumar N (1984) Small-cell carcinoma of the endometrium in a 23-year-old woman: light microscopic and ultrastructural study. Am J Clin Pathol 31:98–101
Lewin K (1987) Carcinoid tumors and the mixed (composite) glandular endocrine cell carcinomas. Am J Surg Pathol 11:71–86
Lloyd RV, Mervak T, Schmidt K, Warner TFCS, Wilson BS (1984) Immunohistochemical detection of chromogranin and neuron-specific enolase in pancreatic endocrine neoplasms. Am J Surg Pathol 8:607–614
Lojek MA, Fer MF, Kasselberg AG et al. (1980) Cushing's syndrome with small cell carcinoma of the uterine cervix. Am J Med 69:140–144
Louka MH, Danoff B, Brodovsky HS, Jahshan AE (1982) Carcinoid tumor of the uterine cervix. Respone to combination chemotherapy and radiotherapy. Am J Clin Oncol 5:487–493
Lundqvist M, Wilander E, Esscher T, Pahlman S (1985) Neuron-specific enolase in mucosal endocrine cells and carcinoid tumours of the small intestine: a comparative study with neuron-specific enolase immunocytochemistry and silver stains. Histochem J 17:323–331
Mackay B, Osborne BM, Wharton JT (1979) Small cell tumor of cervix with neuroepithelial features. Ultrastructural observations in two cases. Cancer 43:1138–1145
Manivel C, Wick MR, Sibley RK (1986) Neuroendocrine differentiation in müllerian neoplasms. An immunohistochemical study of a "pure" endometrial small-cell carcinoma and a mixed müllerian tumor containing small-cell carcinoma. Am J Clin Pathol 86:438–443
Matsuyama M, Inoue T, Ariyoshi Y et al. (1979) Argyrophil cell carcinoma of the uterine cervix with ectopic production of ACTH, β-MSH, serotonin, histamine, and amylase. Cancer 44:1813–1823
Michels S, Swanson PE, Robb JA, Wick MR (1987) Leu-7 in small cell neoplasms. An immunohistochemical study with ultrastructural correlations. Cancer 60:2958–2964
Miles PA, Greenberg H, Herrera GA, Rawding-Patterson G (1982) Primary carcinoid tumor of the uterine cervix presenting as adenosquamous carcinoma. Diagn Gynecol Obstet 4:327–337
Miwa A, Kitagawa M, Terada S (1981) So-called malignant apudoma of the uterine cervix. Postmortem findings and electron microscopic observation. Jpn J Cancer Clin 27:178–184
Mullins JD, Hillard GD (1981) Cervical carcinoid ("argyrophil cell" carcinoma) associated with an endocervical adenocarcinoma: a light and ultrastructural study. Cancer 47:785–790
Muraoka S, Takahashi T, Ando M, Nishikawa Y, Fujita M, Shimoda A (1987) Minute carcinoid tumor of the uterine cervix associated with microinvasive adenocarcinoma, with reference to its histogenesis. Acta Pathol Jpn 37:1183–1198
Oberndorfer S (1907) Karzinoide Tumoren des Dünndarms. Frankf Z Pathol 1:426–429
Okudaira Y, Tateishi R, Sato Y, Saji F, Hayakawa K, Matsui Y, Sawada M (1980) Argyrophil cell of the endometrial adenocarcinoma. Acta Obstet Gynecol Jpn 32:1541–1550
Olson N, Twiggs L, Sibley R (1982) Small-cell carcinoma of the endometrium: light microscopic and ultrastructural study of a case. Cancer 50:760–765
Ooi A, Mai M, Ogino T et al. (1988) Endocrine differentiation of gastric adenocarcinoma. The prevalence as evaluated by immunoreactive chromogranin A and its biologic significance. Cancer 62:1096–1104

Ouchi K, Matsuo Y, Yahata K et al. (1981) A case report of oat cell carcinoma of the cervix, suggested by cytology and confirmed by electronmicroscope. J Jpn Soc Clin Cytol 20:572–577
Paz R, Frigerio B, Sundblad A, Eusebi V (1985) Small cell (oat cell) carcinoma of the endometrium. Arch Pathol Lab Med 109:270–272
Pazdur R, Bonomi P, Slayton R et al. (1981) Neuroendocrine carcinoma of the cervix: implications for staging and therapy. Gynecol Oncol 12:120–128
Pearse AGE (1969) The cytochemistry and ultrastructure of polypeptide hormone-producing cells of the APUD series and the embryologic, physiologic and pathologic implications of the concept. J Histochem Cytochem 17:303–313
Picket RL, Rall LB, Phelps P, Rutter WJ (1976) The neural crest and the origin of insulin-producing and other gastrointestinal hormone-producing cells. Science 191:191–192
Radi MJ, Fenoglio-Preiser CM, Bartow SA, Key CR, Pathak DR (1986) Gastric carcinoma in the young: a clinico-pathological and immuno-histochemical study. Am J Gastroenterol 81:747–756
Reagan JW, Mamonic MS, Wentz WB (1957) Analytical study of the cells in cervical squamous cell cancer. Lab Invest 6:241–250
Said JW, Vimadalal S, Nash G, Shintaku IP, Heusser RC, Sassoon AF, Lloyd RV (1985) Immunoreactive neuron-specific enolase, bombesin, and chromogranin as markers for neuroendocrine lung tumors. Hum Pathol 16:236–240
Sakamoto Y, Kishi Y, Yamamoto Y, Ino H (1982) Carcinoid tumor (argyrophil cell carcinoma) in the uterine cervix: with special reference to cytologic figures. J Jpn Soc Clin Cytol 21:702–708
Satake T, Matsuyama M (1987) Argyrophil cells in normal endometrial glands. Virchows Arch [A] 410:449–454
Satake T, Matsuyama M, Kuzuya K, Suchi T, Sato T (1982) Argyrophil reactive cells in the normal uterus and differentiated endometrial carcinoma. Acta Pathol Jpn 32:1017–1026
Sato Y, Ozaki M, Ueda G, Tanizawa O (1986) Clinical significance of argyrophilia in endometrial carcinomas. Gynecol Oncol 25:53–60
Scully RE, Aguirre P, DeLellis RA (1984) Argyrophilia, serotonin, and peptide hormones in the female genital tract and its tumors. Int J Gynecol Pathol 3:51–70
Seidel R Jr, Steinfeld A (1988) Carcinoid of the cervix: natural history and implications for therapy. Gynecol Oncol 30:114–119
Sheets EE, Berman ML, Hrountas CK, Liao SY, DiSaia PH (1988) Surgically treated, early-stage neuroendocrine small-cell cervical carcinoma. Obstet Gynecol 71:10–14
Silva EG, Kott MM, Ordonez NG (1984) Endocrine carcinoma intermediate cell type of the uterine cervix. Cancer 54:1705–1713
Smith DM Jr, Haggitt RC (1984) The prevalance and prognostic significance of argyrophil cells in colorectal carcinomas. Am J Surg Pathol 8:123–128
Stahl R, Demopoulos RI, Bigelow B (1981) Carcinoid tumor within a squamous cell carcinoma of the cervix. Gynecol Oncol 11:387–392
Stassart J, Crum CP, Yodan EL, Fenoglio CM, Richart RM (1982) Argyrophilic carcinoma of the cervix. A report of a case with coexisting cervical intraepithelial neoplasia. Gynecol Oncol 13:247–251
Stockdale AD, Leader M, Phillips RH, Henry K (1986) The carcinoid syndrome and multiple hormone secretion associated with a carcinoid tumour of the uterine cervix. Case report. Br J Obstet Gynecol 93:397–401
Stratton M, Evans DJ, Lampert IA (1986) Effects of oestrogens on endocrine cells in prostatic carcinoma (abstr). J Pathol 148:83A
Sweeney EC, McDonnell L (1980) Atypical gastric carcinoids. Histopathology 4:215–224
Tateishi R, Wada A, Hayakawa K, Hongo J, Ishii S, Terakawa N (1975) Argyrophil cell carcinomas (apudomas) of the uterine cervix. Light and electron microscopic observations of 5 cases. Virchows Arch [A] 336:257–274
Taxy JB, Tischler AS, Insalaco S-J, Battifora H (1981) "Carcinoid" tumor of the breast. A variant of conventional breast cancer ? Hum Pathol 12:170–179
Tsukamoto N, Hirakawa T, Matsukuma K, Kaku T, Matsuyama T, Kamura T, Saito T (1989) Carcinoma of the uterine cervix with variegated histological patterns and calcitonin production. Gynecol Oncol 33:395–399
Tuji K, Taguchi T, Horinaga T (1978) Fine structural observation of ACTH-producing carcinoid tumor of the uterine cervix. J Clin Electron Microscopy 11:5–6
Turner WA, Gallup DG, Talledo OE, Otken LB Jr, Guthrie TH (1986) Neuroendocrine carcinoma of the uterine cervix complicated by pregnancy: case report and review of the literature. Obstet Gynecol 67:80s–83s

Ueda G (1988) Biological behavior of argyrophil carcinoma of the cervix. J Jpn Soc Gynecol Pathol Colposc 6:47–58
Ueda G, Sato Y, Yamasaki M et al. (1977) Argyrophil cell adenocarcinoma of the endometrium. Acta Obstet Gynecol Jpn 29:1167–1168
Ueda G, Yamasaki M, Inoue M, Kurachi K (1979) A clinicopathologic study of endometrial carcinomas with argyrophil cells. Gynecol Oncol 7:223–232
Ueda G, Yamasaki M, Inoue M, Tanaka Y, Hiramatsu K, Inoue Y, Abe Y (1984a) Immunohistochemical demonstration of peptide hormones in cervical adenocarcinomas with argyrophil cells. Int J Gynecol Pathol 2:373–379
Ueda G, Yamasaki M, Inoue M et al. (1984b) Argyrophil cells in the endometrioid carcinoma of the ovary. Cancer 54:1569–1573
Ueda G, Tanaka Y, Inoue Y et al. (1985) Immunohistochemical demonstration of chromogranin in endometrial carcinomas with argyrophilia. Acta Obstet Gynecol Jpn 37:2853–2854
Ueda G, Yamasaki M, Inoue M, Tanaka Y, Inoue Y, Abe Y, Tanizawa O (1986) Immunohistochemical demonstration of HNK-1-defined antigen in gynecologic tumors with argyrophilia. Int J Gynecol Pathol 5:143–150
Ueda G, Inoue M, Saito J, Shimizu H, Shimizu C, Sasagawa H, Tanizawa O (1987a) Distribution of epithelial membrane antigen in endometrial carcinoma with argyrophilia. Acta Obstet Gynecol Jpn 39:998–999
Ueda G, Nishino T, Saito J, Abe Y, Shimizu H, Tanizawa O (1987b) Detection of chromogranin in argyrophil cells of endometrial carcinoma. Gynecol Oncol 27:159–165
Ueda G, Shimizu C, Shimizu H, Saito J, Tanaka Y, Inoue M, Tanizawa O (1989) An immunohistochemical study of small-cell and poorly differentiated carcinomas of the cervix using neuroendocrine markers. Gynecol Oncol 34:164–169
Ulich TR, Liao SY, Layfield L, Romansky S, Cheng L, Lewin KJ (1986) Endocrine and tumor differentiation markers in poorly differentiated small-cell carcinoids of the cervix and vagina. Arch Pathol Lab Med 110:1054–1057
Van Nagell JR Jr, Powell DE, Gallion HH et al. (1988) Small cell carcinoma of the uterine cervix. Cancer 62:1586–1593
Wake N, Slocum HK, Rustum YM, Matsui S, Sandberg AA (1981) Chromosomes and causation of human cancer and leukemia. XLIV. A method for chromosome analysis of solid tumor. Cancer Genet Cytogenet 3:1–10
Walker AN, Mills SE, Taylor PT (1988) Cervical neuroendocrine carcinoma: a clinical and light microscopic study of 14 cases. Int J Gynecol Pathol 7:64–74
Warner TFCS (1978) Carcinoid tumor of the uterine cervix. J Clin Pathol 31:990–995
Warren WH, Memoli VA, Gould VE (1988) Well-differentiated and small cell neuroendocrine carcinomas of the lung. Two related but distinct clinicopathologic entities. Virchows Arch [B] 55:299–310
Waxman M, Vuletin JC, Pertshuk DO (1979) Lysosomes in Brenner's tumor simulating secretory argentaffin granules. Arch Pathol Lab Med 103:183–186
Wick MR, Stanley M, Cherwitz DL, Savage JE (1986) Concomitant neuropeptide-producing endometrial carcinomas and ileal carcinoid tumors. J Clin Pathol 85:406–410
Yamasaki M, Tateishi R, Hongo J, Ozaki M, Inoue M, Ueda G (1984) Argyrophil small cell carcinomas of the uterine cervix. Int J Gynecol Pathol 3:146–152
Yokota J, Tsukada Y, Nakajima T et al. (1989) Loss of heterozygosity on the short arm of chromosome 3 in carcinoma of the uterine cervix. Cancer Res 49:3598–3601
Yoshida A, Yoshida H, Fukunishi R, Inohara T (1984) Carcinoid tumor of the uterine cervix. A light and electron microscopic study. Virchows Arch [A] 402:331–336

# Flow Cytometry of Ovarian Neoplasms

D.A. BELL



## 1 Introduction

Epithelial carcinomas are the most common malignant tumors of the ovary and are the most common cause of death from genital malignancies in women (BALL et al. 1990). Although advances in therapy have resulted in prolonged disease-free survivals, these intensive treatments are associated with substantial side-effects and the majority of women with advanced stage epithelial carcinoma eventually die of their tumor despite therapy. These factors have resulted in a search for features that would permit greater prognostic accuracy and tailoring of treatment regimens to the biologic behavior of the tumor in an individual patient. The development of a method of DNA analysis on paraffin-embedded tissue by HEDLEY and co-workers (HEDLEY et al. 1983, 1985; HEDLEY 1989) has

Current Topics in Pathology
Volume 85, Ed. N. Sasano

prompted numerous investigations of the prognostic significance of DNA content and cell cycle analysis as possibly more objective and reproducible indicators of tumor behavior. The majority of these studies have examined the relation of flow cytometric analysis to known prognostic factors and to survival in surface epithelial carcinomas; a smaller number of studies have addressed these issues in ovarian neoplasms of other types. This article will briefly summarize the technical aspects of DNA analysis by flow cytometry, concentrating on technical difficulties that may interfere with the analysis, and then review in detail the relation of DNA ploidy and cell cycle data to clinical and histologic features and survival for each tumor type.

## 2 Technical Summary

Flow cytometric determination of DNA content may be defined as the electronic measurement of the relative intensities of fluorescence of various fluorescent dyes that bind stoichiometrically with DNA in thousands of cells over a rapid period of time. To perform the analysis, the flow cytometer must be presented with individual cells or nuclei in suspension (COLVIN and PREFFER 1987; COON et al. 1987). These are obtained from solid tumors by mechanical, detergent, or enzymatic disaggregation techniques. Depending on the method used, either intact single cells or free nuclei are obtained from fresh or deparaffinized tissue. Each tissue source has its proponents; the advantages and disadvantages of each is outlined in Table 1 (COON et al. 1987; HEDLEY 1989). After disaggregation, the cells or nuclei are stained with one of the many fluorescent dyes that intercalate into DNA and the specimen is analyzed by the flow cytometer. In the machine, the single cells or nuclei are presented to the laser beam single file in suspension and detectors measure the amount of light transmitted in a forward direction (forward angle scatter, which correlates with cell volume), the amount of light reflected at an angle (90° angle or side scatter, which correlates with internal"granularity"), and the intensity of excited fluorescence of the fluorescent dye. These data are recorded for each individual cell in a computer and are generally analyzed as various forms of graphic and numerical output including the DNA histogram, scattergram, and cell cycle analysis data (COLVIN and PREFFER 1987; COON et al. 1987). The DNA histogram tabulates the number of cells with relative DNA fluorescent intensities as a frequency distribution (Fig. 1). The relative fluorescent intensities are indicated on the x-axis in arbitrary units (channel numbers) and the number of cells or nuclei with each fluorescent intensity is indicated on the y-axis. Thus, in normal tissue or a diploid tumor, one sees a single large peak of cells ($G_0/G_1$) with a 2N or diploid DNA content, a smaller peak of cells in $G_2$ and M. Just prior to completion of mitosis with twice the normal DNA content, and cells with a DNA content between these peaks that have variable amounts of DNA secondary to DNA

**Table 1.** Comparison of fresh and deparaffinized tissue

*Fresh tissue:*

Advantages:
1. External standards with known ploidy may be used to determine the DNA index of the tumor population
2. Less debris is present, resulting in better histogram resolution
3. Whole cells may be analyzed, allowing identification of cytoplasmic and plasma membrane antigens in addition to DNA content analysis

Disadvantages:
1. Tissue must be obtained prospectively
2. Histologic localization of specific regions of interest is not possible

*Deparaffinized tissue:*

Advantages:
1. May be analyzed retrospectively
2. Histologic examination of tissue sections allows specific sampling of small lesions by trimming the paraffin block

Disadvantages:
1. External ploidy standards cannot be used due to a variable reduction in DNA fluorescence secondary to fixation; normal inflammatory and stromal cells in the block are utilized as the diploid "normal" population
2. Cutting sections from the paraffin block results in debris, which decreases the histogram resolution
3. Only bare nuclei are obtained

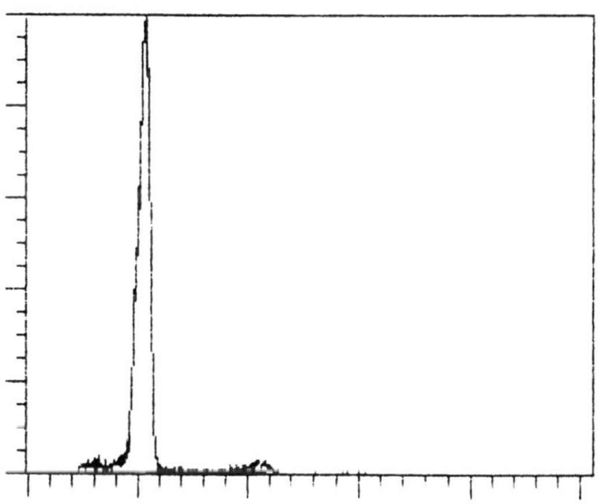

**Fig. 1.** DNA diploid histogram with a single large $G_0/G_1$ peak and a smaller $G_2M$ peak with twice the relative fluorescene (4N) of the $G_0/G_1$ peak (*y axis*, number of cells or nuclei; *x-axis*, relative fluorescent intensities in channel numbers)

synthesis prior to cell division (S-phase fraction, SPF) (Fig. 1). In a specimen that contains abnormal populations with a different DNA content than normal cells, one or more additional large $G_0/G_1$ peaks are present, often associated with their own $G_2M$ peaks with twice the fluorescent intensity of the abnormal stemline (Figs. 2–4). The degree of aneuploidy is expressed as the DNA index,

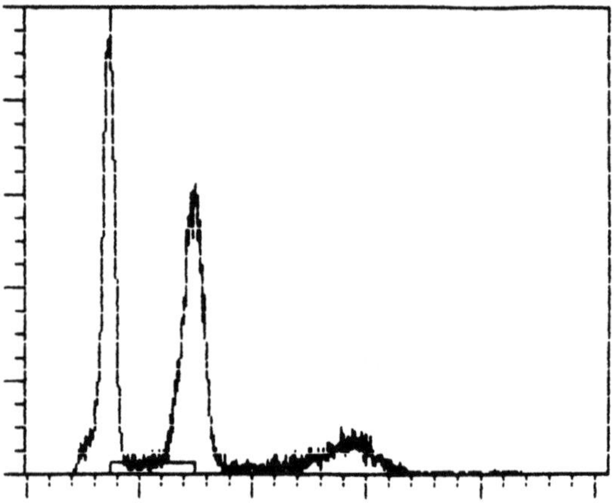

**Fig. 2.** DNA tetraploid histogram with an additional large $G_0/G_1$ peak located in the diploid $G_2M$ region (DNA index of 2.0) and a corresponding $G_2M$ peak in the 8N region, indicating a cycling DNA tetraploid population

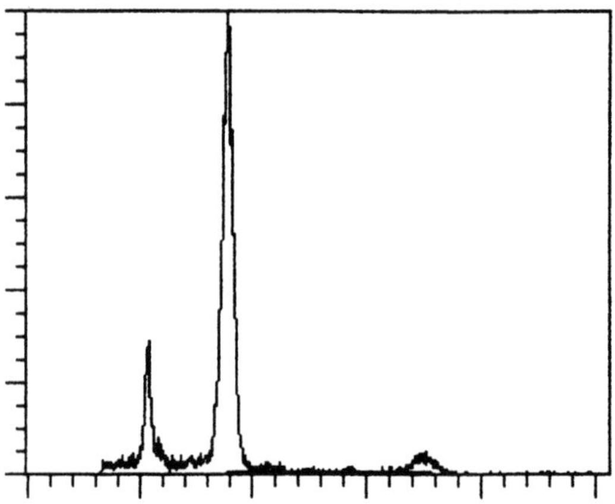

**Fig. 3.** DNA aneuploid histogram with a single additional large $G_0/G_1$ peak with a DNA index of 1.65 and a corresponding small $G_2M$ peak with twice the relative fluorescence of the abnormal $G_0/G_1$ peak, indicating a cycling DNA aneuploid stemline

which is defined as the mean or modal channel of the $G_0/G_1$ peak of the abnormal population or populations over that of the $G_0/G_1$ peak of the normal cells (Figs. 2–4). The percent of cells in the synthetic phase is represented by the area beneath the curve between the $G_0/G_1$ and $G_2M$ peaks, which can be obtained by various mathematical models. The scattergram plots the forward angle scatter and side scatter for each cell or nucleus.

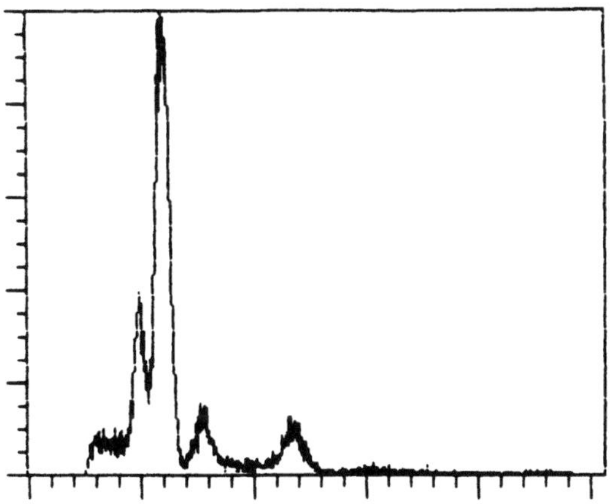

**Fig. 4.** DNA multiploid histogram with multiple additional $G_0/G_1$ peaks with DNA indices of 1.2 and 1.58. A $G_2M$ peak corresponding to the abnormal population with a DNA index of 1.2 is also present

This method of DNA analysis, although quite reliable and reproducible, has a number of technical and interpretation errors that may affect the results of the analysis. Disaggregation of the tumor necessarily creates debris, which can adversely affect the ability to detect peridiploid or small aneuploid peaks (Fig. 5). The resolving power of the histogram may be judged by the coefficient of variation (CV) of the $G_0/G_1$ peak, which is a measure of the width of the curve (i.e., the larger the CV, the less the resolving power). As the specimen passes through the flow cytometer, particles may clump together, creating artifactual peaks at the 4N, 6N, etc. locations (Fig. 6). These artifacts can be reduced by

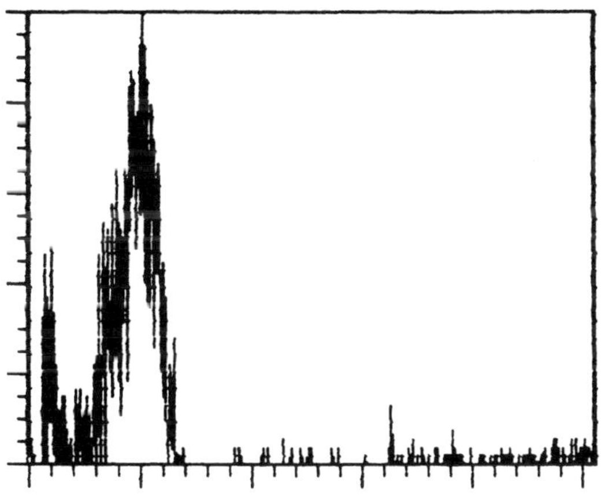

**Fig. 5.** Unsatisfactory histogram composed of debris and few cells

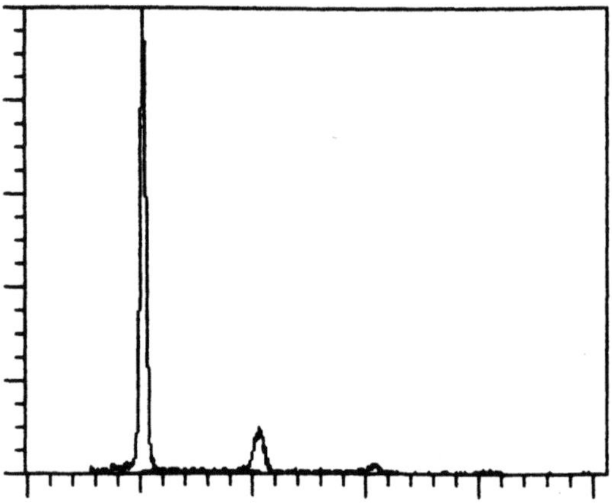

**Fig. 6.** DNA diploid histogram from normal tonsil control showing artifactual peaks at the 4N, 6N, and 8N location caused by clumping of muclei

sonication (GONCHOROFF et al. 1990) or electronic analysis of the data utilizing a pulse processor (COLVIN and PREFFER 1987), or may be excluded by comparison with the scattergram. Finally, although interpretation of histograms is often straightforward, standardized criteria for the "diagnosis" of the curves have not been established and various authorities utilize differing definitions of "DNA diploid" and "DNA aneuploid" (Table 2). An even greater number of methods of analysis of cell cycle data are in use; these utilize different mathematical models of calculating the number of cells that are present beneath the various portions of the curve. Some workers also use computer techniques that subtract presumed debris from the histogram or analyze cell cycle data in overlapping populations by mathematical manipulation of the data. These factors render comparison of data from different laboratories difficult and may explain divergent results in apparently similar studies.

**Table 2.** Definitions of DNA aneuploidy

1. Presence of two or more discrete $G_0/G_1$ peaks
2. DNA index greater than 1.05 (JAKOBSEN et al. 1988) or 1.1 (SAHNI et al. 1989) in fresh tissue when compared to an external diploid standard
3. A single broad $G_1$ peak (MURRAY et al. 1989; ROBEY et al. 1989; RODENBURG et al. 1988)
4. More than 20% of total number of cells in the region of the diploid $G_2M$ peak (4N) with a corresponding $G_2M$ peak in the 8N location (DNA tetraploid) (BLUMENFELD et al. 1987)
5. Diploid tumors with a $G_2/M$ two times greater than SPF and more than 15% of total cell count (DNA tetraploid) (KALLIONIEMI et al. 1988b)
6. "Peak" in the diploid $G_2/M$ region (4N) with another peak at 8N location (KLEMI et al. 1989; MURRAY et al. 1989)

## 3 Surface Epithelial Tumors

### 3.1 Carcinomas

Over 30 studies have reported the results of flow cytometric DNA analysis in ovarian carcinomas from approximately 2500 patients. These studies have generally examined the relation of DNA content with either survival or clinicopathologic features previously shown to be of possible prognostic significance.

#### *3.1.1 Relation of DNA Analysis to Stage and Extent of Residual Tumor*

The majority of studies in the literature are in agreement that the most important clinical prognostic factors in surface epithelial carcinoma are the stage and extent of residual tumor after debulking surgery (DISAIA and CREASMAN 1989). Eleven studies have examined the relation of DNA ploidy and staging in detail (BARNABEI et al. 1990; BLUMENFELD et al. 1987; BRESCIA et al. 1990; FRIEDLANDER

**Table 3.** DNA content and FIGO stage

| Author | Stage 1 | | Stage 2 | | Stage 3 | | Stage 4 | | Sig. |
|---|---|---|---|---|---|---|---|---|---|
| | No. | % Aneupl. | No. | % Aneupl. | No. | % Aneupl. | No. | % Aneupl. | |
| BARNABEI et al. (1990) | 17 | 59 | 13 | 69 | 61 | 80 | 24 | 80 | Yes |
| BLUMENFELD et al. (1987) | 0 | | 7 | 43 | 58 | 50 | 19 | 63 | No |
| BRESCIA et al. (1990) | 17 | 18 | 10 | 60 | 69 | 51 | 3 | 100 | NA |
| ERBA et al. (1989) | | | | | 82 | 77[a] | | | |
| FRIEDLANDER et al. (1988) | 20 | 40[b] | | | 30 | 100[a] | | | Yes |
| HAMAGUCHI et al. (1990) | 4 | 25 | 6 | 17 | 24 | 54 | 8 | 62 | Yes |
| IVERSON and SKAARLAND (1987) | 12 | 8 | 8 | 25 | 26 | 77 | 4 | 100 | Yes |
| JAKOBSEN et al. (1988) | 11 | 45 | 2 | 100 | 15 | 47 | 6 | 67 | No |
| KALLIONIEMI et al. (1988b) | 77 | 48 | 12 | 42 | 48 | 73 | 20 | 70 | NA |
| KLEMI et al. (1989) | 16 | 81[b] | | | 27 | 59 | 27 | 63 | No |
| KLEMI et al. (1989) | 26 | 54 | 20 | 55 | 54 | 63 | 34 | 71 | No |
| MURRAY et al. (1989) | 9 | 44 | 15 | 73 | 15 | 53 | 1 | 100 | No |
| VOLM et al. (1989) | 0 | | 0 | | 20 | 55 | 17 | 65 | No |

NA, not analyzed; Aneupl., DNA aneuploid; Sig., statistically significant
[a] Grades 3 and 4 combined
[b] Grades 1 and 2 combined
[c] Serous carcinomas only

**Table 4.** SPF and FIGO Stage

| Author | Stage 1 | | Stage 2 | | Stage 3 | | Stage 4 | | Sig. |
|---|---|---|---|---|---|---|---|---|---|
| | No. | % SPF | No. | % SPF | No. | % SPF | No. | % SPF | |
| BARNABEI et al. (1990) | 17 | 9.5 | 13 | 10.2 | 61 | 13.1 | 24 | 15.9 | No |
| KALLIONIEMI et al. (1988b) | 77 | 11.4 | 12 | 13.0 | 48 | 16.4 | 20 | 16.5 | NA |
| KLEMI et al. (1989) | 20 | 60[a] | 11 | 27a | 38 | 50[a] | 28 | 75[a] | Yes |
| VOLM et al. (1989) | | | | | 15 | 53[a] | 9 | 67[a] | No |

NA, not analyzed; Sig., statistically significant
[a] % of patients with SPF greater than 11%

**Table 5.** DNA analysis and size of residual tumor

| Author | None | | 2 cm or less | | More than 2 cm | | Sig. |
|---|---|---|---|---|---|---|---|
| | No. | % Aneupl. | No. | % Aneupl. | No. | % Aneupl. | |
| BARNABEI et al. (1990) | 29 | 69 | 43 | 79 | 38 | 79 | No |
| BLUMENFELD et al. (1987) | | | 36 | 44 | 48 | 58 | NA |
| ERBA et al. (1989) | | | 27 | 59 | 66 | 88 | Yes |
| HAMAGUCHI et al. (1989) | | | 25 | 28 | 17 | 71 | Yes |
| KLEMI et al. (1989) | 39 | 54 | 26 | 50 | 65 | 69 | No |
| RODENBURG et al. (1987a) | | | 23[a] | 52 | 51[a] | 92 | Yes |
| | No. | % SPF | No. | % SPF | No. | % SPF | |
| BARNABEI et al. (1990) | 29 | 9.7 | 43 | 13.8 | 38 | 15.0 | Yes |
| KLEMI et al. (1989) | 28 | 46[b] | 18 | 61[b] | 48 | 60[b] | No |

Aneupl., DNA aneuploid; NA, not analyzed; Sig. statistically significant
[a] Less than or greater than 1.5 cm
[b] % of patients with SPF greater than 11%

et al. 1983; HAMAGUCHI et al. 1990; IVERSEN and SKAARLAND 1987; JAKOBSEN et al. 1988; KALLIONIEMI et al. 1988b; KLEMI et al. 1988, 1989; MURRAY et al. 1989 et al. 1989) (Table 3). Although several failed to show a relationship, many of the studies found a greater frequency of DNA aneuploidy in stage 3 or 4 than stage 1 or 2 carcinomas (BARNABEI et al. 1990; FRIEDLANDER et al. 1983; HAMAGUCHI et al. 1990; IVERSEN and SKAARLAND 1987). The four studies (Table 4) which analyzed the relation of SPF and stage all showed an increased percentage of cells in the SPF with increasing stage; however, in one study these differences were not statistically significant (Barnabei et al. 1990), in another they were of marginal statistical significance (Klemi et al. 1989), in the third study the statistical significance of the data was not reported (Kallioniemi et al. 1988b), and in the fourth study only advanced stage tumors were compared (Volm et al. 1989).

The majority of studies have demonstrated a statistically significant association between DNA aneuploidy and bulky postoperative residual disease, as shown in Table 5 (Barnabei et al. 1990; Blumenfeld et al. 1987; Erba et al. 1989; Hamaguchi et al. 1990; Klemi et al. 1989; Rodenburg et al. 1987a). One study found an elevation of SPF with a large amount of residual tumor (Barnabei et al. 1990); another found no association between these factors (Klemi et al. 1989).

### *3.1.2 Relation of DNA Content to Pathologic Features*

A number of studies have suggested that the histologic type and degree of differentiation of surface epithelial carcinomas are important prognostic features (Aure et al. 1971; Sobre et al. 1982); however, others have been unable to confirm these findings. Although the majority of studies have concluded that there is no clear relationship between DNA ploidy and histologic type (Barnabei et al. 1990; Bell et al. in preparation, Blumenfeld et al. 1987; Brescia et al. 1990; Christov and Vassilev 1987; Friedlander et al. 1983, 1984a; Hamaguchi et al. 1990; Heinonen et al. 1988; Jakobsen et al. 1988; Kallioniemi et al. 1988a; Klemi et al. 1988, 1989; Kuhn et al. 1989; Murray et al. 1989; Tase et al. 1987; Volm et al. 1985; Watson et al. 1987), it is apparent from examination of the results of these studies that the majority of serous and undifferentiated carcinomas are DNA aneuploid whereas the frequency of aneuploidy in the other cell types is higly variable (Table 6). These latter results may reflect the substantial intra- and interobserver variation in histologic subtyping that has been amply documented in the literature (Baak et al. 1986b; Cramer et al. 1987; Hernandez et al. 1984). Two studies (Kallioniemi et al. 1988a; Bell et al. in preparation) noted an increased frequency of multiple aneuploid stemlines in carcinomas of clear cell type. Only a small number of articles have included data on unusual types of surface epithelial carcinomas. Of the 20 reported cases of transitional cell carcinoma, ten were DNA aneuploid, six were DNA tetraploid, and the remainder were DNA diploid (Bell et al., in preparation; Robey et al. 1989). Two of the four malignant Brenner tumors were DNA aneuploid (Heinonen et al. 1988; Kuhn et al. 1989; Trebeck et al. 1987). Twenty-four (71%) of the 34 cases of serous surface carcinoma were DNA aneuploid (Brescia et al. 1990; Rutledge et al. 1989). The small number of studies that have examined SPF and histologic type have demonstrated a relatively low SPF among mucinous and endometrioid carcinomas (Barnabei et al. 1990; Kallioniemi et al. 1988a; Klemi et al. 1989; Kuhn et al. 1989) when compared to other histologic types.

**Table 6.** DNA analysis and histologic type

| | Serous | | Mucinous | | EMoid | | Clear cell | | Undiff. | |
|---|---|---|---|---|---|---|---|---|---|---|
| Author | No. | % A | No. | % A | No. | % A | No. | % A | No. | % A |
| Barnabei et al. (1990) | 67 | 84 | 10 | 70 | 23 | 56 | 4 | 50 | 11 | 82 |
| Bell et al. in prep | 64 | 77 | 7 | 43 | 14 | 21 | 7 | 43 | 0 | |
| Blumenfeld et al. (1987) | 60 | 55 | 10 | 70 | 7 | 29 | 4 | 25 | 0 | |
| Brescia et al. (1990) | 50 | 54 | 6 | 33 | 22 | 32 | 3 | 33 | 7 | 57 |
| Christory and Vassilev (1987) | 24 | 67 | 3 | 67 | 2 | 50 | 0 | | 3 | 67 |
| Friedlander et al. (1983) | 24 | 88 | 2 | 100 | 11 | 45 | 3 | 100 | 2 | 100 |
| Friedlander et al. (1984a) | 60 | 72 | 7 | 57 | 7 | 86 | 6 | 83 | 2 | 50 |
| Hamaguchi et al. (1990) | 29 | 48 | 2 | 50 | 5 | 4 | 3 | 33 | 3 | 33 |
| Heinonen et al. (1988) | 4 | 50 | 3 | 33 | 3 | 100 | | | 2 | 100 |
| Jackobsen et al. (1988) | 21 | 57 | 5 | 40 | 5 | 60 | 2 | 50 | 2 | 50 |
| Kallioniemi et al. (1988a) | 59 | 61 | 26 | 38 | 18 | 61 | 13 | 54 | 28 | 75 |
| Klemi et al. (1988) | 90 | 57 | | | | | | | | |
| Klemi et al. (1989) | 69 | 55 | 8 | 62 | 35 | 46 | 19 | 84 | 3 | 100 |
| Kuhn et al. (1989) | 65 | 65 | 8 | 62 | 13 | 77 | 1 | 100 | 12 | 50 |
| Murray et al. (1989) | 16 | 63 | 6 | 33 | 11 | 73 | 0 | | | |
| Tase et al. (1987) | 28 | | 5 | 0 | 5 | 17 | 5 | 100 | 0 | |
| Volm et al. (1985) | 33 | 73 | 0 | | 3 | 100 | 0 | | 3 | 100 |
| Waston et al. (1987) | 36 | 78 | 0 | | | | 0 | | | 0 |

EMoid, endometroid; % A, % DNA aneuploid

Many studies have examined the relation of DNA content to grade as determined by various methods. The majority of these studies have shown an increased frequency of DNA aneuploidy and an elevated SPF with increasing Brother's grade (Erba et al. 1989), nuclear grade (Kallioniemi et al. 1988a), the grade as determined by the percentage of solid tumor (architectural grade) (Barnabei et al. 1990; Brescia et al. 1990; Kallioniemi et al. 1988a; Rodenburg et al. 1988), or the grade as determined by unspecified methods (Erba et al.1989; Friedlander et al. 1983; Blumenfeld et al. 1987; Iverson and Skaarland 1987; Klemi et al. 1989; Rutgers et al. 1987) when all surface epithelial carcinoma types are combined in the analysis. The two studies that examined this feature in serous carcinomas only did not find an association between ploidy and grade (KLEMI et al. 1988; WATSON et al. 1987).

### *3.1.3 Relation of DNA Content to Survival*

Several studies have analyzed the relation of DNA ploidy to the interval to first recurrence with conflicting results. Two studies (BARNABEI et al. 1990; HAMAGUCHI et al. 1990) were unable to document a difference in length of disease-free survival between patients with DNA aneuploid and DNA diploid tumors whereas two other groups (MURRAY et al. 1989; RODENBURG et al. 1987a) found a significantly longer time to first recurrence in patients with diploid rather than aneuploid tumors. BARNABEI and co-workers (1990) also noted that an SPF of less than 18% was association with a longer disease-free survival than an SPF greater than 18%. Other studies did not examine this feature.

The major emphasis of most of the studies in this area has been the relation of DNA analysis and overall survival. Twelve large studies have noted a statistically significant shorter median survival time or a smaller percentage of survivors among patients with DNA aneuploid tumors rather than DNA diploid ones (BAAK et al. 1988; BARNABEI et al. 1990; BLUMENFELD et al.1987; BRESCIA et al. 1990; FRIEDLANDER et al. 1988; GAJEWSKI et al., in preparation; HAMAGUCHI et al. 1990; KALLIONIEMI et al. 1988b; KLEMI et al. 1989; MURRAY et al. 1989; RODENBURG et al. 1987a; VOLM et al. 1989) (Table 7). In a few studies the differences in survival were most marked during the first several years of follow-up (BLUMENFELD et al. 1987; HAMAGUCHI et al. 1990). A small number of studies failed to demonstrate a difference in prognosis between ploidy groups in tumors of all epithelial types (ERBA et al. 1989; RUTGERS et al. 1987), or in serous carcinomas only (KLEMI et al. 1988); however, there was a trend toward a worse prognosis with DNA aneuploidy (P = 0.11) in the study of ERBA and co-workers (1989) and a statistically significant difference in survival between tumors with a low versus high DNA index (less than or greather than 1.3) in the serous carcinomas studied by KLEMI and colleagues (1988). Six of the eight studies that examined the association between SPF and survival found a shorter median survival time or smaller percentage of survivors among those patients whose tumors had a high rather than a low SPF (BARNABEI et al. 1990; KALLIONIEMI et al. 1988b; KLEMI et al. 1989; KUHN et al. 1988, 1989; RUTGERS et al. 1987; VOLM et al. 1989). The SPF that best discriminated between prognostic groups varied from study to study. Two studies (BRESCIA et al. 1990; ERBA et al. 1989) did not find a statistically significant association between these features.

### *3.1.4 Prognostic Significance of DNA Analysis Compared to Other Prognostic Factors*

Nine studies examined the relative importance of DNA ploidy and other possible prognostic factors by multivariate analysis (BAAK et al. 1988; BLUMENFELD

**Table 7.** DNA ploidy and survival

| Author | Stage | Survival length (mo) | | % Survival | | Sig. |
|---|---|---|---|---|---|---|
| | | Diploid | Aneuploid | Diploid | Aneuploid | |
| BAAK et al. (1988) | 3, 4 | NR | 42 | 72 | 46 | Yes |
| BARNABEI et al. (1990) | 1–4 | 36 | 23 | NA | NA | Yes |
| BLUMENFELD et al. (1987) | 2–4 | 48 | 19 | 68 | 24 | Yes |
| BRESCIA et al. (1990) | 1–4 | NA | NA | 50 | 22 | Yes |
| ERBA et al. (1989) | 1–4 | NA | NA | 62 | 32 | No[a] |
| FRIEDLANDER et al. (1988) | 3, 4 | 65 | 13 | NA | NA | Yes |
| GAJEWSKI et al., in preparation | 1–4 | NA | NA | 57 | 25 | Yes |
| HAMAGUCHI et al. (1990) | 1–4 | NA | NA | 74 | 37 | Yes |
| KLEMI et al. (1989) | 1–4 | NA | NA | 49 | 23 | Yes |
| MURRAY et al. (1989) | 1–4 | NA | NA | 74 | 22 | Yes |
| RODENBURG et al. (1987) | 2B–4 | 60 | 24 | 87 | 44 | Yes |
| VOLM et al. (1989) | 3, 4 | 41 | 14 | NA | NA | Yes |

NR, not reached; NA, not available; Sig., statistically significant
[a] $P = 0.11$

et al. 1987; ERBA et al. 1989; FRIEDLANDER et al. 1984a, 1988; KALLIONIEMI et al. 1988b; KLEMI et al. 1988, 1989; RODENBURG et al. 1987a, b; 1988). Five studies (BLUMENFELD et al. 1987; FRIEDLANDER et al. 1988; KALLIONIEMI et al. 1988b; KUHN et al. 1988; RODENBURG et al. 1988) found that DNA ploidy was a major, independent prognostic factor in surface epithelial ovarian carcinomas. Four groups did not document this association (BAAK et al. 1988; BARNABEI et al. 1990; ERBA et al. 1989; KLEMI et al. 1989); however, Klemi and co-workers (1989) noted that a DNA index of greater than or less than 1.3 was independently associated with prognosis. The divergent results in the series by ERBA and co-workers (1989) may be secondary to the inclusion of cases in which the DNA content was determined on ascites only. No obvious explanation for the conflicting results of the other groups (BAAK et al. 1988; BARNABEI et al. 1990) is apparent. Two of the three studies that included SPF in the multivariate analysis found that it was an independent prognostic indicator (BARNABEI et al. 1990; KLEMI et al. 1989). The divergent results of the third study may be due to the inclusion of SPF data on ascites samples, as previously noted (ERBA et al. 1989).

### *3.1.5 DNA Analysis Combined with Other Prognostic Factors*

Several groups have explored the possibility that combinations of prognostic features including the DNA analysis data may allow more precise division of patients into favorable and unfavorable prognostic groups. JAKOBSEN and BICHEL (1989) have shown that a combination of DNA index and a histopathologic grading index that evaluates eight histologic features of the tumor effectively separates patients into low, intermediate, and high risk categories. KALLIONIEMI and co-workers (1988b) and KUHN and co-workers (1989) found an improved prognostic separation when a combination of ploidy and SPF was used. KLEMI and colleagues (1989) found improvement of predictive power utilizing a combination of SPF and DNA index. PUNNONEN and co-workers (1989) found that a combination of DNA ploidy, percentage of cells in SPF, stage, and histologic type provided optimal distinction between low and high risk groups. RUTGERS and co-workers (1987) found that age, grade, stage, and percentage of cells in $G^1$ identified prognostic subgroups most effectively. None of these studies, however, found any combination of parameters which could distinguish absolutely between individual high and low risk patients.

### 3.1.6 Stability of DNA Content

The stability of DNA content and cell cycle parameters in multiple sites from the primary tumor, primary and metastatic tumor, primary and recurrent or persistent tumor, and primary tumor and ascites has been examined in a number of studies (BAKER et al. 1987; BLUMENFELD et al. 1987; BRESCIA et al. 1990; ERBA et al. 1985, 1989; FRIEDLANDER et al. 1984c; HAMAGUCHI et al. 1990; IVERSEN and SKAARLAND 1987; JAKOBSEN et al. 1988; KALLIONIEMI 1988; ROBEY et al. 1989; RODENBURG et al. 1987a; RUTGERSC et al. 1987; VOLM et al. 1985). Some authors have shown a high degree of intratumoral stability of DNA index in up to 93% of tumors (JAKOBSEN et al. 1988); others, in contrast, have noted intratumoral variations in from 22% to 27% of cases (BRESCIA et al. 1990; HAMAGUCHI et al. 1990; KLLIONIEMI 1988). These differences in DNA content may have biologic significance, since the highest mortality in one study was observed in those patients with an unstable DNA content (HAMAGUCHI et al. 1990). There is a very high rate of agreement, varying from 87% to 100%, between the DNA content of primary tumors and their matastases (BLUMENFELD et al. 1987; ERBA et al. 1989; IVERSEN and SKAARLAND 1987; ROBEY et al. 1989; RODENBURG et al. 1987a; VOLM et al. 1985) and primary carcinomas and recurrent or persistent tumor (BLUMENFELD et al. 1987; BRESCIA et al. 1990; FRIEDLANDER et al. 1984c; ROBEY et al. 1989; RODENBURG et al. 1987a; RUTGERS et al. 1987). It has also been shown that the DNA content of ovarian carcinoma remains stable before and after in vitro cultures (ERBA et al. 1985) or implantation into nude mice (FRIEDLANDER et al. 1984c). A single study has noted a high rate of DNA content heterogeneity (31%) among serous surface carcinomas; these data may support a multifocal peritoneal origin of the neoplasms (RUTLEDGE et al. 1989).

FRIEDLANDER and co-workers (1984c) found a substantial intratumoral variation in SPF in 8 of 16 tumors sampled at different sites and ERBA and colleagues (1985) found that the SPF "varied greatly" in 33 tumors before and after in vitro cell cultures. VOLM and co-workers (1985), however, found SPF to be stable in five of five tumors multiply sampled.

### 3.1.7 DNA Content and Response to Therapy

BRESCIA and co-workers (1990) found that 56% of patients with aneuploid tumors had positive second-look laparotomies compared to 27% of those with

DNA diploid tumors and that 71% of patients with DNA aneuploid tumors and negative second-look laparotomies suffered a late recurrence of tumor while this occurred in only 31% of those patients with DNA diploid tumors and negative second-look laparotomies. These data indicate that DNA polidy may identify patients with negative second-look laparatomies who are at greater risk of recurrence. FRIEDLANDER and clleagues (1988) also noted a higher "true response rate" at second-look laparotomy among patients with DNA diploid tumors. This group has also shown that the times to treatment failure were similar in patients with diploid tumors initially treated with either chlorambucil and cisplatin or chlorambucil alone, in contrast to patients with aneuploid carcinomas, in whom combination chemotherapy was superior to chlorambucil alone in prolonging the time to first recurrence. The addition of cisplatin to the treatment regimen of the latter patients with aneuploid tumors resulted in further responses. This at present unconfirmed study indicates that flow cytometry may identify a group of patients with advanced stage diploid carcinoma that have a good prognosis regardless of the type of treatment in whom the initial use of relatively nontoxic therapy may be considered. These findings also strongly support randomization of patients according to DNA content in pros-pective clinical trials (FRIEDLANDER et al. 1988).

### 3.2 Borderline Tumors

Much less information is available on the DNA content of borderline tumors and its biologic significance. Results of DNA analysis have been reported from 114 stage 1–3 serous borderline tumors; 98 (86%) were DNA diploid and 16 (14%) were DNA aneuploid (BELL et al. 1988; HEINONEN et al. 1988; IVERSEN and SKAARLAND 1987; KLEMI et al. 1988; KUHN et al. 1989; WATSON et al. 1987; FRIEDLANDER et al. 1984b). In the only study (FRIEDLANDER et al. 1984b) that separated the results by stage, the ovarian tumors in all of the stage 1 cases were diploid and two of ten stage 3 tumors were aneuploid. Follow-up information was available from four of these series; all but two of the patients with diploid tumors were living and four of 14 patients with DNA aneuploidy in whom follow-up information was available had succumbed to tumor (BELL et al. 1988; FRIEDLANDER et al. 1984b; KLEMI et al. 1988; KUHN et al. 1989). Two of the patients with DNA aneuploid tumors of further histopathologic investigation were found to have invasive peritoneal implants (FRIEDLANDER et al. 1984b). KUHN and co-workers (1989) found a mean SPF of 1.7% (range 0.4–3.4) in ovarian serous borderline tumors and a slightly higher mean SPF of 2.2% (range 1.6–2.8) in their peritoneal implants.

The DNA content of 21 mucinous borderline tumors has been reported; all were DNA diploid, including 13 stage 1 and four stage 3 tumors (FRIEDLANDER et al. 1984b; HEINONEN et al. 1988; IVERSEN and SKAARLAND 1987; KUHN et al. 1989). All of those patients in whom follow-up data were available were living without tumor (FRIEDLANDER et al. 1984b; KUHN et al. 1989). DNA analysis has been reported from three borderline endometrioid tumors and five borderline Brenner tumors; all were stage 1 and DNA diploid (FRIEDLANDER et al. 1984b; TREBECK et al. 1987). These data indicate that the prognostic significance of DNA aneuploidy in borderline tumors has yet to be definitively established.

### 3.3 Benign Tumors

A small number of articles have analyzed the DNA content and SPF of benign tumors of the ovary with divergent results. Thirty-nine benign serous cystadenomas or cystadenofibromas have been analyzed (HEINONEN et al. 1988; IVERSEN and SKAARLAND 1987; KLEMI et al. 1988); three of them were DNA aneuploid with DNA indices ranging between 1.5 and 1.7 (KLEMI et al. 1988). Follow-up data were given on the three aneuploid cases; one woman died without tumor at autopsy 9 years postoperatively, and two were living without evidence of tumor for 10 months and 14 years, respectively (KLEMI et al. 1988). Three simple cysts (HEINONEN et al. 1988), 11 mucinous cystadenomas (HEINONEN et al. 1988; IVERSEN and SKAARLAND 1987), and six benign Brenner tumors (IVERSEN and SKAARLAND 1987: TREBECK et al. 1987) reported were all DNA diploid. Thus, although DNA aneuploidy may occur in benign tumors, it is a rare finding.

## 4 Sex Cord/Stromal Tumors

### 4.1 Granulosa Cell Tumors

Six studies have examined the DNA content of granulosa cell tumors in 117 women (CHADHA et al. 1990; CHRISTOV and VASSILEV 1987; HITCHCOCK et al. 1989; SWANSON et al. 1990; SUH et al. 1990; Jacoby et al., in preparation). DNA aneuploidy was detected in 2 of 10 and 3 of 17 women with adult granulosa cell tumors (HITCHCOCK et al. 1989; SUH et al. 1990). 21 of 45 with juvenile granulosa cell tumors (SWANSON et al. 1990), and 2 of 40 granulosa cell tumors of unspecified subtype (CHADHA et al. 1990). The DNA indices of the DNA aneuploid tumors ranged from 1.33 to 1.98 in the adult granulosa cell tumors (HITCHCOCK et al. 1989; SUH et al. 1990), from 1.2 to 2.4 in the juvenile granulosa cell tumors (SWANSON et al. 1990), and from 1.16 to 1.20 in the granulosa cell tumors of unspecified type (CHADHA et al. 1990). One of the aneuploid juvenile granulosa cell tumors had multiple abnormal stemlines (SWANSON et al. 1990). DNA ploidy did not correlate with the presence of metastatic or recurrent tumor in adult granulosa cell tumors (HITCHCOCK et al. 1989; SUH et al. 1990) and the presence of DNA aneuploidy or multiploidy was not associated with aggressive behavior in juvenile granulosa cell tumors confined to the ovary (stage 1A) (SWANSON et al. 1990; Jacoby et al., in preparation). DNA aneuploidy did correlate with nuclear atypia in both adult and juvenile granulosa cell tumors (HITCHCOCK et al. 1989; Jacoby et al., in preparation; SWANSON et al. 1990) and high mitotic activity in one study of adult granulosa cell tumors (SUH et al. 1990). A single report found DNA aneuploidy in 80% (four of five) "malignant" granulosa cell tumors; however, the latter entity was not defined and clinical and follow-up information was not given on these patients (CHRISTOV and VASSILEV 1987). In the largest series, three of five aneuploid tumors were reclassified as undifferentiated carcinomas on review of the hematoxylin-eosin stained sections and after immunohistochemical stains for keratin and epithelial membrane antigen were found to be positive (CHADHA et al. 1990). Thus, undifferentiated carcinoma should be excluded when a putative granulosa cell tumor, especially in an adult, has an aneuploid DNA content.

### 4.2 Thecomas/Fibromas

The DNA content of 12 fibromas (FEICHTER et al. 1985; IVERSEN and SKAARLAND 1987) and two thecomas (CHRISTOV and VASSILEV 1987) have been examined; all were DNA diploid.

### 4.3 Sertoli–Leydig Cell Tumor

Only one tumor has been analyzed and was DNA diploid (BAKER et al. 1987).

## 5 Germ Cell Tumors

### 5.1 Dysgerminomas

All of the 31 dysgerminomas discussed in the literature have been DNA aneuploid (OUD et al. 1988; KUHN et al. 1989; CHRISTOV and VASSILEV 1987; TASE et al. 1987). No correlation between the DNA index of the abnormal stemlines and stage or clinical behavior was noted in the single study that examined these features (OUD et al. 1988).

### 5.2 Yok Sac Tumors

Only rare yolk sac tumors have been analyzed and have been DNA diploid (KUHN et al. 1989).

### 5.3 Teratomas

The three "benign" teratomas (IVERSEN and SKAARLAND 1987) and four "metastasizing" teratomas (KUHN et al. 1989) that have been reported were DNA diploid.

## 6 Small Cell Carcinomas

Eighteen small cell carcinomas of the type associated with hypercalcemia have been analyzed; surprisingly, all were DNA diploid. Neither ploidy nor SPF was associated with survival (EICHHORN et al., in preparation).

## 7 Malignant Mesodermal Mixed Tumors (Carcinosarcomas) and Sarcomas

Seven of the nine carcinosarcomas or malignant mesodermal mixed tumors (BLUMENFELD et al. 1987; BRESCIA et al. 1990; FRIEDLANDER et al. 1983) and one of the two pure sarcomas (KUHN et al. 1989) reported were DNA aneuploid. No follow-up data were available on these patients.

## 8 Conclusions

The data summarized in the chapter indicate that DNA content analysis by flow cytometry correlates with known prognostic factors, such as stage, extent of residual disease, and grade, and provides additional, independent prognostic information in patients with ovarian surface epithelial carcinomas. It may also supply important information regarding responses to therapy that may allow greater individualization of treatment. The clinical value of DNA content analysis in borderline and malignant nonepithelial tumors of the ovary remains to be established by larger studies with adequate follow-up data.

## References


Aure JC, Hoeg H, Kolstad P (1971) Clinical and histologic studies of ovarian carcinoma: long term follow-up of 900 cases. Obstet Gynecol 37:1–9

Baak JPA, Delemarre JFM, Langley FA, Talerman A (1986a) Grading ovarian tumors. Evaluation of decision making by different pathologists. Anal Quant Cytol Histol 8:349–353

Baak JPA, Langley FA, Talerman A, Delemarre JFM (1986b) Interpathologist and intrapathologist disagreement in ovarian tumor grading and typing. Anal Quant Cytol Histol 8:354–357

Baak JPA, Schipper NW, Wisse-Brekelmans ECM, Ceelen T, Bosman FT, van Geuns H, Wils J (1988) The prognostic value of morphometrical features and cellular DNA content in cis-platin treated late ovarian cancer patients. Br J Cancer 57:503–508

Baker VV, Haskill S, Fowler WC, Walton LA, Currie JL (1987) Cellular DNA content and CA-125 antigen expression in ovarian carcinomas. Oncology 44:283–286

Ball HG, Bell DA, Griffin TW (1990) Cancer of the ovary. In: Osteen RT (ed) Cancer manual, 8th edn. American Cancer Society Massachusetts Division, Boston, pp 266–270

Barnabei VM, Miller DS, Bauer KD, Murad TM, Rademaker AW, Lurain JR (1990) Flow cytometric evaluation of epithelial ovarian cancer. Am J Obstet Gynecol 162:1584–1592

Bell DA, Pestel-Levy C, Flotte TJ (1988) DNA content in serous borderline tumors. Lab Invest 58:8A

Bell DA, Flotte, TJ, Preffer F, Colvin RB (in preparation) DNA content stability and histopathological features of ovarian carcinoma

Blumenfeld D, Braly PS, Ben-Ezra J, Klevecz RR (1987) Tumor DNA content as a prognostic feature in advanced epithelial ovarian carcinoma. Gynecol Oncol 27:389–398

Brescia RJ, Barakat RA, Beller U, Frederickson G, Suhrland MJ, Dubin N, Demopoulos RI (1990) The prognostic significance of nuclear DNA content in malignant epithelial tumors of the ovary. Cancer 65:141–147

Chadha S, Cornelisse CJ, Schaberg A (1990) Flow cytometric DNA ploidy analysis of ovarian granulosa cell tumors. Gynecol Oncol 36:240–245

Christov K, Vassilev N (1987) Flow cytometric analysis of DNA and cell proliferation in ovarian tumors. Cancer 60:121–125

Colvin RB, Preffer FI (1987) New technologies in cell analysis by flow cytometry. Arch Pathol Lab Med 111:628–632

Coon JS, Landay AL, Weinstein RS (1987) Advances in flow cytometry for diagnostic pathology. Lab Invest 47:453–479

Cramer SF, Roth LM, Ulbright TM et al. (1987) Evaluation of the reproducibility of the World Health Organization classification of common ovarian cancers. With emphasis on methodology. Arch Pathol Lab Med 111:819–829

DiSaia PJ, Creasman WT (1989) Clinical gynecologic oncology, 3rd edn. C.V. Mosby, St. Louis, p 349

Eichhorn JE, Flotte TJ, Preffer F, Bell DA (in preparation) DNA content of small cell carcinoma of the ovary.

Erba E, Vaghi M, Pepe S et al. (1985) DNA index of ovarian carcinomas from 56 patients: in vivo in vitro studies. Br J Cancer 52:565–573

Erba E, Ubezio P, Pepe S et al. (1989) Flow cytometric analysis of DNA content in human ovarian cancers. Br J Cancer 60:45–50

Feichter GE, Kuhn W, Czernobilsky B et al. (1985) DNA flow cytometry of ovarian tumors with correlation to histopathology. Int J Gynecol Pathol 4:336–345

Friedlander ML, Taylor IW, Russell P, Musgrove EA, Hedley DH, Tattersall MHN (1983) Ploidy as a prognostic factor in ovarian cancer. Int J Gynecol Pathol 2:55–63

Friedlander ML, Hedley DW, Taylor IW, Russell P, Coates AS, Tattersall MHN (1984a) Influence of cellular DNA content on survival in advanced ovarian cancer. Cancer Res 44:397–400

Friedlander ML, Russell P, Taylor IW, Hedley DW, Tattersall HN (1984b) Flow cytometric analysis of cellular DNA content as an adjunct to the diagnosis of ovarian tumors of borderline malignancy. Pathology 16:301–306

Friedlander ML, Taylor IW, Russell P, Tattersall MHN (1984c) Cellular DNA content—a stable feature in epithelial ovarian cancer. Br J Cancer 49:173–179

Friedlander ML, Hedley DW, Swanson C, Russell P (1988) Prediction of long-term survival by flow cytometric analysis of cellular DNA content in patients with advanced ovarian cancer. J Clin Oncol 6:282–290

Gajewski W, Bell DA, Flotte TJ, Preffer F, Colvin RB (in preparation) DNA content in ovarian surface epithelial carcinoma.

Gonchoroff NJ, Ryan JJ, Kimlinger TK, Witzig TE, Greipp PR, Meyer JS, Katzmann JA (1990) Effect of sonication of paraffin-embedded tissue preparation for DNA flow cytometry. Cytometry 11:642–646

Hamaguchi K, Nishimura H, Miyoshi T, Miyahara K, Tateno N, Yakushiji M, Yokoyama MM (1990) Flow cytometric analysis of cellular DNA content in ovarian cancer. Gynecol Oncol 37:219–223

Hedley DW (1989) Flow cytometry using paraffin-embedded tissue: five years on. Cytometry 10:229–241

Hedley DW, Friedlander ML, Taylor IW, Rugg CA, Musgrove EA (1983) Method for analysis of cellular DNA content of paraffin-embedded pathological material using flow cytometry. J Histochem Cytochem 31:1333–1335

Hedley DW, Friendlander ML, Taylor IW (1985) Application of DNA flow cytometry to paraffin-embedded archival material for the study of aneuploidy and its clinical significance. Cytometry 6:327–333

Heinonen PK, Morsky P, Aine R, Koivula T, Pystynen P (1988) Hormonal activity of epithelial ovarian tumors in post-menopausal women. Maturitas 9:325–338

Hernandez E, Bhagavan BS, Parmley TH, Rosenshein NB (1984) Interobserver variability in the interpretation of epithelial ovarian cancer. Gynecol Oncol 17:117–123

Hitchcock SL, Norris HJ, Khalifa MA, Wargotz ES (1989) Flow cytometric analysis of granulosa tumors. Cancer 64:2127–2132

Iversen O-E, Skaarland E (1987) Ploidy assessment of benign and malignant ovarian tumors by flow cytometry. A clinicopathologic study. Cancer 60:82–87

Jacoby A, Flotte TJ, Young RH, Preffer F, Bell DA (in preparation) DNA content of juvenile granulosa cell tumors.

Jakobsen A, Bichel P (1989) Ploidy level, histopathological differentiation and response to chemotherapy in serous ovarian cancer. Eur J Cancer Clin Oncol 25:1589–1593

Jakobsen A, Hansen V, Poulsen HS (1988) DNA profile and steroid receptor content of human ovarian cancer. Eur J Gynaecol Oncol 6:461–463

Kallioniemi O-P (1988) Comparison of fresh and paraffin-embedded tissue as starting material for DNA flow cytometry and evaluation of intratumor heterogeneity. Cytometry 9:164–169

Kallioniemi O-P, Mattila J, Punnonen R, Koivula T (1988a) DNA ploidy level and cell cycle distribution in ovarian cancer: relation to histopathological features of the tumor. Int J Gynecol Pathol 7:1–11

Kallioniemi O-P, Punnonen R, Mattila J, Lehtinen M, Koivula T (1988b) Prognostic significance of DNA index, multiploidy, and S-phase fraction in ovarian cancer. Cancer 61:334–339

Klemi PJ, Joensuu H, Kiilholma P, Mäenpää J (1988) Clinical significance of abnormal nuclear DNA content in serous ovarian tumors. Cancer 62:2005–2010

Klemi PJ, Joensuu H, Mäenpää J, Kiilholma P (1989) Influence of cellular DNA content on survival in ovarian carcinoma. Obstet Gynecol 74:200–204

Kuhn W, Kaufmann M, Feichter GE, Schmid H, Hanke J, Rummel HH (1988) Psammomabody content and DNA-flow cytometric results as prognostic factors in advanced ovarian carcinoma. Eur J Gynaecol Oncol 9:234–241

Kuhn W, Kaufmann M, Feichter GE, Rummel HH, Schmid H, Heberling D (1989) DNA flow cytometry, clinical and morphological parameters as prognostic factors for advanced malignant and borderline ovarian tumors. Gynecol Oncol 33:360–367

Murray K, Hopwood L, Volk D, Wilson JF (1989) Cytofluorometric analysis of the DNA content in ovarian carcinoma and its relationship to patient survival. Cancer 63:2456–2460

Oud PS, Soeters RP, Pahlplatz MMM, Hermkens HG, Beck HLM, Reubsaet-Veldhuizen J, Vooijs GP (1988) DNA cytometry of pure dysgerminomas of the ovary. Int J Gynecol Pathol 7:258–267

Punnonen R, Kallioniemi O-P, Mattila J, Koivula T (1989) Prognostic assessment in stage I ovarian cancer using a discriminant analysis with clinicopathological and DNA flow cytometric data. Gynecol Obstet Invest 27:213–216

Robey SS, Silva EG, Gershenson DM, McLemore D, El-Naggar A, Ordonez NG (1989) Transitional cell carcinoma in high-grade high-stage ovarian carcinoma. An indicator of favorable response to chemotherapy. Cancer 63:839–847

Rodenburg CJ, Cornelisse CJ, Heintz PAM, Hermans J, Fleuren GJ (1987a) Tumor ploidy as a major prognostic factor in advanced ovarian cancer. Cancer 59:317–323

Rodenburg CJ, Ploem-Zaaijer JJ, Cornelisse CJ et al. (1987b) Use of DNA image cytometry in addition to flow cytometry for the study of patients with advanced ovarian cancer. Cancer Res 47:3938–3941

Rodenburg CJ, Cornelisse CJ, Hermans J, Fleuren GJ (1988) DNA flow cytometry and morphometry as prognostic indicators in advanced ovarian cancer: a step forward in predicting the dinical outcome. Gynecol Oncol 29:176–187

Rutgers DH, Wils IS, Schaap AHP, van Lindert ACM (1987) DNA flow cytometry, histological grade, stage and age as prognostic factors in human epithelial ovarian carcinomas. Pathol Res Pract 182:207–213

Rutledge ML, Silva EG, McLemore D, El-Naggar A (1989) Serous surface carcinoma of the ovary and peritoneum. A flow cytometry study. Pathol Annu 24:227–236

Sahni K, Tribukait B, Einhorn N (1989) Flow cytometric measurement of ploidy and proliferation in effusions of ovarian carcinoma and their possible prognostic significance. Gynecol Oncol 35:240–245

Sobre B, Frankendal B, Veress B (1982) Importance of histologic grading in the prognosis of epithelial ovarian carcinoma. Obstet Gynecol 59:567–582

Suh K-S, Silverberg SG, Rhame JG, Wilkinson DS (1990) Granulosa cell tumor of the ovary. Histopathologic and flow cytometric analysis with clinical correlation. Arch Pathol Lab Med 114:496–501

Swanson SA, Norris HJ, Kelsten ML, Wheeler JE (1990) DNA content of juvenile granulosa tumors determined by flow cytometry. Int J Gynecol Pathol 9:101–109

Tase T, Oikawa N, Toki T, Wada Y, Yajima A (1987) Flow cytometric DNA analysis of gynecologic malignant tumors using paraffin-embedded tissue. Acta Obstet Gynaecol Jpn 39:87–91

Trebeck CE, Friedlander ML, Russell P, Baird PJ (1987) Brenner tumors of the ovary; a study of the histology, immunohistochemistry and cellular DNA content in benign, borderline and malignant ovarian tumors. Pathology 19:241–246

Volm M, Brüggemann A, Günther M, Kleine W, Pfleiderer A, Vogt-Schaden M (1985) Prognostic relevance of ploidy, proliferation, and resistance-predictive tests in ovarian carcinoma. Cancer Res 45:5180–5185

Volm M, Kleine W, Pfleiderer A (1989) Flow-cytometric prognostic factors for the survival of patients with ovarian carcinoma: a 5-year follow-up study. Gynecol Oncol 35:84–89

Watson JV, Curling OM, Munn CF, Hudson CN (1987) Oncogene expression in ovarian cancer: a pilot study of c-myc oncoprotein in serous papillary ovarian cancer. Gynecol 28:137–150

# Oncogenes in Gynecological Tumors

H. SASANO and C.T. GARRETT



## 1 Introduction

Recent scientific and technical advances in molecular biology have provided a new understanding of the basis of various diseases, especially malignant neoplasms. These techniques and knowledge are not only tools of medical research but are becoming increasingly utilized in the fields of clinical medicine, including both anatomic and clinical pathology.

In oncology there has been a remarkable advancement in understanding of the molecular basis of cancer. Our growing knowledge of oncogenes and their possible role in the etiology and biologic behaviour of human malignant neoplasms can contribute to improving the diagnosis and classification of neoplastic diseases. In turn, this should enhance our ability to predict a tumor's clinical behaviour and response to therapy. Also, direct monitoring of drug resistance in individual primary and recurrent tumors may soon be possible. Thus, it is becoming increasingly necessary for those who are engaged in the management of cancer patients, including surgical pathologists and clinical oncologists, to be familiar with the basic tools and concepts of molecular biology.

In this chapter we will focus on genes directly involved in the tumorigenesis of human gynecological malignancies, including oncogenes and tumor suppressor genes. We will explore the relationship between oncogene activation and the clinical and pathologic features of the tumor, including various histopathologic and other prognostic factors. For further reading on general aspects of

Current Topics in Pathology
Volume 85, Ed. N. Sasano

molecular biology and oncogenes, one can refer to other general reviews. (Brodeur 1987; Buck et al. 1988; Freifelder 1985; Garrett 1986; Haluska et al. 1987; Masuda et al. 1987; Stanbridge 1988; Williams and Fenoglio-Preiser 1987).

## 2 Oncogenes

### 2.1 General Characteristics of Oncogenes

Advances in the basic molecular biology of neoplasia have led to the identification of dominantly acting genes whose expression seems to be associated with conversion of normal cells to cancer cells. Expression of these genes may also play an important role in tumor progression. These genes are known as oncogenes and were first identified in the genomes of acutely transforming rodent and avian retroviruses. Subsequent analysis revealed these so-called viral oncogenes were actually of mammalian or avian origin and had been incorporated into the genome of the retrovirus by the process of transduction during the period of infection of the host by the virus. The homologous genes present in mammalian or avian DNA are generally referred to as cellular oncogenes or proto-oncogenes, and it appears that their protein products play critical roles in cellular differentiation and division. In addition, actual viral genes have been identified in some human retroviruses that are not homologous to genes present in eukaryotes and that are responsible for an oncogenic activity by the virus (Haseltine et al. 1984). New cellular and viral transforming genes are continuing to be detected and characterized. Moreover, many of the cellular transforming genes, that is, proto-oncogenes and transforming growth factors, have been identified directly from the DNA of human tumors and are not present in any known retrovirus (Brodeur 1987).

### 2.2 Structure and Function of Oncogenes

The primary function of proto-oncogenes in humans and other mammals appears to regulate steps of cellular differentiation and proliferation. These proto-oncogenes can be classified into five categories based on the location and function of their gene products (Brodeur 1987; Hunter 1984). The first and largest class of proto-oncogenes encodes protein kinases. This group can be further subclassified into oncogenes encoding tyrosine-specific kinases, including *src*, *abl*, *fes*, *fgr*, *ros*, *rel*, *yes*, and *syn*, and proto-oncogenes encoding proteins that have a kinase-like domain but do not possess detectable tyrosine kinase activity in vitro, which include *raf*, *pks*, *kit*, *mos*, and *sea* (Brodeur 1987). The next class of proto-oncogenes is the so-called *ras* proto-oncogene family and consists of H-*ras*, K-*ras*, and N-*ras*. Members of the *ras* proto-oncogene family that contain activating point mutations are generally capable of transforming cell lines. The *ras* proto-oncogenes encode proteins with a molecular weight of 21000 that are referred to as p21. p21 binds GTP and GDP and has a GTPase and autokinase activity. It is located on the plasma membrane when active. The third class of proto-oncogenes encodes growth factors. The most well-studied example is *sis*, which produces a protein identical to the β-chain of platelet-derived growth factor (PDGF) (Brodeur 1987). The fourth class encodes polypeptide growth factor receptors or proteins with the characteristic transmembrane structure of a growth factor receptor. This group of proto-oncogenes includes *erb*-A, *erb*-B, *fms*, and *kit*. Typically, these proteins span the cell membrane and posseess an intracellular cytoplasmic domain and an extracellular domain. Binding of ligands to the extracellular domain of these growth factor receptors leads to the activation of the intrinsic tyrosine kinase activity of the intracellular cytoplasmic domain of the receptor molecule, resulting in the induction of cellular proliferation. The last class of proto-oncogenes encodes proteins located in the nucleus. These proteins may regulate gene expression and include the *myc* group of proto-oncogenes (c-*myc*, N-*myc*, and L-*myc*), *myb*, *foc*, *ets*-1, *ets*-2, *fos*, and *ski*.

## 2.3 Oncogene Activation

In order for proto-oncogenes to play a role in neoplastic transformation and progression, they must be "activated." Activation of proto-oncogenes occurs as a result of structural changes in the gene that result in qualitative or quantitative changes in the encoded protein. The types of structural changes that can cause activation include point mutations, chromosomal rearragements, and amplification. These changes in the DNA can lead to increased expression of the protein, enhanced activity of the protein, and/or deregulation of expression of the protein. All of these modes of activation have been demonstrated in different types of human neoplasms. Similar changes have also been demonstrated in experimentally induced animal tumors and in tissue culture model systems, where these changes appear to be at least in part responsible for the neoplastic transformation of these tissues. Although the possibility remains that such changes in primary human tumors merely reflect an increased level of genetic instability of these neoplasms, the consistent association between several of these activating genetic alterations and particular types of human neoplasia makes the possibility of a fortuitous association between proto-oncogene activation and human neoplasia unlikely. In addition, proto-oncogenes are considered as the molecular targets for environmental mutagens and carcinogens. However, in most naturally occuring human tumors, activation of a single proto-oncogene probably does not lead to immediate malignant transformation. Various experiments have pointed out that naturally occuring cancer results from multiple events that may involve activation of more than one proto-oncogene, as well as loss of other cellular genes that suppress the development of the tumor cell type, i.e., tumor suppressor genes.

## 2.4 Tumor Suppressor Genes in Neoplasms

Genes that predispose individuals to the development of cancer by loss of their function have been termed "tumor suppressor genes." Loss of function may occur through mutation or deletion of these genes and has been demonstrated to be associated with a number of different malignant phenotypes (KLEIN 1987; SAGER 1986; STANBRIDGE 1988; WILLIAMS and FENOGLIO-PREISER 1987). These genes have also been called recessive oncogenes, antioncogenes, and cancer predisposition genes (BRODEUR 1987). Studies using somatic cell hybridization and monochromosomal transfer indicate that tumor suppressor genes play an important role in the control of malignant expresson, and loss of putative tumor suppressor genes has been found to be associated with an increasing number of human cancers (HALUSKA et al. 1987). The best studied of these putative tumor suppressor genes is the retinoblastoma (RB) gene, which is located on the long arm of chromosome 13 (13q14). Expression of this gene is altered in virtually all cases of retinoblastoma (FRIEND et al. 1986; FUNG et al. 1987; LEE W-H et al. 1987) and in some other tumors (FRIEND et al. 1987). Another putative tumor suppressor gene, referred to as p53, is located on chromosome 17p. This gene was initially considered a nuclear proto-oncogene rather than a tumor suppressor gene, since transfection of mutant variants into cells along with *ras* oncogenes leads to malignant transformation. It was subsequently learned, however, that the mutant p53 protein accomplished its part in the transformation process through inactivation of a tumor suppressor function of the wild type p53 gene (BAKER et al. 1989). Increasing numbers of new tumor suppressor genes are being identified.

## 2.5 Oncogenes in Diagnostic Application

The first step in learning whether a proto-oncogene may be involved in the biologic behaviour of a human neoplasm is to determine whether or not it has been activated through one of the process previously mentioned (mutation, gene rearragement, or amplification). Major tools to detect these changes are summarized in Table 1. Among these procedures, transfection assays are still tools of the basic science laboratories. Nucleotide sequencing is becoming an important method through introduction of the polymerase chain reaction (PCR) and direct sequencing methods. These newer techniques are available in some diagnostic laboratories but are still considered as a state of the art. The techniques that have the most widespread use in diagnostic laboratories at this juncture are DNA/mRNA hybridization systems and immunologic detection systems. The hybridization systems include dot/slot blot, Southern, Northern,

**Table 1.** Major methods of detecting changes of cellular oncogenes in the laboratory

1. Transfection assays
2. Nucleotide sequencing
3. Restriction fragment length polymorphism; Southern blot hybridization
4. Northern blot hybridization
5. Dot/slot blot hybridization
6. In situ hybridization
7. Immunologic detection of oncogene products

and in situ hybridization. Immunologic detection systems include Western blot analysis and immunohistochemistry.

Among the processes that activate proto-oncogenes, amplification is of particular interest because it has never been detected in benign disorders. Moreover, its presence has been correlated inversely with clinical outcome in a variety of human neoplasms (MASUDA et al. 1987). Amplification can be detected by slot/dot blot or by Southern blot hybridization. However, it is best examined by Southern blot hybridization after extracting DNA from tumors and digesting with restriction enzymes as shown in Fig. 1. A similar analysis using dilutions of DNA from the samples of tumor can also be useful in quantitating the degree of amplification present (Fig. 2). Amplification of proto-oncogenes

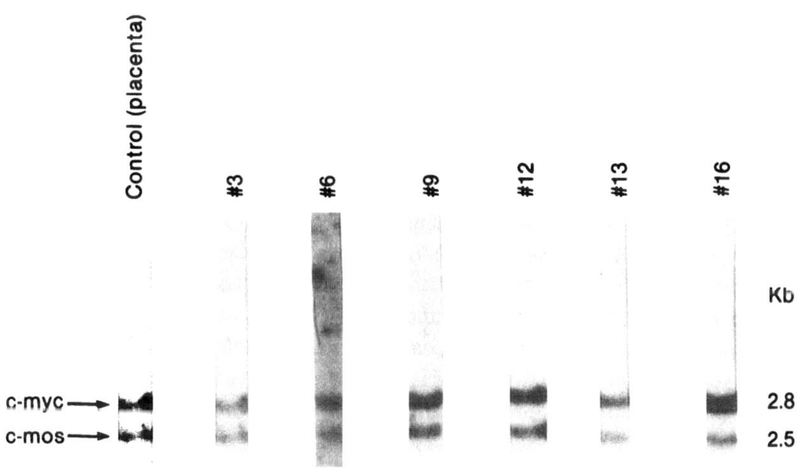


**Fig. 1.** Amplification of c-*myc* in six cases of ovvarian carcinoma. Lanes are from an autoradio graph of a Southern blot of HindIII digested DNA from normal placenta and six ovarian carcinomas. The intensity of signal of c-*myc* relative to that of c-*mos* (control probe used to monitor efficiency of DNA transfer) for each of the six tumors is greater than that for the placental control DNA, indicating amplification of the c-*myc* oncogenes in the tumors. (SASANO et al. 1990b)

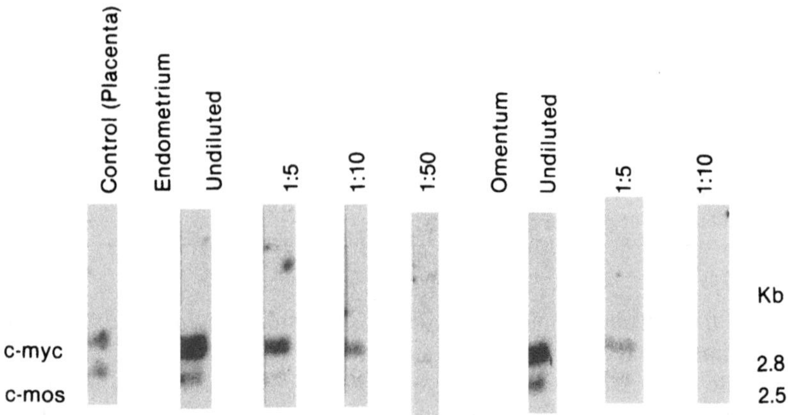


**Fig. 2.** Dilutional study of c-*myc* Amplification in DNA extracted from endometrial and omental tumors analyzed by Southern blot hybridization. The DNA from the endometrial tumor exhibited approximately tenfold and that from the omental lesion approximately fivefold c-*myc* amplification. (SASANO et al. 1990c)

can enhance their expression by increasing the amount of DNA available for production of mRNA.

The clearest example of a relationship between oncogene amplification and prognosis is the presence of N-*myc* amplification in neuroblastoma (MASUDA et al. 1987). N-*myc* amplification is now considered as an independent marker of rapidly progressive disease in patients with neuroblastoma. Breast cancer has also been extensively studied, and amplification of either the c-*erb*B-2, *int*-2, or c-*myc* proto-oncogene has been suggested in different studies to imply a less favourable prognosis (MACHOTKA et al. 1989; SLAMON et al. 1989).

*Ras* activation has been studied in human neoplasia and experimental carcinogenesis. Activation of *ras* occurs by point mutation (BRODEUR 1987; GARRETT 1986; MASUDA et al. 1987; WILLIAMS and FENOGLIO-PREISER 1987). Known carcinogens have been shown to cause point muations in *ras* genes in animal models. With the advent of PCR, a number of human neoplastic and preneoplastic conditions have been examined for point mutations of *ras* proto-oncogenes. Activation of K-*ras* and N-*ras* proto-oncogenes appears to occur early in the development of some cases of colonic cancer (VOGELSTEIN et al. 1988, 1989) and acute myelogenous leukemia (AML) (YUNIS et al. 1989). Detection of activated *ras* proto-oncogenes in the premalignant phase of AML may actually be of prognostic value (YUNIS et al. 1989).

A large number of immunohistochemical or immunochemical studies of expression of normal *ras* p21 have been performed on various human tumors, but results, especially those of immunohistochemistry, are still controversial. Extra care should be taken when assessing enhanced expression of oncogene products in immunohistochemistry or in situ hybridization, because definitive quantitation is very difficult and many benign conditions have been known to cause increased expression of these products.

Analysis of tumor suppressor genes is still not useful diagnostically except for the RB gene in immediate family members of patients with retinoblastoma. Analysis of tumor suppressor genes will become more important in the future as more of these genes are identified and the role which they play in the development of cancer at other sites becomes more clear.

## 3 Oncogenes in Gynecological Tumors

At this juncture there has been no definitively established correlation between abnormalities of cellular oncogenes and the development and/or prognosis of gynecological malignancies. However, an increasing number of studies in this field are now being reported, though findings are somewhat conflicting. The results of these investigations seem to indicate, however, that activated proto-oncogenes are involved in the pathogenesis and/or progression of some gynecological cancers. It is probable that in the near future the role of activated proto-oncogenes in gynecological tumors will be clarified and the results will be applied at the diagnostic level as in cancers of other sites.

### 3.1 Ovarian Cancer

Of all gynecological malignancies, ovarian carcinoma has the highest mortality in most of the developed countries. However, recent advances in chemotherapy following debulking surgery have improved the response rate, even in patients with advanced ovarian cancer. On the other hand, side-effects or complications of chemotherapy are significant. Thus, at present, it is very important to evaluate carefully different factors affecting prognosis and, accordingly, to individualize the therapy of ovarian cancer patients. In this regard, there have been an increasing number of studies that suggest that activated proto-oncogenes should be considered among the factors which determine clinical outcome.

Results from major studies on abnormalities of proto-oncogenes are summarized in Table 2. As shown in this table, conflicting results were obtained regarding the involvement of the *ras* group of oncogenes and the c-*erb*B-2 oncogene. Concerning c-*erb*B-2, SLAMON et al. (1989) found a relatively high incidence of amplification of this proto-oncogene in ovarian malignancies, and both amplification and overexpression were associated with decreased survival. Other reprots, however, have observed neither the frequncy nor the correlation with clinical course as did SLAMON, including our investigations of histopathologically proven ovarian carcinoma (SASANO et al. 1990b). On the other hand,

**Table 2.** Summary of major studies on abnormalities of proto-oncogenes in ovarian cancer

| Author | Oncogenes examined | Type of abnormality | Summary of results |
|---|---|---|---|
| SASANO et al. (1990b) | c-*erb* B-2 *int*-2 | Amplification | 0/12 |
| | | Amplification | 1/12 |
| | c-*myc* | Amplification | 6/12 |
| ZANG et al. (1989) | c-*erb* B-1 | Amplification | 0/15 |
| | c-*erb* B-2 | Amplification | 3/15 |
| BERCHUK et al. (1990) | c-*erb* B-2 | Overexpression (immunohistochemistry) | Intense staining is associated with poor survival |
| SLAMON et al. (1989) | c-*erb* B-2 | Amplification | 31/20[a] |
| ZHOU et al. (1988) | c-K-*ras* | Amplification | 3/7 |
| | c-H-*ras* | Amplification | 1/12 |
| | c-*myc* | Amplification | 3/12 |
| | c-*erb*B-2 | Amplification | 1/12 |
| MASUDA et al. (1987) | c-*myc* | Amplification | 3/11 |
| | c-*erb*B-2 | Amplification | 1/11 |
| | c-*erb*B-1 | Amplification | 0/5 |
| | c-K-*ras* | Amplification | 2/5 |
| | c-H-*ras* | Amplification | 1/11 |
| | myb | Amplification | 0/8 |
| | N-*myc* | Amplification | 0/4 |
| | sis | Amplification | 0/6 |
| VAN'T VEER et al. (1988) | c-K-*ras* | Amplification | 3/37 |
| | | Point mutation | 0/30 |
| FUKUMOTO et al. (1989) | c-K-*ras* | Amplification[b] | 2/8 |
| | | Point mutation | None |
| BOLTZ et al. (1989) | c-K-*ras* | Amplification | 2/81[c] |
| HAAS et al. (1987) | *ras* group | Transfection | 1/18 active in serous papillary carcinoma |
| WASTON et al. (1987) | c-*myc* | Overexpression (flow cytometry) | Overexpression in serous papillary carcinoma |
| POLACARZ et al. (1989) | c-*myc* | Overexpression (immunohistochemistry) | Difference of staining pattern among mucinous neoplasms |
| RODENBURG et al. (1988) | *ras* group | Overexpression (immunohistochemistry) | More intensive staining in carcinoma than normal ovary[d] |
| SLAMON et al. (1984) | *abl* | Overexpression | 0/6 |
| | *fes* | (m-RNA) | 0/6 |
| | *fos* | Overexpression | 6/6 |
| | *fms* | Overexpression | 4/6 |
| | c-*myc* | Overexpression | 6/6 |
| | myb | Overexpression | 0/6 |
| | c-H-*ras* | Overexpression | 6/6 |
| | c-K-*ras* | Overexpression | 4/6 |
| LEE et al. (1989) | c-H-*ras* | Rearrangement | 1/17 |
| | | Allele loss | 5/17 |

[a] Overexpression generally correlated with amplification
[b] Amplification was examined by in gel renaturation assay
[c] Specimen consisted of 26 patients and seven xenografted overian cancer cell lines
[d] No correlation of *ras* expression with histologic type of ovarian cancer, tumor ploidy, or clinical outcome

c-*myc* activation and/or overexpression have been shown in 25% (ZHOU et al. 1988) to 100% (SLAMON et al. 1984) of ovarian cancers. In correlating proto-oncogene activation with established morphologic prognostic factors in ovarian carcinoma, we found that the presence of c-*myc* amplification was associated with a higher degree of nuclear atypia and high mitotic count (SASANO et al. 1990b). Both nuclear grade and mitotic index are known to be important prognostic factors in human ovarian cancer (SILVERBERG 1989). The correlation between nuclear atypia and c-*myc* amplification could reflect in part the fact that gene amplification entails physical alteration of chromosomal DNA in the nucleus, and that physical alteration of chromosomal DNA also probably leads to the morphologic changes in the nucleus associated with atypia. c-*myc* amplification might also be expected to be associated with high mitotic count, since it codes for a factor believed to facilitate transition from $G_0$ to $G_1$ in the cell cycle (KACZMARE et al. 1985). Also, a relatively strong association was observed between the presence of oncogene amplification and the presence of serous differentiation in our study (SASANO et al. 1990b).

Oncogene amplification probably reflects a step in tumor progression rather than an initiating event in early neoplastic transformation (MACHOTKA et al. 1989). However, some evidence suggests that at least in ovarian cancer, amplification of c-*myc* may occur at an early stage of progression. WATSON et al. (1987) showed that elevation of the protein product of c-*myc*, p62, preceded the development of aneuploidy in the evolution of ovarian cancer. In our study, tow of three cases which showed c-*myc* amplification but not aneuploidly were clinically in stage I (SASANO et al. 1990b). Moreover, three cases of ovarian carcinoma which showed both aneuploidy and c-*myc* amplification demonstrated a higher degree of amplification than the cases which did not show aneuploidy. These observations suggest that at least for some ovarian carcinomas, c-*myc* amplification occurs before development of aneuploidy and that c-*myc* amplification may be involved in the early progression of these tumors.

Interestingly, carcinoma of low malignant potential (LMP), which generally has a better prognosis even at an advanced clinical stage, has not shown any oncogene amplification (SASANO et al. 1990b). Also, the presence of aneuploidy, which has been associated with an unfavorable prognosis, has not been observed in ovarian carcinoma of LMP (FRIEDLANDER et al. 1984; SASANO et al. 1990b). Moreover, the number of nucleolar organizer regions per nucleus, which reflect the overall level of cellular metabolism and proliferative activity, is less in ovarian carcinoma of LMP than in invasive ovarian carcinoma (SASANO et al., unpublished observations). These results utilizing recently developed techniques reinforce the importance of histopathologic examiniation, including assessment of nuclear grade and morphologic separation of ovarian carcinoma of LMP from invasive ovarian carcinoma.

DNA ploidy and proto-oncogene activation are both relatively new prognostic factors in oncology. Generally, the presence of increased oncogene copy number through amplification or other mechnisms and/or aneuploidy would be expected to have an adverse effect on tumor behavior and prognosis. As discussed earlier, proto-oncogenes are involved in the induction of cell growth and cell division. Amplification would be expected to enhance these features within the tumor cells. Aneuploidy is considered to contribute to neoplastic transformation or progression through deletion of chromosomes containing important tumor suppressor genes (BAKER et al.1989; KACZMARE et al. 1985). Aneuploidy and gene amplification are probably independent prognostic factors, however, in ovarian carcinoma. The presence of aneuploidy has not been correlated with oncogene amplification (SASANO et al. 1990b) or *ras* p21 expression (RODENBURG et al. 1988). Moreover, aneuploidy refelcts major changes in DNA content, due mostly to abnormalities in chromosome replication during cell division (BLUMENFELD et al. 1987; SASANO et al. 1990b). Gene amplification detects relatively minor changes in DNA, which can result in little or no detectable change in the amount of DNA present in the nucleus (BLUMENFELD et al. 1987; SASANO et al. 1990b).

### 3.2 Uterine Cervical Carcinoma

A number of reports have appeared regarding oncogene activation and expression in carcinomas of the uterine cervix, and the results of these studies are summarized in Table 3. Most of the studies have focused on c-*myc*, and the data from both amplification and overexpression studies are conflicting. Further investigations will be required to clarify any possible relationship between c-*myc* activation or overexpression and development of cervical carcinoma.

Of particular interest has been the observed association between human papilloma virus (HPV) and the development and/or progression of cervical neoplasms. HUGHES et al. (1989) have demonstrated that HPV antigen positive specimens in human normal and neoplastic epithelium contain more dividing cells than HPV negative specimens. Studies by DURST et al. (1987) suggested that one mechanism by which HPV might induce neoplasia was through integration into cellular DNA in the proximity of c-*myc* and induction of c-*myc* expression. However, the recent evidence that E6 protein produced by HPV binds to the RB gene product and presumably inactivates it suggests that HPV's tumor-inducing properties may be related more to inhibition of cancer suppressor genes than to activation of proto-oncogenes (DYSON et al. 1989).

### 3.3 Uterine Endometrial Cancer

Studies of endometrial carcinoma for proto-oncogene activation and expression are less numerous than for uterine cervical and ovarian carcinoma. Reported findings are summarized in Table 4. Of particular interest was the absence of oncogene amplification in classical endometrioid carcinoma but high degree of c-*myc* amplification in endometrial serous papillary adenocarcinoma SASANO

**Table 3.** Summary of major studies on abnormalities of proto-oncogenes in uterine cancer

| Authors | Oncogenes examined | Type of abnormality | Summary of results |
|---|---|---|---|
| RIOU et al. (1988) | c-H-*ras* | Locus analysis | Loss of one allele in 36% |
| | | Point mutation | 24% [a] |
| DILUCA et al. (1989) | c-*myc* | Amplification | 0/14 |
| OCADIZ et al. (1987) | c-*myc* | Amplification | 17/35 |
| BAKER et al. (1988) | c-*myc* | Amplification | 14/44 |
| HENDY-IBBS et al. (1987) | c-*myc* | Overexpression (flow cytometry) | Normal cervix higher than carcinoma |
| RIOU et al. (1987) | c-*myc* | Overexpression (Northern and slot blot) | 25/72 |
| HUGHES et al. (1989) | c-*myc* | Overexpression (immunohistochemistry) | Normal cervix more positive than carcinoma |
| SAGAE et al. (1989) | *ras* (p21) | Overexpression (immunohistochemistry) | 57.1% [b]<br>54.2% [c]<br>38.7% [d] |

[a] Mutation at codon 12
[b] Keratinizing type of squamous cell carcinoma
[c] Large cell nonkeratinizing type
[d] Small cell type

**Table 4.** Summary of major studies on abnormalities of proto-oncogenes in uterine endometrial cancer

| Authors | Oncogenes examined | Type of abnormality | Summary of results |
|---|---|---|---|
| SASANO et al. (1990c) | c-*myc* | Amplification | 1/4 |
| | *int*-2 | Amplification | 0/4 |
| | c-*erb* B-2 | Amplification | 0/4 [a] |
| KACINSKI et al. (1988) | *fms*<br>*fos*<br>c-*erb* B-2<br>c-K-*ras* | Overexpression (in situ hybridization) | High levels of expression |
| LONG et al. (1988) | *ras* group (p21) | Overexpression (immunohistochemistry) | Higher rate of positivity in high-grade carcinoma |

[a] Amplification was seen only in serous papillary carcinoma, not in classical endometrioid carcinoma
[b] Positivity of p21 was also seen in stromal cells

et al., unpublished observations). This histologic subtype of carcinoma is known to be associated with an aggressive biologic behavior and poor prognosis HENDRICKSON et al. 1982). This tumor is likely to behave like serous papillary carcinoma of the ovary rather than classical endometrioid carcinoma, as shown in spreading over the peritoneal surface and response to chemotherapy. We have demonstrated a relatively strong association of c-*myc* amplification with serous differentiation in ovarian carcinoma (SASANO et al. 1990b). Thus, these findings emphasize the concept of an "extended müllerian system" and provide still further evidence of the similarity between neoplasms arising in primary Müllerian duct derivatives such as the endometrium and the peritoneal surface of the ovaries (LAUCHLON 1968).

Two studies have noted high levels of *ras* gene expression in endometrial cancer (KACINSKI et al. 1988; LONG et al. 1988) Moreover, in the study by KACINSKI et al., the level of c-*fms* expression was found to correlate closely with the degree of aggressive behavior of the tumor as judged by high FIGO histologic grade, high FIGO clinical stage, and deep myometrial penetration (KACINSKI et al. 1988). KACINSKI et al. proposed that prehysterectomy endometrial curretings of FIGO stage I patients be assayed for c-*fms* expression to identify preoperatively those patients with deep myometrial penetration or other local or regional spread.

### 3.4 Tumor Suppressor Genes in Gynecological Tumors

There have been very few studies to date on possible cancer suppressor genes in gynecological tumors. However, the known genetic predisposition of some women to develop these types of malignant tumors strongly implies the involvement of cancer suppressor genes in their pathogenesis (LYNCH et al. 1982). The postulated mechanism for the genetic transmission of cancer is that the patient inherits one defective cancer suppressor gene from one parent and then inactivates the other gene through spontaneous mutation or deletion in cells that give rise to the tumor (SAGER 1989). In tumors that arise in individuals without a genetic predisposition, the cells undergoing malignant transformation must inactivate or lose both normal alleles (SAGER 1989). This is generally detected by observing that a tumor contains only one of the two alleles for a given gene that are present in the normal tissue. Thus, allelic deletion in tumor cells usually reflects the loss of a functioning cancer suppressor gene on the deleted allele and retention of a mutated nonfunctional cancer suppressor gene on the remaining allele (SAGER 1989). There have been very few studies to date on possible cancer suppressor genes in ovarian tumors. Evidence that a cancer suppressor gene located on chromosome 11p may be involved in ovarian tumorigenesis has been reported by LEEJH et al. (1989). In that study, deletion of DNA from chromosome 11p in the region of the c-Ha-*ras* gene was observed in five out of ten cases of ovarian carcinoma. A study by EHLEN and DUBEAU (1990) has also demonstrated allelic deletion of DNA on chromosome 11p in ovarian cancers. In addition, their study showed that cancer suppressor genes involved in ovarian tumorigenesis may also be present on chromosome 3p and on 6q (EHLEN and DUBEAU 1990). RIOU et al. (1988) found 10 of 28 cases of carcinoma of the uterine cervix with allelic deletions of 11p.

We have recently demonstrated that possible involvement of the RB gene in an ovarian carcinoma of low malignant potential. We examined 24 ovarian neoplasms and three cases of endometrial carcinoma for evidence of homozygous deletion of the RB gene. One of 16 cases of ovarian carcinoma demonstrated such as lesion (Fig. 3), and, interestingly, in occurred in a tumor that by morphologic criteria would be classified as being of low malignant potential. Of additional interest was the fact that this borderline tumor behaved in an unusually aggressive fashion and resulted in the death of the patient 8 months following diagnosis (SASANO et al. 1990a). The possibility that the observed deletion of the RB gene in our case was an incidental finding cannot be completely ruled out. However, based on current knowledge regarding the biology of this gene this seems unlikely, and we speculate that structural alterations of the RB gene in our case did contribute to its aggressive clinical behavior.

Information regarding a role for potential cancer suppressor genes in endometrial carcinomas is also quite limited. However, YOSHIDA et al. (1986) have demonstrated rearrangements of chromosomes 1 and 11 in recurrent endometrial carcinoma, and cell fusion studies using an endometrial carcinoma cell line have implicated chromosomes 1, 6, and 9 as bearing cancer suppressor genes (SAGER 1989).

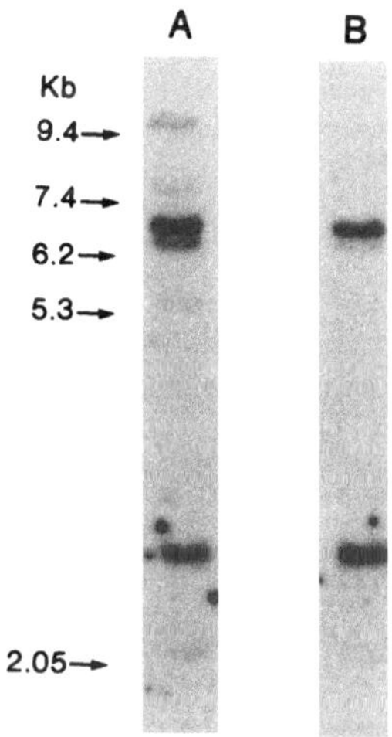


**Fig. 3.** Southern blot analysis of control DNA (*lane A*) and endometrioid carcinoma of LMP (*lane B*) by a probe to the RB gene and a probe to monitor DNA transfer. The intensity of the band monitoring the amount of DNA present on the filter (two intensive bands in this figure) was nearly identical in the control and tumor tissue. Compared to the control tissue in lane A, the 9.4-kb and 7.4-kb bands detected by the probe to the RB gene were deleted in lane B. (SASANO et al. 1990a)

## 4 Summary

Evidence is increasing that proto-oncogenes and cancer suppressor genes are involved in the development and/or progression of gynecological malignancies. While histopathologic examination remains an indispensable tool of the surgical pathologist in the diagnosis and evaluation of patients with gynecological malignancies, the advancement to technology and the development of new knowledge regarding neoplastic transformation are providing a basis for new opportunities to improve patients care. These new opportunities will depend on the use of the skills and reagents developed in the basic medical science laboratories. Thus, it is important for those in the field of diagnostic pathology to begin to acquire a knowledge of proto-oncogenes and cancer suppressor genes as well as a basic understanding of the techniques used to detect and evaluate them.

## References


Baker SJ, Fearon ER, Nigro JM, et al. (1989) Chromosome 17 deletions and p53 gene mutations in colorectal carcinoma. Science 244:217–221

Baker VV, Hatch KD, Shingleton HM (1988) Amplification of c-*myc* proto-oncogene in cervical carcinoma. J Surg Oncol 39:225–228

Berchuck A, Kamel A, Whitaker R, Kerns B, Olt G, Kinney R, Soper JT, Dodge R, Clarke-Pearson DL, Marks P, McKenzie S, Yin S, Bast RC Jr (1990) Overexpression of HER-2/nev is associated with poor survival in advanced epithelial ovarian cancer. Cancer Res 50:4087–4091

Black MM, Spear FD (1957) Nuclear structure in cancer tissues. Surg Gynecol Obstet 105:97–102

Blumenfeld D, Braly PS, Ben-Ezra J, Klevecz RR (1987) Tumor DNA content as a prognostic feature in advanced epithelial carcinoma. Gynecol Oncol 27:389–398

Boltz EM, Kefford RF, Leary JA, Houghton CR, Friendlander ML (1989) Amplification of c-*ras*-ki oncogene in human ovarian tumors. Int J Cancer 43:423–430

Brodeur GM (1987) The involvement of oncogenes and suppressor genes in human neoplasia. Adv Pediatr 34:1–44

Buck KB, Liu ET, Larrick JW (1988) Oncogenes. Springer, New York Heidelberg Berlin

DiLuca D, Costa S, Monini P et al. (1989) Search for human papilloma virus, herpes simplex virus and c-*myc* oncogene in human genital tumors. Int J Cancer·43:570–577

Durst M, Croce CM, Grissman L, Schwartz E, Huebner K (1987) Papilloma virus sequences integrate near cellular oncogenes in some cervical carcinomas. Proc Natl Acad Sci USA 84:1070–1074

Dyson N, Howley PM, Munger K, Harlow E (1989) The human papilloma virus–16E7 oncoprotein is able to bind to the retinoblastoma gene product. Scinece 243:934–940

Ehlen T, Dubeau L (1990) Loss of heterozygosity on chromosomal segments 3p, 6q, and 11p in human ovarian carcinomas. Oncogene 5:219–224

Freifelder D (1985) Essentials of molecular biology. Jones and Bartlett, Boston

Friedlander ML, Russell P, Taylor IW, Hedley DW, Tattersail MHN (1984) Flow cytometric analysis of cellular DNA content as an adjunct to the diagnosis of ovarian tumors of borderline malignancy. Pathology 16:301–306

Friend SH, Bernard SR, Rogelj S, Weinberg RA, Rapaport JM, Albert DM, Dryja TP (1986) A human DNA segment with properties of the gene that predisposes to retinoblastoma and osteosarcoma. Nature 323:643–646

Fukumoto M, Estensen RD, Sha L et al. (1989) Association of ki-*ras* with amplified DNA sequences detected in human ovarian carcinomas by a modified in-gel renaturation assay. Cancer Res 49:1693–1697

Fung Y-KT, Murphree AL, T'Ang A, Qian J, Hinrichs SH, Benedict W (1987) Structural evidence for the authenticity of the human retinoblastoma gene. Science 244:217–221

Garrett CT (1986) Oncogenes. Clin Chim Acta 156:1–40

Haas M, Isakov J, Howell SB (1987) Evidence against *ras* activation in human ovarian carcinomas. Mol Biol Med 4:265–275

Haluska FG, Tsujimoto Y, Croce CM (1987) Oncogene activation by chromosome translocation in human malignancy. Ann Rev Genet 21:321–345

Harbour JW, Lai S-L, Wang-Peng J, Gazdar AF, Minna JD, Kaye FJ (1988) Abnormalities in structure and expression of the human retinoblastoma gene in SCLC. Science 241:353–357

Haseltine WA, Sodroski J, Patarca R, Briggs D, Perkins D, Wang-Staal F (1984) Structure of 3' terminal region of type II human T lymphotrophic virus; evidence for a new coding region. Science 225:419–421

Hendrickson M, Ross J, Eifel P, Martinez A, Kempson R (1982) Uterine papillary serous carcinoma. A highly malignant form of endometrial carcinoma. Am J Surg Pathol 6:93–108

Hendy-Ibbs P, Cox H, Evan GI, Watson JV (1987) Flow cytometric quantitation of DNA and c-*myc* oncoprotein in archival biopsies of uterine cervix neoplasia. Br J Cancer 55:275–282

Hughes RA, Neill WA, Norval M (1989) Papilloma virus and c-*myc* antigen expression in normal and neoplastic cervical epithelium. J clin Pathol 42:46–51

Hunter T (1984) Oncogenes and proto-oncogenes: How do they differ? JNCI 73:773–786

Kacinski BM, Carter D, Mittal K et al. (1988) High level expression of *fms* proto-oncogene mRNA is observed in clinically aggressive human endometrial adenocarcinoma. Int J Radiat Oncol Biol Phys 15:823–829

Kaczmare KL, Hyland JK, Watt R, Rosenburg M, Baserga R (1985) Microinjected c-*myc* as a competence factor. Science 228:1313–1315

Klein G (1987) The approaching era of the tumor suppression genes. Science 2338:1539–1545

Lauchlon SC (1968) Conceptual unity of the müllerian tumor group: a histological study. Cancer 22:601–610

Lee EY-HP, To H, Shew J-Y, Bookstein R, Scully P, WH (1988) Inactivation of the retinoblastoma susceptibility gene in human breast cancers. Science 241:218–221

Lee JH, Kavanagh JJ, Wharton JT, Wildrick KDM, Blick M (1989) Allele loss at the c-Ha-*ras*1 locus in human ovarian cancer. Cancer Res 49:1220–1222

Lee W-H, Bookstein R, Hong F, Young L-J, Shew J-Y, Lee EY-H (1987) Human retinoblastoma susceptibility gene: cloning, identification and sequence. Science 235:1394–1399

Long CA, O'Brien TJ, Sanders MM, Bard DS, Quirk JG Jr (1988) A *ras* oncogene is expressed in adenocarcinoma of the endometrium. Am J Obstet Gynecol 159:1512–1515

Lynch HT, Albano WA, Lynch JF, Lynch PM, Campbell A (1982) Surveillance and management of patients at high genetic risk for advanced ovarian carcinoma. Obstet Gynecol 59:589–596

Machotka SV, Garrett CT, Schwartz AM, Callahan R (1989) Amplification of the proto-oncogenes *int*-2, c-*erb*B-2 and c-*myc* in human breast cancer. Clin Chim Acta 184:207–218

Masuda H, Battifora H, Yokota J, Meltzer S, Cline MJ (1987) Specificity of proto-oncogene amplification in human malignant diseases. Mol Biol Med 4:213–227

Merkel DE, Mcguire WL (1988) Oncogenes and cancer prognosis. In: Davis VT Jr, Hellman S, Rosenberg SA (eds) *Important advances in oncology*. J.B. Lippincott, Philadelphia, pp 103–117

Ocadiz R, Sauceda R, Cruz M, Graef AM, Gariglio P (1987) High correlation between alterations of c-*myc* oncogene and carcinoma of the uterine cervix. Cancer Res 47:4173–4177

Polacarz SV, Hey NA, Stephenson TJ, Hill AS (1989) c-*myc* oncogene product $p62^{c\text{-}myc}$ in ovarian mucinous neoplasms: immunohistochemical study correlated with malignancy. J Clin Pathol 42:148–152

Riou G, Barrois M, Le MG, George M, Le Doussal V, Hale C (1987) c-*myc* protooncogene expression and prognosis in early carcinoma of the uterine cervix. Lancet I (8536) 761–763

Riou G, Barrois M, Sheng ZM, Duvillard P, Lhomme C (1988) Somatic deletion and mutations of c-Ha-*ras* gene in human cervical cancers. Oncogene 3:329–333

Rodenburg CJ, Koelma IA, Nap M, Fleuren GJ (1988) Immunohistochemical detection of the *ras* oncogene product p21 in advanced ovarian cancer. Arch Pathol Lab Med 912:151–154

Sagae S, Kuzumaki N, Hisada T, Mugikura Y, Kudo R, Hashimoto M (1989) *Ras* oncogene expression and prognosis of invasive squamous carcinoma of the uterine cervix. Cancer 63: 1577–1582

Sager R (1986) Genetic suppression of tumor formation: a new frontier in cancer research. Cancer Res 46:1573–1580
Sager R (1989) Tumor suppressor genes: the puzzle and the promise. Science 246:1406–1412
Sasano H, Comerford J, Silverberg SG, Garrett CT (1990a) Analysis of abnormalities of the retinoblastoma gene in human ovarian and endometrial carcinoma. Cancer 66:2150–2154
Sasano H, Carrett CT, Wilkinson DS, Silverberg SG, Comerford J, Hyde J (1980b) Protooncogene amplification and tumor ploidy in human ovarian neoplasms. Hum Pathol 21:382–391
Sasano H, Comerford J, Wilkinson DS, Schwartz A, Garrett GT (1990c) Serous papillary adenocarcinoma of the endometrium: protooncogene amplification, flow cytometry, estrogen and progesterone recepros and immunohistochemical analysis. Cancer 65:1545–1551
Silverberg SG (1989) Prognostic significance of pathologic features in ovarian carcinoma. Curr Top Pathol 78:85–109
Slamon DJ, de Kernion JB, Verma IM, Cline MJ (1984) Expression of cellular oncogenes in human malignancy. Science 224:256–262
Slamon DJ, Godolphin W, Jones LA et al. (1989) Studies of the HER-2/*neu* protooncogene in human breast and ovarian cancer. Science 244:707–712
Stanbridge EJ (1988) Genetic analysis of human malignancy using somatic cell hybrids and monochromosome transfer. Cancer Surv 7:317–324
van't Veer LJ, Hermens R, van der Bakker LAM et al. (1988) *ras* oncogene activation in human ovarian carcinoma. Oncogene 2:157–165
Vogelstein B, Fearon ER, Hamilton SR et al. (1988) Genetic alterations during colorectal-tumor development. N Engl J Med 319:525–532
Vogelstein B, Fearon ER, Kern SE, Hamilton SR, Presinger AC, Nakamura Y, White R (1989) Allotype of colorectal carcinomas. Science 244:207–211
Watson JV, Curling OM, Munn CF, Hudson CN (1987) Oncogene expression in ovarian cancer: a pilot study of c-*myc* oncoprotein in serous papillary ovarian cancer. Gynecol Oncol 28:137–150
Williams CL, Fenoglio-Preiser CM (1987) Oncogenes, suppressor genes, and carcinogenesis. Hum Pathol 18:895–902
Yavner D, Rice L, Weinberg D, Mendoza A, Lage J (1989) DNA analysis of borderline (BL) ovarian tumors. Lab Invest 60:107A
Yoshida MA, Ohyashiki K, Piver SM, Sandberg AA (1986) Recurrent endometrial adenocarcinoma with rearrangement of chromosomes 1 and 11. Cancer Genet Gytogenet 20:218–220
Yunis JJ, Boot AJM, Mayer MG, Bos JL (1989) Mechanism of *ras* mutation in myeolodysplastic syndrome. Oncogene 4:609–614
Zang X, Silva E, Gershenson D, Hung M-C (1989) Amplification and rearrangement of c-*erb*-proto-oncogenes in cancer of human female genital tract. *Oncogene* 4:985–989
Zhou DJ, Gonzalez-Cadavid N, Ahuva H, Battifora H, Moore GE, Cline MJ (1988) A unique pattern of proto-oncogene abnormalities in ovarian adenocarcinoma. Cancer 62:1573–1576

# Subject Index

## Index of Volumes 82–84 Current Topics in Pathology

**Volume 84/1: Reaction Patterns of the Lymph Node.**
Edited by E. GRUNDMANN, E. VOLLMER



**Volume 84/2: Reaction Patterns of the Lymph Node.**
Edited by E. GRUNDMANN, E. VOLLMER

MIX
Papier aus verantwortungsvollen Quellen
Paper from responsible sources
FSC® C105338

If you have any concerns about our products,
you can contact us on
**ProductSafety@springernature.com**

In case Publisher is established outside the EU,
the EU authorized representative is:
**Springer Nature Customer Service Center GmbH**
**Europaplatz 3, 69115 Heidelberg, Germany**

Printed by Libri Plureos GmbH
in Hamburg, Germany